The Director's Story

Mamoulian on Garbo and Dietrich:

"As for Dietrich . . . she and Garbo are opposite poles. Garbo is intuitive, she's a natural phenomenon, like a geyser, or a stream or a flower; if you touch the right spots—of course I'm talking intellectually now!—she comes through. Dietrich is not like that, she's a tremendous trooper; no one works harder, no one is more disciplined, and once she's accepted she does exactly what you ask her. With her it's all calculated: with Garbo it's all instinctive."

Billy Wilder's account of Louis B. Mayer's reaction to Sunset Boulevard:

"And I still remember Mr. Louis B. Mayer shaking his fist and saying, 'We should horsewhip this Wilder! We should throw him out of this town! He has dirtied the nest! He has brought disgrace on the town that is feeding him!'
. . . Louis B. Mayer lived in a kind of dream world, unfortunately."

Robert Aldrich on working with Bette Davis and Joan Crawford:

"The two stars didn't fight at all on *Baby Jane*. I think it's proper to say they really detested each other. . . ."

Frankenheimer on making his first Hollywood film:

"I swore I was never going to put myself through anything like that again as long as I lived. And I was going to have a film my way or I wasn't going to do it at all . . . I have to have complete control. And I didn't on *The Young Stranger*. It's a *lousy* movie. RKO cut it, and I thought, 'Who has to take that kind of crap?'"

SIGNET and MENTOR Titles
of Special Interest

The Celluloid Muse

HOLLYWOOD DIRECTORS SPEAK

by
Charles Higham and Joel Greenberg

A SIGNET BOOK from
NEW AMERICAN LIBRARY
TIMES MIRROR

SIGNET TRADEMARK REG. U.S. PAT. OFF. AND FOREIGN COUNTRIES
REGISTERED TRADEMARK—MARCA REGISTRADA
HECHO EN CHICAGO, U.S.A.

SIGNET, SIGNET CLASSICS, SIGNETTE, MENTOR AND PLUME BOOKS
are published by The New American Library, Inc.,
1301 Avenue of the Americas, New York, New York 10019

FIRST PRINTING, SEPTEMBER, 1972

PRINTED IN THE UNITED STATES OF AMERICA

For Don Prince

Contents

Introduction

The real Hollywood is a place the casual visitor, or even the rabid tourist, seldom sees. Coming to this fabled Dreamland, the fan is fobbed off with the foot and hand prints of Grauman's Chinese Theatre, hideously celebrating the immortals, or the golden names of yesterday's idols that stud Hollywood Boulevard's paving-stones ("*Mary Pickford,*" a child muses, gazing at her name on a plaque outside the theatre, "I've heard of her somewhere . . .").

In the great Hollywood restaurants, usually designed in padded black or scarlet leather, studded with great brass knobs, where telephones are brought to the table and plugged in, where martinis and Bloody Marys are lethally powerful (restaurants like Chasen's and the Brown Derby, or more elegant places like Perino's and the Scandia), the angels and monsters of Hollywood can be watched, like exotic beasts in an expensive menagerie, and heard—very loud and clear—in language laced with *craps,* and *sons-of-bitches* and *Oh Christs, baby.* Hollywood language has a barbaric toughness—even pretty women talk like marines— and the gossip is of divorces and scandals and who is making love to whom. Yet often conversation is witty, sharp, acute, full of brilliant wisecracks.

On the telephone, one aspect of the place, hard, brutal and merciless, comes through. Operators' voices are like chips of steel, unwilling to brook the slightest hesitation on the part of the caller. Flesh is cheap, and easily traded, for ambition is the central fact of the environment. American materialism here offers its most enticing possibilities to the lucky or the unscrupulous, the beautiful or the damned.

9

Beyond the pushing street crowds, tense and restless, the screaming squabbles in lobby or bar, the Bourbon breakfasts and the shuttered rooms, the endless pale pink or beige boulevards, with their shabby palms stretching to the seal-grey Pacific past a seedy bristle of electric signs, the atmosphere is not wholly corrupt. Civilization survives on the edge of this desert, this crumbling oasis, where houses are apt to topple from their precarious stilts as the ground shifts constantly. For to this strange place came great exiles from the European cinema and intelligentsia to work and flourish. And here, too, men of the generous humanism of a Ford, a Frankenheimer, a Milestone have survived without sacrificing their values, fighting bitterly against studio front offices to preserve their decent vision intact. For the interested visitor, lucky enough to gain entrée to this world, life can be wholly pleasant. And always there is the irresistible tourist lure, the knowledge, most intoxicating of all, that the figures which have haunted the world's dreams are just around the corner.

Behind Hollywood Boulevard, with its sucker-bait tourist-traps, its tacky souvenir shops, its gaudy five-and-ten-cent stores, its quietly desperate legions of hustlers and pomaded drag queens, is the Hollywood Bowl, splendid by night, sad and lacklustre by day; behind it, again, the Hollywood Hills, with winding tortuous roads leading up, up past comfortable, slightly sinister-looking villas guarding their many secrets behind firmly closed venetian blinds. And not far away, the Hollywood Cemetery, where so many of the veterans are pretentiously and gaudily interred.

Further west, towards the sea, is the area the foldout maps still call Glamorland: Bel Air, secluded behind its massive black metal gates; Beverly Hills, with its succession of picturebook residences behind level flanking palm-guarded lawns, each trying to look more opulently Home Beautiful than its immediate neighbour. Here you walk alone at your peril, risking questioning by motor police patrols constantly cruising the streets, for in this district the only recognized mode of transportation is the car. Here are houses, you feel, designed not so much to be lived in as to be admired.

Do real people, you cannot help wondering, actually live in these places? If Loretta Young is real, yes. Sometimes a busload of tourists, passing the gilded residence of some superstar, may be blessed with a visit from its gracious occupant, emerging from the marble and chintz of an imitation French château to bestow a smile and a wave, and perhaps an autograph or two, on grateful fans who will return to Ohio or Wisconsin to treasure the memory of that supreme moment till the end of their days.

Innocent of sidewalks, the streets of Glamorland disclose vista upon vista of immaculate residential splendour, the foliage tended down to the last leaf, the grass greener than green. Lawns or ivied mounds run up to paths, then more rolling lawns to the door. Inside, the "homes" are apt to boast glittering chandeliers, Spanish-style stone floors, lush and leathery cocktail-bars full of chunky glassware, cosy dens with matching books, bathrooms with fur-lined toilet seats and multi-coloured soaps piled decoratively on top of each other in tall transparent containers, on rows of glittering glass shelves. Everything is shining, seemingly virginal and new and untouched. The *décor* is very frequently in beige and white, in a style that has remained practically unchanged since the late nineteen-thirties: vintage Cedric Gibbons or Hans Dreier. House after house is the kind of thing in which Greta Garbo or Norma Shearer queened it in the depths of the depression. Real estate deals here seldom run into sums of less than six figures, while local rates and taxes match land prices in being among the world's highest. It isn't uncommon, attending a Hollywood party, to hear someone saying, "I told (Paul Newman) he couldn't have it for $350,000."

If Glamorland, where the stars and moviemakers live and play, is a shopgirl's idea of heaven (and an Oxford don's idea of hell), the studios where they toil from early morning till late afternoon (and very often beyond) more closely resemble Detroit automobile plants or Pittsburgh steel-mills in their strictly utilitarian functionalism. To gain admission to the film factories (unless you are taking the standard guided tour) you must submit to scrutiny by a cop or a receptionist controlling electronically-operated doors. A call to your contact, a frosty smile, and Open Sesame. Once in, it is difficult to reconcile preconceived notions of glitter or razzmatazz with the humdrum reality before you: endless corridors in grey or muted green, containing none too luxurious offices housing publicists, script girls, administrative officials, junior executives. (Offices of the magnificence of, say, that of Hal B. Wallis at Paramount are rare.) It is all very sobering, and so are the sound-stages where the actual film-making occurs: tall dark caverns strewn with cables and lighting fixtures, steamily airless in the brutal Californian sun, whose heat is supplemented by the fierce white blaze of the arcs.

These twin *milieux*—the sumptuous magnificence of Glamorland and the plain, straightforward non-architecture of the major studios—are the settings for the interviews which follow. Our enquiry began as research for a previous joint volume, *Hollywood in the Forties,*[1] during which we interviewed numerous American film-makers, including those in this book. Gradually we found the scope of our enquiry expanding to cover not only these men's careers, their films and the people with whom they had been associated, but also the entire role of the director in American films; involuntarily, it became group autobiography by the film-makers themselves, illuminating the relationships between the directors and their studios, producers, writers, agents, and stars; the director's historical role in Hollywood from silent days to the present; and the way in which certain major films had reached the screen in the forms in which we now know them.

The interviews thus told us more than just the historical circumstances of the genesis of movies like *All Quiet on the Western Front*, more than the steps by which the directors had made their respective transitions from editing, art direction, the stage, or television to motion picture direction; they enriched our understanding of the film-making process and helped to define more clearly than ever before the precise nature of the director's contribution.

We were intrigued by authentic and hitherto unrecorded pieces of movie lore and memorabilia of the stars: Bette Davis nearly drowning while making *A Stolen Life* or weeping at the sight of her own image on the screen in *Whatever Happened to Baby Jane?*; Garbo elucidating her approach to the character of Marguerite Gautier in *Camille*; Dietrich striving to look ever younger in *Rancho Notorious*; the comic ingenuity with which John Garfield was made to seem a professional on-camera violinist in *Humoresque*; the secret, reluctantly disclosed for the first time by the director, of the one-take transforma-

[1] Zwemmer, London, and A. S. Barnes, New York, 1968.

tion of Fredric March from Dr Jekyll into Mr Hyde in Rouben Mamoulian's 1932 film.

But beyond the mere preservation of the past, beyond their contribution to a more complete record of Hollywood's heyday—valuable as these things are—the directors, we felt, raised other issues of equal importance to the student of cinema and the ordinary filmgoer: the extent to which motion-picture directors can be considered creative artists, and the ways in which the truly original creative artists among them can be distinguished from gifted interpreters of other people's work, and from able but unoriginal craftsmen.

Leaving aside the implications of the French critical theory, first propounded in the influential magazine *Cahiers du Cinéma*, of the *politique des auteurs*—according to which a film's artistic success must be judged by the extent to which a single creative mind, or *auteur,* can be discerned in it—we find among the fifteen directors here assembled archetypal artists, interpreters, and craftsmen.

The artists are those whose films make some kind of statement about the human condition, or express some deeply-held outlook on life, in a recognizably individual style. The interpreters, or middle-men, are those who bring technical expertise and dramaturgical mastery to the screen translation of other people's original material, be it novel, play, or whatever. The craftsmen are film-makers with an agreeable flair for the language of the screen, whose skills might equally well be applied to one kind of subject as another: they are strictly entertainers.

Thus it is clear by his own admission and definition here that Hitchcock, for example, cannot be considered an artist (*pace* Truffaut, etc.) because his films do not reveal a valid and strongly held *Weltanschauung,* but are simply vehicles for personal self-indulgence, expertly engineered. Similarly, Vincente Minnelli does have a recognizable personal visual style, elegant, glossy and decorative, but he has nothing to say, and the diffidence with which he discussed his films with us makes this fact entirely clear.

In our present selection, those who may unequivocally be claimed as artists number four: Fritz Lang, Billy Wilder, Lewis Milestone, and King Vidor.

Throughout Lang's films runs his belief in the inescapability of Fate, his conception of human destiny as a continual flight from Death. This theme can be traced as far back as his silent German picture *Der Muede Tod* and throughout his American period also (to which the present interview is confined) in films like *Fury, Scarlet Street,* and *The Big Heat.* His is a cinema of shadow and darkness, its chief setting the nocturnal city, the work of an oppressive, remarkably single-minded genius.

Billy Wilder's strain of bitterly amused misanthropy emerged in the screenplays he wrote with Charles Brackett for Mitchell Leisen and Ernst Lubitsch before he entered direction himself—as, incidentally, a fully-fledged *auteur,* being both writer and director on all his films. The bitterness became increasingly pronounced in movies like *Double Indemnity* and *The Lost Weekend,* where people were shown as weak, vicious and selfish, and reached perhaps its most intense expression in *Ace in the Hole* (also called *The Big Carnival*), in which the plight of a man trapped in an almost inaccessible cave was made the occasion for an ambivalent attack on mass hysteria and sensation-seekers. Wilder's outlook is depressing, but it has resulted in some of the American cinema's most acerbic and individual films, often technically and stylistically superior also.

Lewis Milestone and King Vidor belong to an older generation than Wilder, having started their careers in the silent era. Each has shown himself in his films to be a lyricist, and a humanist, Milestone in his famous studies of men in war and in his adaptations from the work of John Steinbeck, Vidor in his numerous cinematic tributes to a bygone pastoral America. Each has made major contributions to screen language and technique; each is a master of motion picture mechanics; each has been put firmly on the shelf in Hollywood.

These, then, are the artists. What of the interpreters, the middle-men? They are often no less skilled in the manipulation of images and sound than the four men whose work we have just discussed—sometimes perhaps even more so—but they have no world-view to propound, no artistic statements to make, which might raise their films from the level of enormously skilful artefacts to that of works of art.

This category includes some of the American cinema's most celebrated names. Among our interviewees in this group are no less than seven: Alfred Hitchcock, Rouben Mamoulian, George Cukor, Robert Aldrich, John Frankenheimer, Jacques Tourneur, and Vincente Minnelli. To some it may come as a surprise to find one or two of these individuals denied the title of artist, but applying our previous test—technical mastery allied to a discernible world outlook expressed in a majority of a director's films—it will be seen that Hitchcock, for example, gifted and ingenious prestidigitator though he is, brings little more to the screen than his own delight in its mechanics, together with some private psychological preoccupations.

The distinction becomes clearer in the case of George Cukor, middle-man *par excellence*. Sophistication and technical adroitness notwithstanding, he is principally an interpreter of other people's creations—novels, plays, even original screenplays—and not a director with a philosophy to convey or with a systematized outlook for which his films are made the vehicle. Like Minnelli, he was significantly reluctant to discuss them in intellectual terms. Similar limitations exist in the case of the other five. While it is true that the subjects to which they are most frequently drawn do betray certain preferences and predilections, these are mainly clues to the individual directors' temperaments rather than evidence of any coherent or cohesive world-view.

Finally we come to the craftsmen, frequently men of considerable accomplishment whose skills are applied to any and almost every kind of subject that may present itself. Their films can, and often do, give enormous pleasure, but they work within an altogether smaller emotional and intellectual compass than the occupants of our two previous categories. We interviewed four such filmmakers: Curtis Bernhardt, Irving Rapper, Jean Negulesco, and Mark Robson. At their best estimable dreammerchants (the first three neglected today), they bring formidable taste, craftsmanship, and mechanical flair to their films but seldom, if ever, make anything other than strictly formula movies—women's pictures, melodramas, Westerns, or romantic comedies—without transcending the conventions of any of these *genres*. They are represented here as absolutely typical examples of Hollywood men, modest craftsmen happiest in a rigid industry setup.

The combined testimonies of these fifteen movie-makers told us much about Hollywood and its *mores*: about the former roles of the big studios in the days when they held almost everyone under contract; about professional relationships among various branches of the industry; and about the vicissitudes through which many a film must pass before it finally reaches the public screen.

The passing of the heyday of the big, all-powerful studio and its big, all-powerful boss was lamented by at least three directors. Curtis Bernhardt sighed for the days when Jack Warner ruled Burbank with what he calls "an iron fist", and even the most exalted stars (with one exception) had to conform to studio discipline or risk suspension. This was an atmosphere in which professional film-makers could—and did—contribute to an annual studio output of some forty features; not just assembly-line formula films, but in many instances works of permanent value which the system was large and flexible enough to accommodate.

The studio chiefs—men like Warner, Louis B. Mayer, Harry Cohn—were, as Robert Aldrich reminds us, picture-makers first and businessmen second. Cohn "wasn't in the money business," Aldrich says. "He was in the movie business"—meaning that Cohn's primary concern, unlike that of the New York financiers who really run the film industry, was with the making of good pictures. Certainly the more profitable they were the better, but he represented an all but extinct breed—the executive film-maker—and the Hollywood scene is the poorer for its passing (the new chain-store mentality is scarcely to be welcomed). Billy Wilder puts it another way when he remarks that today eighty per cent of a director's time is spent making deals and the remaining twenty per cent making films, whereas in the nineteen-thirties and forties that ratio was reversed. Freedom, it seems, creates even more problems than it solves.

The great producers of Hollywood's golden era figure prominently in the directors' narratives. The most frequent complaint is of excessive producer interference. Goldwyn emerges least creditably here, for both Mark Robson and Lewis Milestone found their periods spent with him among the unhappiest of their careers. Many producers, in fact, habitually tinkered with the directors' handiwork, sometimes—like Hal Wallis and Selznick—even after the director had finished shooting the film and had left the lot.

The producer who seems omnipresent in many of the directors' lives is the late David O. Selznick, who emerges as perhaps the most important independent producer of his time. Hitchcock, whose first American film, *Rebecca*, was a Selznick production, appears to have coped best with the producer's rather wayward temperament, perhaps because he was equally strong-willed. Others were less fortunate: George Cukor's long-standing association with Selznick came to an inglorious end when—as he relates here—he was taken off the direction of *Gone With the Wind* in 1939 and replaced after one month of shooting. King Vidor complains bitterly of Selznick's profligacy and extravagance, of his impossible behaviour on *Duel in the Sun,* which resulted in a quarrel with the director, who walked out two days before the shooting of the film was due to end. And, in a private letter, William Dieterle confirms that Selznick thought nothing of retaking a scene, regardless of expense, if he thought it could thereby be improved. All agree on one point only: that Selznick had a maddening habit of elaboration, of adding more and more sequences to a film after it had seemingly been finished; ironically, Dieterle himself became a party to this practice when he shot the opening bar-room sequence in *Duel in the Sun* months after its director left the lot.

From all this, we receive a portrait of Selznick as piecemeal and contradictory as the composite portrait of Charles Foster Kane in the Orson Welles film, a portrait which yet coheres and gives us a rounded, three-dimensional figure, one of the most gifted, unpredictable, and stimulating ever to have worked in American films, and one whom Frankenheimer, for instance, can describe as his greatest mentor in the cinema.

A producer on whom all who knew him are agreed in their praise and liking is the late Jerry Wald. Ebullient, brimming with enthusiasm, utterly movie-struck, a fan to his finger-tips, this short-lived *Wunderkind* infected all his associates with his passion for celluloid. Curtis Bernhardt and Mark Robson speak of him with affection, and so does Jean Negulesco, many of whose most memorable Warners films were made with Wald as producer.

Negulesco speaks somewhat less affectionately—although certainly with more respect—of the two great studio heads, Jack Warner and Darryl F. Zanuck. Both could strike terror into their subordinates, directors included. Both were virtual dictators, seldom benevolent, and, as such, responsible for their studios' overall story selection, casting, and choice of directors. They also habitually had a large say in their pictures' cutting. Constantly uppermost in their minds was their responsibility to the companies' stockholders and Eastern money-men.

In their respective *milieux* they were second only to God. Mamoulian, still awestruck, tells the story of a joke at Zanuck's expense, perpetrated during the making of the Tyrone Power version of *The Mark of Zorro*, which conveys some idea of the fear and trembling with which the production head of Twentieth Century-Fox was regarded in the nineteen-forties. Lewis Milestone, too, had ample experience of Zanuck's ways: "He can be good," he says, "but, boy, oh boy, he can also be very, very bad."

Jean Negulesco respectfully relates how Zanuck became indignant when Negulesco attempted to apologize for making a picture which flopped: it was, the producer insisted, just as much the fault of the studio and of himself—they had jointly approved choice of story, cast, location, and script—as of the director; more, if anything.

From the foregoing we may deduce that, while producers and directors were not always happy with each other, they both recognized—often reluctantly—that each was mutually necessary to the creation of motion pictures. To what extent the finished films represent the personalities of producers or directors must necessarily vary from film to film but, in the case of those we have characterized as major artists, we may state quite confidently that the end product always bore unmistakably the stylistic stamp of the director.

Hollywood without its stars would cease to exist (it already practically has). Dominating them all, through sheer talent and force of personality, is the formidable Bette Davis, with whom no less than five of our directors found themselves professionally involved at various stages of their careers.

To Irving Rapper she is unapproachable, regal, remote; in conversation he disclosed that although he and Miss Davis are often in Los Angeles simultaneously he has not actually spoken to her in person for years, deeming it prudent to communicate only by telephone or letter at precisely judged times. Even today, it seems, the mistress of the Warner lot of the nineteen-forties can still have a devastating effect on directors who once had the temerity to give her instructions.

One man she could not scare was King Vidor, who directed her last film of the forties at Warners, *Beyond the Forest*. The decade's close marked also the close of her reign as Queen of Hollywood, but the years had been marvellously rewarding. Curtis Bernhardt, director of perhaps her best Warners starring vehicle, *A Stolen Life*, began his association with her in a quarrel, but afterwards came to admire her professionalism and sharp intelligence. Jean Negulesco, too, is full of praise for her appearance as a bed-ridden invalid in his underrated *Phone Call from a Stranger*.

But it is Robert Aldrich, who staged her vastly successful "comeback" film *Whatever Happened to Baby Jane?* and followed it up with *Hush, Hush, Sweet Charlotte*, who seems to have experienced Davis at her most temperamental and vulnerable. Reading his remarks on the Davis personality, or on her relationships with co-workers and other stars, we seem confronted with a real-life Margo Channing, the actress she impersonated so memorably in Joseph L. Mankiewicz' *All About Eve*.

Both Aldrich and Bernhardt had ample opportunity to compare Davis *vis à vis* Joan Crawford, for many years her runner-up and rival as Hollywood's greatest post-Garbo star. Bernhardt defines the difference between the two stars by characterizing Davis's talent as wholly cerebral and Crawford's as principally intuitive, while Jean Negulesco considers Crawford a full-time actress off-screen as well, throwing herself into her daily roles of mother, wife, corporation executive, and public glamour symbol with all the drive and energy and dedication she habitually brings to her screen parts.

Garbo, Dietrich, Garland, Ava Gardner, Marilyn Monroe: they are all here, seen through the eyes of the men who helped to create their myths. Barbara Stanwyck is here, too, the subject of flattering and enthusiastic tributes from Fritz Lang and Curtis Bernhardt. Billy Wilder's opinion, if he has one—he directed Stanwyck in one of her best remembered roles in *Double Indemnity*—remains undisclosed (though a note of waspishness shows in the memory of her kissing Gloria Swanson's skirt in homage at the *Sunset Boulevard* preview).

A measure of vanity in men of proven talent is forgivable, and in movie directors—if they are to survive in the gilded jungle—essential. Over and over again they claim credit as innovators, as being the first to introduce a new device or technique. Often their immodesty is justified; sometimes it is not, but the high-pressure image, the proud boast, must always be sustained.

Lewis Milestone correctly claims credit for being the first to have a theme song running continuously throughout a movie (*A Walk in the Sun*), while Fritz Lang, acknowledging this, reminds us that his *Rancho Notorious* was the first such Western.

Rouben Mamoulian takes great delight in recalling how the Paramount technicians, in the early days of sound, balked at attempting many of the convention-shattering devices which he, a newcomer to films from the theatre, successfully introduced at that time. King Vidor asserts that his experiments with cinematographic time in *Street Scene* and *H.M. Pulham Esq* foreshadowed many of the stylistic practices of the *nouvelle vague,* while Curtis Bernhardt believes he was among the first to use genuine travelling shots in silent films and also describes an ingenious flashback technique of his own invention which he introduced in *Payment on Demand*.

Though by no means all of them enjoy universal critical esteem, these are clearly men of many talents, several of them having come to the cinema from professional careers in other media—most frequently, the stage. George Cukor, Vincente Minnelli, Irving Rapper and Curtis Bernhardt all came to films from the theatre, with distinguished records. Lewis Milestone, concurrently with his cinema career, has directed several Broadway plays. But that the cinema has perhaps even more affinities with the plastic arts than with the performing arts is suggested by the number of directors who have entered it through painting, or who have since begun painting.

Jean Negulesco came to America in the late nineteen-twenties, after beginning as a painter in Paris, and today he still paints and draws (his Beverly Hills homes are full of his portraits and sketches). Vincente Minnelli's musicals, no less than his comedies and melodramas, clearly owe much of their surface sheen to his background as stage artist and designer, and, in an early nineteen-fifties edition of the *Memoirs of Casanova,* his illustrations reveal a graphic black-and-white style not unlike that of Aubrey Beardsley.

King Vidor's paintings echo his films also, mainly in their formalized feeling for landscape. And Alfred Hitchcock, who began his film career as an art director and set designer, has always placed the utmost emphasis on the "look", the visual ambience of his films; as is well known, he preplans them setup by setup in a series of drawings, as does Lewis Milestone, who does not draw himself but works in very close collaboration with the art director.

Artists, interpreters, craftsmen: all have helped mould the nature and history of the American screen, have contributed to its splendour and vitality. They have also lived through some staggering changes in Hollywood. In the late nineteen-forties the studios were still intact, producing their massive annual quotas of films, run by figures like Jack Warner, Louis B. Mayer, Harry Cohn and Darryl F. Zanuck under instructions from New York. Through the theatre chains they controlled, the majors, as these great studios were known, could send out a flood of celluloid, much of which was sure to earn handsome box-office returns. Stars, groomed and fêted under individual studio policies, were glamorous clock-in, clock-out employees. Directors were hired to direct totally preordained subjects, teased out by writers under a producer's careful guidance. Working in Hollywood was like working for a bank, except that you were paid in solid gold.

Today everything has altered, and not entirely for the better. By anti-monopoly government action in the nineteen-fifties, studios were deprived of theatre-chains and, through this disaster and the upsurge of television, were forced to cut their staffs, firing even distinguished directors and stars. Stars became independents, and the pattern of setting up a picture changed completely. Today, a producer with a property—a novel, or original story—prepares a package including an interested star or stars, director and screenwriter. This package is taken to a distributor and, with distribution guaranteed, work can begin in a specially hired studio-space.

Thus the independents obtained power over the majors, so that firms like Seven Arts, designed to release whole sets of package deals, finally moved in and consolidated with the majors themselves. Other groups were financed by chain-grocers or oil companies or real-estate complexes. Nowadays Paramount is merged with Gulf and Western Industries, Warner Brothers with the Kinney Service Corporation, United Artists with Transamerica, and the pattern is spreading.

Along with the breakdown of the major studios into fragments, the wreckage of the star system, there has been an overall decline in production standards. Laboratories that once produced flawless prints now turn out many that are shoddy and substandard. (The Technicolor Laboratories can be exonerated from this charge.) The unions, rigid and exclusive, keep out new talent—a fact which has meant a tragic lack of new, vital blood in the Hollywood mainstream in recent years. Old men rule too much of Hollywood, and it is only in the last two years that some striking figures of under forty-five—men like Theodore Flicker, Norman Jewison, and Noel Black—have broken through to start a new, stimulating trend, notably in the field of comedy, while relatively youthful production heads like Richard Zanuck and Robert Evans are gradually filling their elders' places.

Nearly all the surviving senior men are represented here, with three major exceptions: Frank Capra, creator of sociological morality plays and "message" comedies of the thirties and forties, brilliant technician and master of the art of editing, was, alas, unavailable for interview. John Ford, arguably the greatest American director of all, did agree to see us but jovially sent us up, playing his role of cornpone pioneer to the hilt, and Howard Hawks was out of town during our visit. It would have been pleasant to include these three, and their absence is regretted; so is William Wyler's.

Our thanks go finally to those whose generosity and kindness made many of these encounters possible: Don Prince, Twentieth Century-Fox; Robert Vogel, Metro-Goldwyn-Mayer; Louis Blaine, Universal Pictures. And to the directors themselves.

Robert Aldrich

Follow the long plain corridors of the MGM Administration Building, climb a flight of prosaic stairs and turn several corners and you will eventually reach an office which sometimes serves as the temporary headquarters of Aldrich and Associates, Inc. An inner room, rather murky and cluttered, its main furnishings a mountainous desk and a number of big black leather chairs, discloses a burly, bespectacled man who looks as if he might have been a formidable college footballer. This is Robert Aldrich, and he was indeed a formidable college footballer. He is now an even more formidable veteran of countless Hollywood in-battles, and creator of a body of films which at their best reflect his own urban-American energy and his pre-occupation with the morality and ethics of violence in an amoral, violent world. He offers us Coca Cola, talking briskly and often pungently of the vicissitudes of a movie director's career. After the interview—although it is now well past normal office hours and the building is practically deserted—he will confer long into the evening with a colleague on the preparation of their new film. Movie-making, for Robert Aldrich, is clearly a twenty-four-hours-a-day activity: not just a profession, more a way of life.

I got into the film business in 1941, just as I was about to leave the University of Virginia. I couldn't see myself in either banking or publishing like my father, but he had a brother who was involved in some New York banks and also had some movie interests in California. So I went to this uncle and told him I would like to get into films.

He pointed out that there were three divisions, produc-

23

tion, exhibition, and distribution, and making up my mind quickly I naturally plumped for production. He gave me a job for six weeks at $25 per week saying, "I never want to see you again." And that's how I entered films.

My first job was as a production clerk, a position that's since been done away with. It was the lowest form of human life here, the guy below the bookkeeper and below the tea-boy. It was the guy who'd be sent running if anybody needed anything or who had to fill out all the actors' time-cards and production reports at the end of the day or before the company started its day's shooting. They were finally unionized about 1942 or 1943 and became third or fourth assistants, but at that time it was the lowest job in existence on a sound stage.

From third or fourth assistant you'd generally progress to second assistant, which is quite important in the production setup, and then you'd make the big jump to first assistant. I made that jump rather hurriedly thanks to World War II. I was in the Air Corps for about a day and a half and was thrown out because of some old football injuries. By then the war had created a need in the movie industry—as in every industry—for manpower, particularly young, energetic, ambitious manpower, and owing to the lack of good first assistants I got the opportunity to be one. From there I rose to the position of production manager.

I was terribly lucky in my assignments. I worked with Lewis Milestone on four or five pictures when he was just about at the peak of his career—although *he* mightn't consider it the peak. Anyhow, he had recently done some really great films. I worked with Chaplin, with Joseph Losey and Bill Wellman, and also with some terribly bad directors whom there's no point in naming—but you learn just as much from the bad ones as you do from the good ones, strangely. And, perhaps most notably, I worked at Enterprise Studios with people like Abraham Polonsky and Robert Rossen.

Enterprise embodied a really brilliant idea of a communal way to make films. It was a brand new departure, the first time I can remember that independent film-makers had all the money they needed. David Loew was a partner. He had unlimited bank finance from the Bank of America. But we wasted—that's presumptuous—the *company* wasted an awful lot of money, energy, and effort on bad material, on improperly developed material, because its story selection and picture execution were not what they should have been.

The studio, in fact, had everything in the world in its favour except one thing: it didn't have anybody in charge who knew how to make pictures. There's an ethnic saying here: "A fish stinks from the head." Well, there was no head of that studio. There were a lot of very talented, experienced, intelligent people among its various branches, but there was no knowledgeable guy to run the shop.

But, for about two and a half or three years before it went down the drain, I would guess that it had a better *esprit de corps,* and more interest and excitement going for it among its employees, from the labourer to the star, than any place in Hollywood. When, as they inevitably must, people began to realize that the end product wasn't worth all this extra care and concern, the bubble burst and the dream faded. But I think it will be tried again some day.

For example, just by going to work there you got a life insurance policy—not terribly large, but it was paid for by the company. You got a guaranteed vacation, which wasn't enacted industry-wide for about ten years afterwards. You got all the free coffee and doughnuts and Coca Cola that you could eat and drink. That mightn't mean an awful lot now but in those days it meant a great deal—it just wasn't being generally done. Personal relations between the employees and management were extraordinary, and they paid the top dollar to all technicians. Thus they got the best technicians from every major studio in town. It was an unequalled organization.

While Enterprise did have an orientation towards stories with "social significance", I think it would be unfair to say that that was its "aim". As the Irish say, this was just before the "troubles", and the talented people in that period—there were always exceptions, of course—tended to be more liberal than the untalented people, and, because they were more liberal, they got caught up in social processes that had political manifestations which later proved to be economically difficult to live with. In its search for talented and interesting people, Enterprise hired a great many followers of that persuasion and its pictures consequently began to acquire more and more social content.

The studio's main problem was that it had one hit and about nine disasters. The hit was *Body and Soul.* It cost

$2.2 million—today the equivalent of $6 million—whereas it should have cost $1.1 million. John Garfield, the star, was a full partner, Bob Roberts was a full partner, Rossen—although he got *some* money—was a full partner. There was no over and above the line cost.

The picture cost a million dollars more than it should have cost because Rossen was given his head. Polonsky, although he'd written a marvellous script, really interfered too much. Roberts, who was a dear and good friend, never really pretended to be a producer, and, as I said, there was nobody at the head of the studio to bring us all up short.

Despite what has sometimes been said, I didn't direct any of *Body and Soul* myself. I was the first assistant director; Don Weis, who is now an exceptionally good television director and who occasionally does good features, was the script clerk; Bob Parrish was the cutter; James Wong Howe was the cameraman. We all tried to help—particularly James—and came up with many suggestions that were absorbed and used. But, although I think he could have done things better, it was all Rossen's work.

On *Force of Evil* I was production manager *and* assistant director. Abraham Polonsky, who wrote and directed it, is a terribly talented and gifted man. One could have gotten to him if he had had someone he respected to listen to, someone to say: "Hey, wait a minute, maybe that isn't the way, maybe we should re-examine it, perhaps there is another approach." But there was no one like that available, which tended to compound the mistakes in *Force of Evil* that were not inherent in Ira Wolfert's *Tucker's People*, the book from which it came.

Polonsky is now back in town and has done work at Universal for Norman Lloyd. I haven't seen him in several years. In the interim he wrote a couple of novels, one of which was quite well received critically but not commercially, and the other was not well received critically. He went to Canada to work with the man who runs the National Theatre as his kind of general creative artistic assistant. Then, during what we laughingly refer to as the "dark days", his work was to be found on television under a considerable variety of different names. But now that most people say those days are over he's back working: a delightful, very talented man.

You are led to believe that most of the formerly blacklisted people are back. It's not quite true. The rehabilitation process varies in direct proportion to their talent or their need. If they were marginal, or if they were sporadic in their output, you just find that they're not working.

My work on *Caught* was short and abrasive. I had taken over the job of studio production manager from Joe Gilpin who was seriously ill, whereas on *Force of Evil* I was production manager for only that one picture. Max Ophüls, the director of *Caught*, had gotten shingles and John Berry, a very good friend of mine, was brought in—as he and I thought—to finish the film.

Long before, however, there had been a secret deal between management and Ophüls designed to satisfy the banks because by that time we—the studio, that is—were in big financial trouble. According to this deal, Berry was to be engaged only for the duration of Ophüls' illness. But that's not what Berry was told. About two-thirds of the way through filming I began to hear whispers to the effect that sketches and models of forthcoming sets and costumes yet to be photographed were being taken to Ophüls at night and that he was approving them and changing the script and so forth.

Then, about that time, Ophüls recovered and they used the fact that Berry was running two or three days behind schedule—which is not, God knows, a crime on a picture like that—to fire him so they could bring Ophüls back. As studio manager I had to go and tell Berry, my friend, that he was fired; I was the instrument. I couldn't tell him then—I told him about a year afterwards—why he was fired. It was a very unpleasant period. I would guess that between a third and half of the finished film is Berry's. He had been dealt with in a very shabby fashion.

However, four or five months later, Ophüls had to come back for some retakes. We were really out of money then, so I was first assistant on *Caught* as well as studio production manager. I must say that it was with some sadistic delight that I gave Mr Ophüls a very bad couple of days because the bank had vested in me much of the power of deciding what retakes to do or not to do. I never got even for the injustice Mr Berry suffered but it was a pleasant two days.

My first feature film as director was *The Big Leaguer* at Metro-Goldwyn-Mayer. At that studio they'd formed a unit jokingly called "sons of the pioneers" in which sons of producers who'd worked with Louis B. Mayer were producing tiny little features. Dore Schary, who didn't have a very outstanding record here, was nevertheless a pretty wise fellow, and he recognized—in his capacity as studio production head—that with fellows like that as producers you had to have directors who knew what they were doing.

They were accordingly on the lookout for "bright young men" to come in and direct these pictures. At that time I was directing television film—not live—in New York. The only reason I got that job was that it was too tough, unglamorous, and poorly endowed technically to attract anyone else from Hollywood. Herbie Baker, who wrote the screenplay for *The Big Leaguer,* a baseball story, had been with Carl Foreman at Enterprise and suggested my name to Schary. That's how I got to direct features.

Among the television shows I did were a lot of the *China Smith* series starring the late Dan Duryea, a friend of long standing. The photographer was Joe Biroc, who's since worked with me a lot, and the producer was Bernie Tabakin. It was a fun show—we were knocking these episodes out in two days each—and one day I had an idea: "Why not make a feature the next time we close down?" Bernie, who was a great hustler, a great promoter, went and raised about $80,000, which was approximately $40,000 less than we needed.

So, during ten spare days, another fellow and I sat down and wrote a story which became *World for Ransom*. We made it in nine and a half days, at the end of which we ran out of money. To get enough money to finish the film we took on a couple of commercials, a beer commercial and an Eversharp commercial, and interrupted the picture to shoot them. It was a strange and very enjoyable experience and—except for the end results— a marvellous collaboration. It really had no sets, and thanks to Joe Biroc we had reflections in water where there was no water, and all kinds of silly things. I've always looked back on that film with a wistful kind of happy feeling.

My association with Hecht-Lancaster goes back earlier than *World for Ransom*, to the time when they were still kind of sprawling and struggling and had gone to Columbia on a two-picture deal. One was *Ten Tall Men* and the other was one of Frank Tashlin's early films, *The First Time*.

They needed someone to watch the store because

Hecht had never really produced. I don't mean that his contribution on *The Flame and the Arrow* wasn't substantial; I have no way of knowing. But he wasn't too well acquainted with the physical and financial side of picture-making and needed an experienced production manager. I went there as "assistant to the producer", which was really just a glorified way of paying me more money so that I could be their production manager.

Later—after television stuff in New York, after MGM and *World for Ransom*—I got to do *Apache* for them because they wanted a "bright young man" they didn't have to pay much money to. *Apache* was an inexpensive Red Indian epic that could have been better. A great deal of what I wanted to say about the Red Indians in it was lost. The original script ended with the hero, Massai (played by Burt Lancaster), going back up to a shack to be shot needlessly in the back by Federal troops. That was the script I'd been given, that was the script I'd approved, and that was the script I'd shot.

Two or three days before shooting on the picture was due to finish, United Artists prevailed upon Hecht to shoot two endings. I don't know how it is in other countries but in this country when you have somebody suggest two endings you know they're going to use the other one. So I refused to shoot the alternate ending, and for about two days Burt agreed that the original ending was what this picture was all about.

Then, for reasons best known to himself, he changed his mind. Now once Burt had changed his mind it made little difference if I refused to direct the other ending because the next day they could have got someone who would. The point was lost because a $500-a-week director had no hope of prevailing against Hecht-Lancaster and United Artists.

If Burt had stood firm, I think the picture would have been more—"significant" is a pompous word—but I think it would have been more important. It was seriously compromised. You make a picture about one thing, the inevitability of Massai's death. His courage is measured against the inevitable. The whole preceding two hours become redundant if at the end he can just walk away.

Jean Peters, who played Nalinle, Massai's wife, was a delight to work with, very responsive and courageous. She was deeply embroiled with Howard Hughes at the time. That broke off temporarily right in the middle of the picture, obviously causing her great concern. It made no difference to her performance, however. The film involved an awful lot of physical work. When someone's done something that's *almost* good enough you don't want to make them go through all that again just to improve it that one little bit, because who will know, except you, and maybe the actress later? And she would never cop out on that kind of thing. "I didn't do it quite right, did I?" she'd say. "I'd like to do it again." It's not easy to bring yourself to ask someone to do that kind of thing repeatedly, because it was terribly strenuous, and she was marvellous.

Burt Lancaster is not an easy man to get along with, but quite responsive, and we had a much better relationship, I think, than either of us anticipated on *Apache*. That led on to *Vera Cruz*. I think on that picture we probably had a less amicable relationship than we anticipated. This was because Burt, until he directed *The Kentuckian*, thought he was going to be a director, and when you're directing your first great big picture you don't welcome somebody else on hand with directorial notions. There were also a few differences of opinion about concepts and about action. Since Burt directed *The Kentuckian* I think he's probably a more valuable actor.

I'd just finished *Vera Cruz* when Victor Saville, who owned the film rights to all Mickey Spillane, came to me and asked if I would direct one. I'm not being critical of the first two Mickey Spillanes when I say that I thought they were not very good films. I guess they did what they were supposed to do. However, I agreed to do it provided he would let me make the kind of movie I wanted and provided I could produce it. "By all means," he said, and from then until the preview I think he came on the set only twice. I've been told he's a very unpleasant guy to work with but that was never my experience. It was an ideal situation; there was no interference at all.

The original book, *Kiss Me Deadly*, had nothing. We just took the title and threw the book away. The scriptwriter, A. I. Bezzerides, did a marvellous job, contributing a great deal of inventiveness to the picture. That devilish box, for example—an obvious atom bomb symbol—was mostly his idea. We worked a long time to get the sound it made, the ticking and hissing. We finally used the sound of an airplane exhaust overdubbed with the sound made by human vocal cords when someone breathes out noisily, so that it became a subdued "jet roar", a "sonic box" type of thing. You hear it every time the box opens.

I was very proud of the film. I think it represented a whole breakthrough for me. In terms of style, in terms of the way we tried to make it, it provided a marvellous showcase to display my own ideas of moviemaking. In that sense it was an enormous "first" for me.

I've never denied that. I think what irritates some people—and I've been misquoted about this so many times —is that they think I've disowned the importance of the film. I haven't. What I have said is that it has an importance juxtaposed against a particular political background, an importance that's not justified if it's juxtaposed against another one that by accident happens to fit.

It did have a basic significance in *our* political framework that we thought rather important in those McCarthy times: that the ends did not justify the means. Once you got outside the United States, the whole importance of that disappeared and the French—who particularly liked the film—and others read into it all sorts of terribly profound observations. Now, the moment you denied that alleged profundity they thought you were discrediting your own work and their opinion of it. That really wasn't the case. It had a local—meaning American—political application which lost its special kind of importance when applied to other places.

In certain foreign countries they had their own particular sets of circumstances to which they tried to give it an identical application. I'd like to say that I was smart enough to have made a film in which all these bromides applied to all countries under all kinds of pressures. But I wasn't; the film had no such universal application.

I anticipated that we might run into censorship trouble with *Kiss Me Deadly*, but when we did it was not on brutality as I'd expected, not on the usual sexual-salacious morality rap, but only on one particular scene, and why I'll never know.

There's a scene in the picture of a Negro songstress in downtown Los Angeles, an actress by the name of Maddie Comfort, singing a song. She's singing into a white microphone and handling the microphone in an—I guess— overtly suggestive fashion. The Code people of the Motion Picture Association of America passed it; no problem. Strangely, in fact, I've never had any trouble with them. But the Legion of Decency—with whom I've had a lot of trouble—just screamed. Bill Heineman, who was vice-president in charge of distribution for United Artists, willy-nilly made all the cuts that the Legion insisted on, which I felt he didn't have to do. He could have bargained and, while sacrificing some of it, kept the rest.

Most of the actresses in the picture had never been in films. We made it in the very short time of twenty-two days and we wanted unusual, interesting girls. That brings you back to the old bromide: What's an interesting girl? At that time it was very voguish in this country to consider a girl with an over-large bust automatically attractive. That never happened to be my particular point of view and I thought that if we could find some ladies who'd not been seen before and who had other interesting attributes than large breasts, it might be worthwhile. We tried it. Some afterwards stayed on in movies, others retired to be housewives.

At the close of *Kiss Me Deadly* I formed my own company, The Associates and Aldrich, retaining many of the people—film editor Michael Luciano, cameraman Joe Biroc, propmen, assistants—who had been with me before on most of the television stuff, certainly on *World for Ransom*.

By the time I came to make *The Big Knife,* it was an established operation. People here were very upset over what I was saying about Hollywood in that picture. It would have been marvellous if the film had been a success economically. It did very well critically; economically it was, to say the least, a disappointment.

I'd love to be able to say it failed commercially because it was too uncompromising; that would make me out to be a courageous guy. But there were other factors. I found, for example, that lay audiences could not believe that Jack Palance was a movie star. They didn't associate him with a guy who could or could not decide to take $5000 per week. Also, I felt that we had licked the problem that I thought Clifford Odets hadn't licked in the play: to understand that the taking or not taking of $5000 per week was not primarily a monetary problem; it was a problem of internal integrity such as you or I or the guy at the gas station might have.

We didn't communicate that, however. My father, who at that time was a very elderly gentleman, not particularly profound but reasonably smart, and who certainly had every reason to want to like the picture, really spelled out what most people thought about it in this country when he said: "If a guy has to take or not to take $5000 per week, what the hell is the problem?"

Well, the problem was enormous, and for all our honesty we undoubtedly failed to communicate it to the mass audience—not to the critics, not to selective audiences —but to the mass audience. They didn't understand it. I think they found the film credible, but they couldn't identify. Palance wasn't sufficiently good-looking and they couldn't believe that the problem of compromising and selling out was *their* problem. To them it was an alien problem.

I don't know that this dilemma could have been resolved anyhow. The original play had been done on Broadway with John Garfield. If you'd had an electric, charming guy like Garfield in the lead you'd have solved half the problem, but I don't think you'd ever have solved the other half.

As you know, Garfield was dead by the time we came to do the picture. To begin with, we hardly had any money. I thought then—still do, although Palance and I hardly speak any more—that Palance is a wonderful, wonderful actor. He has that kind of intensity and burning integrity that I thought the part required. It's hindsight to say that it never occurred to me that people wouldn't accept him as a movie star.

The rest of the cast was more or less exactly what I wanted. Rod Steiger, who'd never played the part on the stage, based the crying and pleading in his characterization of the producer on L. B. Mayer, but the other elements— the rages and tantrums—were pretty much based on Harry Cohn.

I guess self-survival made me do *Autumn Leaves.* People were getting collective in their criticism of the violence and anger and wrath in my pictures, although these things weren't intentional, and I thought it was about time I made a soap opera—firstly, because I wanted to do one anyway, and secondly, because this seemed a pretty good one. I was also a great fan of the Butlers—Jean Rouverol and the late Hugo Butler—and this was her original story. I didn't think it would turn out to be quite as soap opera-ish as it did. I regret that now. I didn't have the foresight to see it then.

I had always been a Joan Crawford fan and I thought the thing would work. We had big problems from the beginning. It was a joint venture between Bill Goetz and myself. He was the nominal producer but we had certain built-in guarantees of non-interference. About a week before work on the picture began, Miss Crawford wanted her own writer to come in and rewrite, which I refused to allow her to do. Up until the night before shooting on the film was due to commence there was a continued harassment about the possibility of her not showing up. I got a call at two o'clock that very night saying that she wouldn't be there in the morning unless her writer could attend, to which I responded that if her writer showed up we would not shoot.

Looking back, I really think that's the only way you can properly deal with Miss Crawford. The writer didn't show up, but she did, and we proceeded. But she didn't talk to me for about four or five days. She took direction, she did what she was supposed to do, but there was no personal communication. Then one day she was doing a scene terribly effectively—I don't remember which one. I was really touched, and when she looked up after finishing it I tried not to be obvious in wiping away a tear. That broke the ice, and from then on we were good friends for a long long time.

I'm very proud of *Attack!* I never saw *The Fragile Fox*, the play on which it's based, but I read it and thought that it said through the characters many things that I would like to have said about anti-war attitudes.

We had just been through a cycle of markedly unsuccessful preachment pictures in California and I thought that, if you could make this film really honestly and with a good cast, the characters saying what you'd like to say by just playing the parts, it would be a welcome change.

It worked that way, and the picture got a marvellous reception, less gratifying than one hoped economically, but it did make money. Many people prophesied that it wouldn't, but it did. The problem was that it was cross-collateralized against *The Big Knife* so nobody ever saw any of the money.

My main anti-war argument was not the usual "war is hell", but the terribly corrupting influence that war can have on the most normal, average human beings, and what terrible things it makes them capable of that they wouldn't be capable of otherwise.

The casting was mostly what I wanted but I did make a terrible mistake—mine, not the actor's. We talked earlier of what you learn from good directors and bad directors: When we were making *"M"*, Losey was doing a sensational job. You might argue that it should never have been made at all, but if you accept its being made it must be acknowledged that Losey did a marvellous job.

We came to the final scene where David Wayne as the child-killer is cornered, as in the Fritz Lang original. Luther Adler had to deliver this defensive eulogy of Wayne. Adler did it in a rehearsal and it was just brilliant. There wasn't a dry eye on the sound-stage. Everybody applauded. But he never, never got it again; didn't come close to it; didn't come half-way towards getting it. One would have thought that anybody with half a goddamned brain would have remembered that always. I should have been smarter.

We came to the scene in *Attack!* where Eddie Albert has to break down and grab the slippers. I made the same mistake as Losey: he left the performance in the rehearsal-hall. It never got on film. What's there is quite good— we cut and edited it to make it look as good as possible. But he was brilliant in rehearsal. The actor has a right to expect the director to know his limitations sufficiently well to know what he's capable of and to be sure that his best work is captured on film, because he might not have the particular kind of talent that can do it over and over and over again.

The Garment Jungle was a strange experience. I don't remember another case of a guy getting fired for wanting to shoot the picture that he'd been assigned. Usually, if you're fired, it's for wanting to change the script. I have never seen the finished film, although I'm told that about half or two-thirds of it are mine.

The picture's producer, Harry Kleiner, had written a great script. But it was terribly tough, controversial stuff and, as we started getting into it—it was shaping up as a pretty good picture—they suddenly realized that they had no intention of making that kind of a document; they wanted to make "boy meets girl in the dress factory."

I was pretty stubborn, and Harry Cohn, the head of Columbia Pictures, was pretty stubborn, and they wanted to change the focus, the force, the direction of the picture. I wouldn't do it, and Cohn fired me.

I had a great fondness for Cohn. Naturally I think he was wrong in firing me but that's beside the point. I think he ran a marvellous studio; I think that system is better, I

think he did it as well as anybody could do it. He wasn't
in the money business, he was in the movie business. I had
a chance to have a reconciliation with him later and I
didn't go. I've always regretted it.

The reconciliation I mean was in terms of doing other
work. It's pretty silly for grown men not to speak. There
was a rather strong romance between us at one time
because I didn't want to come to Columbia and he said he
liked my work. But he never spoke about *The Big Knife*. I
didn't consider it prudent to mention it, and he chose not
to bring it up.

The Angry Hills is a disappointing picture—not because
it's not good but because it *could* have been good. MGM
and the film's producer, Raymond Stross, had retained
Robert Mitchum as star, specifying a starting date and a
rather heavy salary.

Came the time to start shooting and we weren't ready,
the script wasn't done. But Metro insisted, and Stross—
looking back I don't say it was wrong—chose the easy
way out: "All right," he said, "let's begin it, we'll catch
up." That turned the scriptwriter, A. I. Bezzerides, right
off, and what could have been a rather extraordinary
piece of material became just another story. Bezzerides is
a strange man. To get him to creatively concentrate—he
sits in the room, he types, he does the pages all right,
that's not what I mean—but to get him to turn that thing
off, turn the other thing on, and zero in and focus is
terribly tough. That's the difference between just any
script and an exceptional script.

The Angry Hills had a potential that was never even
remotely realized. *Ten Seconds To Hell,* on the other
hand, is a bad picture. Why, I've never been quite sure.
Some of it has to do with my writing, some of it has to do
with the story, some of it with the fact that United Artists
didn't know what kind of picture it was. If it's bad, it's
bad, but that's as good as you could make it.

Thus, you feel embarrassed maybe about *Ten Seconds
To Hell,* but you feel sad about *The Angry Hills.* No
matter if I did *Ten Seconds To Hell* tomorrow I wouldn't
know how to make it any better. I'd know how to make
The Angry Hills better in a thousand ways.

The Last Sunset was a very unpleasant experience. I
was dead broke at the time, having just come back from
Europe, after spending all I had trying to put *Taras
Bulba*—not the one that you saw—together. I had just

done two bad pictures and had to sell my interest in *Taras Bulba* merely to get the taxes paid.

Dalton Trumbo had done a screenplay. He had yet— this was just towards the end of the McCarthy period—to be given a screen credit, and Preminger had promised him one for *Exodus*. He quit his concentration on *The Last Sunset* to concentrate on the Preminger picture, and by the time he came back to our film, it was too late to save it.

Now I think that, all things considered, Trumbo was two thousand per cent right. But that didn't solve the problem of making *The Last Sunset* any better. However, there was an enormous principle involved here. He was the first writer to break through the blacklist; he was going to force a change in the whole Californian concept of blacklisted writers. That was certainly much more important than making Kirk Douglas look well.

And Kirk was impossible. He knew the screenplay wasn't right. The whole thing started badly, went on badly, ended up badly. Rock Hudson, of all people, emerged from it more creditably than anyone. Most people don't consider him a very accomplished actor, but I found him to be terribly hard-working and dedicated and very serious: no nonsense, no "I've got to look good" or "Is this the right side?" If everybody in that picture, from producer to writer to other actors, had approached it with the same dedication it would have been a lot better. That's not my way of saying that Mr. Hudson is Laurence Olivier, but he was certainly much more honestly involved in the venture than anybody else I can think of.

While I was working in Italy on *Sodom and Gomorrah*, a secretary I had had in England on *Ten Seconds to Hell* found a novel called *Whatever Happened to Baby Jane?* and brought it to my attention. I immediately flipped for it. To buy it, however, would have cost $60,000 and I no more had $60,000 than a hawk in the wind.

Joe Levine, producer of *Sodom and Gomorrah*, and I were then going through the customary romantic honeymoon and he put up the $60,000 needed to buy *Baby Jane* from some scavenger-type fellows who'd acquired it and commissioned some guy to do a screenplay; he never did one. Levine and I had an agreement that, if we couldn't go forward together by a certain date, I had to buy it back from him.

When the time came to do the film, the honeymoon was

long since over. He'd taken a considerable amount of money out of *Sodom and Gomorrah* and left me—so to speak—holding the baby, because the Italians were ready to kill all of us and I felt that as long as I could continue to play Levine off against the Italians it would all be pretty clear sailing.

In the end, the Italians got the worst of the deal and there was nobody left to take their wrath out on but me. Consequently relations between Levine and me became so strained that I arranged to buy *Baby Jane* back from him and made it myself.

As screenwriter I engaged Lukas Heller. Lukas had done a BBC kinescoped teleplay called *Cross of Iron* that his brother-in-law, an ex-friend of mine who had been head of United Artists publicity in New York and was now occupying the same position in England, had drawn my attention to. I found *Cross of Iron* fascinating, bought an option on it, and brought Lukas to Mexico to write a screenplay of it when we were doing *The Last Sunset*.

That occasioned a particularly abrasive collision between Kirk Douglas and myself. We were up in Aguas Calientes, on the northern Mexican plateau, terribly rural, primitive, unsophisticated country. One day three men arrived on the set: Peter Berg, a small Berlin intellectual with *pince-nez* and grey hair who was doing the German version of *Cross of Iron*; Mr. Heller, with his long, flowing, Edwardian locks, who was doing the English version; and a marvellous Negro actor who'd written an English teleplay.

Things had been going so badly on *The Last Sunset* that, knowing I could make a much better picture than that, I'd brought these three writers down to prepare my next projects. When Douglas turned around and caught sight of this trio in the middle of the Mexican wilderness, he went berserk; he just went crazy. So we had to send them to Mexico City where they continued to write; we couldn't have them in Douglas's presence.

Heller did a marvellous job on *Cross of Iron*. Much to my chagrin and his embarrassment we found out that many of the villains of that piece—although it had been done in England and occasioned no comment—still existed in Germany. It concerned a German submarine that was sunk by its own commander. When he was sent to a prisoner-of-war camp, he was executed by his fellow-countrymen.

We had a deal with Artur Brauner to make this picture, but the Germans took legal action against us. If you're a non-German litigant, you have to put up bonds as you appeal to higher courts. Eventually we ran out of bond-money. I think we probably would have lost anyway; I don't know any more. Anyhow, we never made the film.

I did get to know and like Heller's work very much, though. He was in Rome when we lost our final court case on *Cross of Iron*. By then I'd acquired *Baby Jane* and I asked him to do it. We worked together very closely. I think he's a terribly gifted man. I also like to think that many of the turns the story took and the nuances it acquired in its translation to the screen were devised by Heller and myself.

Right from the beginning, Bette Davis and Joan Crawford were my first choices for the two main parts. I'd never met Davis. I did write her a letter saying that she might not want to do the picture, but I thought she'd have to admit it was the best role she'd ever had, and, if she didn't feel that way, she shouldn't see me. After two weeks she wrote back in longhand declaring that it was rather presumptuous of me to say that, but it was certainly a good enough role to warrant discussion.

The two stars didn't fight at all on *Baby Jane*. I think it's proper to say that they really detested each other, but they behaved absolutely perfectly. There was never an abrasive word in public, and not once did they try to upstage each other. Nor did Miss Davis allow her enmity with Miss Crawford to colour her playing of the scenes in which she was supposed to torment her. People who loved the violence of it read that into it and thought it was inherent, but it wasn't. They both behaved in a wonderfully professional manner.

I'd seen Victor Buono on television in an *Untouchables* episode playing a large cameo character called Mr Moon. He was fabulous. Davis didn't like him at first: she thought he was too grotesque. Victor obviously sensed her attitude, but he never commented, and it was never openly displayed. Half-way through the film—we don't really get along, but this is a small instance of the kind of lady she can be when she wants to—she smiled at him and said: "I want you to know that at the beginning of this picture I did everything I could to persuade Bob not to use you and I'd like to apologize because you're just marvellous." And he was.

Miss Davis was wonderful in it, too. She, more than I, decided on her Baby Jane makeup, that ugly chalky mask. I'd say it was eighty per cent Davis and twenty per cent Aldrich, whereas on *Hush, Hush, Sweet Charlotte* it was very close to fifty-fifty, maybe fifty-five per cent Aldrich and forty-five per cent Davis. She did not realize, I think, what the cumulative effect of seeing herself like that would be. Thus she was not prepared for Cannes, where she saw the complete film for the first time among lots of people.

About five minutes into the picture I heard this quiet but kind of desperate sobbing beside me and turned to her wondering what the hell was the matter. "I just look awful," she wept. "Do I really look that awful?"

Miss Davis is a strange lady. She's been misled so many times, and placed her confidence so many times in situations and/or people that didn't pay off, that she's naturally terribly hesitant to trust anybody. You could cite a thousand reasons why this should be so. Once she trusts you, however, she's marvellous.

Consequently *Baby Jane* was not without its difficulties in having her take direction. You always prevailed, but it wasn't easy. By the time we came to do *Hush, Hush, Sweet Charlotte*, she understood my methods and there was never any argument. I thought—the public won't agree, and certainly the critics won't agree—that the job she did in *Charlotte*, because it was a much more difficult, narrow-edged part, and took much more talent and time and thought and care, was a better performance than *Baby Jane*, which was such a bravura, all-out Gothic eye-catcher that everybody thought it superior.

Charlotte came from a three- or four-page original idea by Henry Farrell, author of the *Baby Jane* novel, that I found very exciting. I also wanted to re-team Davis and Crawford. But for all their professional propriety on *Jane*, it couldn't have been more the opposite on its successor. A terribly hostile atmosphere prevailed until Miss Crawford fell ill and was replaced by Olivia de Havilland.

There's no doubt in the world that Crawford was sick, seriously sick. If she'd been faking, either the insurance company would never have paid the claim or she would never have been insurable again. Insurance companies here are terribly tough, there's no such thing as a made-up ailment that they pay you off on.

While Crawford was in hospital we finished all Davis's

scenes in which Crawford didn't appear. When she came back to work she was so exhausted that she could only do about two or three hours' filming a day. Even that proved too much; she returned to hospital and became worse. At that stage, the insurance company offered us the alternatives of finding a replacement for Miss Crawford within two weeks or scrapping the picture.

As you can well imagine, there were great arguments about whom we should get. A number of ladies were considered, all of whom for a variety of reasons were not acceptable to all parties. There was also a contractual problem in that Davis had star approval. Until then it had been academic because she had approved Crawford, but it now became vitally important.

Obviously the ideal candidates would have been Vivien Leigh and Katharine Hepburn. Now it's not necessary that it should become a matter of public record why Davis didn't want either of those ladies. It is fair to say however that it had nothing to do with their talent. But there are deep-seated personal and historical reasons why she didn't want them. I won't say that Olivia was the third choice, but Olivia was the first choice that was acceptable.

I guess if Davis has a friend who's a real lady, it's de Havilland; they're very close. She tried to persuade Olivia to do the part, helped me talk to her on the phone. No good. So I went off to Switzerland to try to convince de Havilland in person. It was terribly difficult. I'm not quite sure why, but I think it has to do with Miss de Havilland's opinion of what her image is vis à vis of what it *may* be. If you look at her career you'll see that, except for *The Snake Pit* and *The Dark Mirror*, she's played mainly "good" women. Although I think she's a marvellous villainess, she dislikes playing them. Such shortcomings as *Charlotte* had in that department were not hers, they were shortcomings in the balance of the parts in the script.

I thought *4 for Texas* could be a "fun" picture, a satire on Westerns, a kind of high-style comedy. Mr. Sinatra and I didn't get along, and I guess I never should have thought that he had the kind of vigour that it takes to do it. You can't do this sort of thing with your left hand, you have to work very hard at it—as evidenced by Dean Martin's enormous success. He worked hard at being casual, and he's really a delight to work with.

The art director William Glasgow did a marvellous job on *4 for Texas*. He did an even better job on *Charlotte* which doesn't show because it's in black-and-white. I believe I gave him his first credit as an art director, and we've been associated ever since. I give him a concept. He comes back with the drawings. It's very subtle. Sometimes it gets terribly complicated when we use a model, but very rarely. We did use one on *Charlotte* and *The Legend of Lylah Clare*. As I approve or disapprove of his suggestions, his ideas snowball and gradually become better and better.

It might seem a silly thing to say, but one preplans one's pictures if there's time. What you find is that you run out of time. You can't let other things intrude on rehearsals, even though you'll pay for it later. You concentrate on rehearsals at the expense of other things so you often have to do a certain amount of improvising while shooting.

Ideally, I'd like to preplan my pictures in their entirety, and on some there's time to do that. Hitchcock is said to do it. Milestone did it. I think it's too rigid. We used to have terrible problems with Milestone. He's a marvellous cutter and director, but he would preplan and pre-sketch a scene so much that, if an actor wanted to depart from it by even one little bit, the whole preparation went for nothing.

Although *The Dirty Dozen* became a big, terribly successful movie, with a marvellous cast, we had difficulties with it during its conception. Metro-Goldwyn-Mayer and the producer Kenneth Hyman had bought the property, a novel by E. M. Nathanson, after I had tried to acquire it when it wasn't even in galleys, just a step outline. Then they had about four or five scripts, the last one written by Nunnally Johnson. This would have made a very good, very acceptable 1945 war picture. But I don't think that a 1945 war picture is necessarily a good 1967 war picture.

That's where the problems started. They continued when, unknown to me, and although I had arranged with Hyman to do the casting and the cutting, Metro hired John Wayne. Now I'm a Wayne fan. His politics don't bother me, that's his mother's problem. In certain kinds of films I think he's marvellous. But you don't get John Wayne to play a Lee Marvin part. Anyhow, after a lot of unnecessary, unpleasant abrasion, Wayne himself decided not to play the part.

The next problem was to try to get a new script. Metro must have had about $300,000 tied up in aborted *Dirty Dozen* scripts by then, and I wanted a whole new concept.

So I called in Lukas Heller. Well, despite considerable resistance, we *got* a whole new concept, and, with the exception of Bosley Crowther, I think you will discover that most people adored—that's a pretty rich word—were fascinated by the anarchy of the picture's first two-thirds, and tolerated and were excited and/or stimulated and/or entertained by the last third. The first two-thirds were Mr Heller's contribution towards making it a 1967 picture and not a 1947 picture, and the last third was a pretty high-class, well-done war adventure.

The Legend of Lylah Clare came from a television Du-Pont "Play of the Month", with Tuesday Weld and Alfred Drake in the parts respectively played in the movie by Kim Novak and Peter Finch. Jean Rouverol and Hugo Butler developed it into a script; we were four years on that monster. We tried to avoid making it *Marienbad Revisited*. It got terribly disjointed, and the big problem was to make it legitimately disjointed and not arty-crafty disjointed. Since then I've done, of course *The Killing of Sister George,* a film about lesbians, and *Too Late the Hero* with Cliff Robertson, a war picture shot in the Philippines.

Among contemporary European directors, I love Godard and Chabrol. I happen to think that Chabrol is terribly underrated in terms of the New Wave. He's a much better director than most people give him credit for. He sometimes chooses unfortunate material, but I think he's just as profound, knowledgeable, aware and talented as Truffaut or some of the more popular French film-makers.

In Hollywood today we have a problem that is hopefully going to be solved, but until it is we're going to go through a frightfully difficult period. I could be wrong, this is not a nationalistic point of view, but it's my opinion that we have just as many talented directors and actors here as anywhere else in the world.

What has happened is that this industry has gone into the money business and not into the film business, and, since they are in the money business, they tend to look for guarantees and protections and things like that before everything else. Because of the inundation of the more honest, more frank European pictures, we were breaking away from that tendency for quite a while, but now that's been offset owing to the enormous revenues that American films can make through being sold to television. All of a sudden there's a fresh inundation of this conservative, play-it-safe, let's-sell-it-by-the-foot, very average mundane material.

And I don't know the answer to that. We have such staggering labour costs here. I don't say that they're unfair but they are high. You can't make a good film without taking time over it. *Morgan* cost no money, but Karel Reisz took sixty-six days to make *Morgan*. Well, you just can't shoot sixty-six days in this country for under two million dollars.

I don't know how you're going to break through at the idea level. A guy comes to you and says he wants to r˙˙ke a daring, controversial piece of material. Now, to make that well, to make it competitive, to make it as well as the Europeans make it, he's got to take the same amount of time. But he can't do that because the Americans in charge of handing out the money aren't going to give him the required amount. They might give him—if he's an extremely talented, well-known guy and the ideas aren't too explosive—one-tenth of the money he needs. But one-tenth of the money he needs is not going to buy him one-third of the time he needs, so he can't come over with a good picture. And I don't know the solution.

Pay-television is certainly part of the answer. But even though it was proved unconstitutional, the public in the State of California were so misled by the avalanche of publicity and pressure from the distributors and the exhibitors as to what pay-television really was they willy-nilly voted against it.

It'll happen again and again, maybe not in that kind of fatalistic fashion. Sure, pay-television is going to come and when it does it will be a solution, but I don't think it is going to come half as quickly as a lot of people think.

Curtis Bernhardt

*Shadybrook Drive, Beverly Hills, is not particularly shady
nor is there a brook. Instead, there are pleasantly luxurious houses, not too ornate or elaborate, and certainly not
ostentatious. If there is wealth here, it is discreet, restrained, without vulgarity. By not calling attention to itself
it becomes subtly omnipresent, apprehended almost sub-
liminally. Curtis Bernhardt's house, set well back from the
roadway, is among the most agreeable on Shadybrook
Drive: large but not overpowering, without the massive,
chunky quality of so many Bel Air or Beverly Hills
homes, it reflects its owner's cosmopolitan good taste, the
civilized and quietly cultivated personality that one senses
in his films. Waiting for him on the front lawn, we look,
he says on returning from a dentist's appointment, as if we
had been delivered by the postman; and during the
interview we are joined by his wife, a remarkably handsome woman to whom he has been married less than ten
years. His speech, clear, precise, and carefully articulated,
reflects the discipline of an old-fashioned German background, tempered by a Jewish geniality and charm, his
slight German-American accent lending it added savour.
This is one of our happiest Hollywood encounters, relaxed
and without fuss. Not a major figure, perhaps, not a Ford,
or a Lang, or a Hitchcock, but nevertheless a fine crafts-
man, an expert storyteller, an accomplished, thoroughly
experienced dealer in celluloid artifice.*

I had a German background. I started out as an actor and
then went on to direct a couple of plays in Berlin. One
day someone came to me after seeing a play I had
directed and asked—this was in the days of silents—

whether I could make a motion picture for sixty thousand marks; that, of course, represented the complete budget, not just the director's salary.

I had no idea whether a motion picture cost sixteen thousand, sixty thousand, or six hundred thousand marks, but I said: "Yes." This was during the twenties, a time of strong pacifist feeling throughout Europe, a feeling I naturally shared. The film was called *War* and starred some very good actors, now unknown.

In it I used what I think must have been one of the first travelling shots ever attempted: during a big Berlin public demonstration I put the camera in a taxi and had it photograph the demonstrators through the rear window as they followed the vehicle on their march.

For a while after that I didn't direct anything, although I was anxious to get away from the theatre and make films. So, with an up-and-coming playwright friend named Carl Zuckmayer, in whose regiment I had been during World War I and who had just had his first big stage success, I collaborated on a story that we developed just for fun.

Someone bought it immediately and I directed it. William Dieterle acted in it together with quite a number of subsequently famous people. That film established me as a director in Germany.

In 1926 I made a version of *Jane Eyre* called *The Orphan of Lowood*. Olaf Foenss, a prominent Scandinavian star of the time, played Rochester, and the title role was played by an actress whose career ended very quickly. An elderly lady now, she lives here in Los Angeles with her husband; I've forgotten her stage name. I tried to give the film a grey, Gothic kind of mood as demanded by the story, although it's not as sombre as, say, *Wuthering Heights*. Later, of course, I was to do the story of the Brontë sisters in Hollywood.

I kept on making silent films until the great day came when they sent me to England saying: "They have pictures in London that speak. We want you to look at them and then make an all-talking film using our Klangfilm system." So, knowing hardly a word of English, I went to London and saw *The Jazz Singer* and all the early talkies.

Returning to Germany, I made for UFA a picture which later became a classic—it is still played there today—called *The Last Company*. Conrad Veidt played the lead in it, and it was a huge success.

That was the first major German sound film, shot simultaneously with *The Blue Angel*. Sternberg shot *The Blue Angel* on one stage and I shot *The Last Company* on an adjoining stage. I looked at Sternberg's rushes and Sternberg looked at my rushes, and I sometimes took his advice because he came from America, and he had made talkies and I had not; this was my first.

Marlene Dietrich, whom I had had in my last silent move, *Die Frau nach der man sich sehnt* (*The Woman One Desires*), sort of commuted between the sets because of our friendship from the previous film. Several years ago, when I made my only postwar German picture, I met Marlene at a big reception for her at the UFA studios. It was attended by hundreds of people to mark her return to Germany, which she was visiting for the first time since the nineteen-thirties.

She saw me, came rushing over and kissed me, and whispered in my ear: *"Die Frau nach der man sich nicht sehnt!"*—"The woman one does *not* desire!"

I agree with her. I don't think the film was very good and I'm not proud of it. However, no matter what Marlene may say about never having appeared in films before *The Blue Angel*, she can't deny that she was in it. In fact she played the lead opposite Fritz Kortner.

After *The Last Company* came several more talkies in quick succession. They included *Der Mann der den Mord Beging* (*The Man Who Killed*), also starring Conrad Veidt. This was based on a well-known French novel by Claude Farrère. It took place among the international diplomatic set in pre-World War I Constantinople. Veidt played a French attaché who kills an English lord (powerfully acted by Heinrich George), after having seduced the lord's wife Mary, played by Trude von Molo. Because the lord had been mistreating his wife an understanding Turkish minister of police allows the attaché to return to Paris at the end scot-free.

The Man Who Killed is one of my favourite films—not necessarily one of my most successful—because it had a certain romantic, brooding mood. There was exotic Constantinople, with eternal danger behind it, and beautiful women, and elegance—all the action occurred in a supremely elegant hotel—and you felt the whole time: "When is this situation going to explode?"

Then came a film called *The Tunnel*, based on the novel by Bernhard Kellermann. I made it rather reluctantly because by that time—this was 1933—Nazism had broken out in Germany. I'd been warned and fled to Paris where I had a contract to do *The Tunnel* in French; Jean Gabin was in it, people like that.

In Paris they received me with great joy saying: "We have a wonderful surprise for you: we're going to make this film in two versions, German and French, shooting in Munich."

"I'm not going back to Germany," I said. "I'm on their blacklist."

"Oh," they said, "we've got a special permit from the ministry of propaganda and you'll be perfectly safe. We insist. If you don't agree we'll see to it that you don't work in the French industry"—and, in those days, that would have been almost catastrophic for a refugee German director.

So I went back and did shoot the picture in two versions. Promptly after it was finished I was arrested by the Gestapo. Then came a big rigmarole: I bluffed my way out of the arrest, was rearrested and fled. Four weeks later I was out of the country, not to return for twenty-five years. That was, so to speak, the end of my German career.

In France I called in my assistant whom I had had for six years and whose name is now Henry Koster, and with him wrote a film called *L'Or dans la Rue* (*Gold in the Street*), which starred Albert Préjean and a young girl of sixteen or seventeen called Danielle Darrieux. I also directed it.

I think that was my first comedy. It was a very funny, sweet picture and a success. Then I was called over to England by a financial associate of Alexander Korda called Ludovico Toeplitz, an Italian with a German name whose father was the president of the Banca Commerciale d'Italia. They wanted me to supervise—not direct—a first production that this man intended to make because in those days the English industry was embryonic and they didn't have any experienced film-makers.

The film was a costume epic called *The Dictator*, which starred Clive Brook as Struensee, the eighteenth-century adventurer in Denmark. It had two directors: Alfred Santell, who later did *Winterset*, began it but created so much antagonism that he was taken off in the middle of it and replaced by Victor Saville, who finished it. That was the only time in my life I did not actually direct a film but merely supervised it technically.

After that the same man, Toeplitz, hired me to direct *The Beloved Vagabond,* starring Maurice Chevalier, who had just come back from Hollywood. It was made in two versions—in French it was called *Le Vagabond Bien Aimé*—and with two casts, except that Chevalier was, of course, in both. Opposite him was a little sixteen-year-old girl called Margaret Lockwood, who later became a star for a time in England. The film was a nice little romantic story about a bum who goes through France and a girl who attaches herself to him.

Then I went back to Paris and made a picture—I hope I'm not confusing my dates—called *Carrefour,* later re-made twice, once in England and once in America: here under the title of *Crossroads* with William Powell and Hedy Lamarr, and in England under the title of *Dead Man's Shoes.*

I had nothing to do with either remake. The original starred Suzy Prim, a star then in France, and Jules Berry, a wonderful actor. Following that, I did another French picture called *La Nuit de Décembre,* with Pierre Blanchard as a pianist. This was also a kind of romantic story with a woman playing two parts, herself and her own daughter twenty years later.

Then the war broke out and found me in an unfortunate predicament: for the Germans I was a Jew, and for the French and the English I was a German. So, at the end of 1939 or the beginning of 1940, I came to the United States and immediately signed with Warner Brothers.

The first thing that hit me here, and hit me hard, was that I no longer had the authority that I had had before. In Germany, France, and Italy before World War II, the director was in charge of the whole artistic side of the film including the script and the choice of the story. The producer had very little influence on actual film-making; he was only the business head of the organization.

In America, I found that the producer was the number one man and that the director was supposed to take a script, make a few changes if he felt like it, and then shoot it. My earliest memory of Warner Brothers in 1940 is of somebody handing me a script and saying: "You start shooting Monday." And I was used to having three, four, or five months' preparation: selecting the story, writing one shooting-script with the writers and then a second shooting-script, and when I was ready I went on the stage and started shooting.

Here the producer said to me: "You start Monday!" When I declined, he took me up to see Jack Warner who said: "Well, if you can't do it, take your release." That was my first impression of Hollywood.

Fortunately I fell sick and didn't have to do that particular film, which turned out miserably in somebody else's hands and hurt *his* career. Eventually, sheer insistence on my part won me the authority really to prepare a film, and my first one was *My Love Came Back*, written by Walter Reisch and featuring Olivia de Havilland, Jane Wyman, Rudy Vallee, and Jeffrey Lynn. A remake of an Austrian original, it was an immediate success.

Then I made *The Lady with Red Hair*, about the career of Mrs Leslie Carter, a famous American actress. It starred Miriam Hopkins as Mrs Carter and Claude Rains as David Belasco. Claude and I became very close friends.

I had a wonderful time making that picture. Although I liked Miriam Hopkins's performance—she conveyed the hysterics and tenseness of a temperamental stage actress very effectively—she was terribly difficult to work with. In fact, she was so tense that it overlapped into real life.

That gave rise to Claude Rains's favourite story. We had a scene in a theatre in which Mrs Carter had to come out and bow two or three times to an audience after the curtain had come down on a play in which she'd appeared: the usual thing. After she'd bowed a few times, the audience had to shout "Belasco!" and then Claude had to come out.

This is a case of that funny phenomenon of an actress identifying too much with her role. I sat at the back with a button in my hand to raise or lower the curtain. At the second curtain the extras clapped and shouted Mrs Carter's name, the curtain went down and up again and then somebody shouted "Belasco!"

Hopkins flew into a rage at that because she had to have at least two curtain calls *without* Belasco. She strode to the footlights shouting, "Who is the idiot who called out 'Belasco!'?" Gazing at the poor extra who had made an unwitting mistake, she began to abuse him. She screamed so much that I pressed the button, bringing the curtain down in front of her nose, and all you could hear were muffled sounds coming from behind it. I never made another film with Miss Hopkins.

Then came a few things with our present governor here, Mr Reagan. He was then sort of an unimportant, pleasant, typical, healthy American boy. You couldn't go wrong with him in that kind of part. I don't like these films, and not only because of Mr Reagan. One was called *Juke Girl,* a sort of semi-Western laid among fruit-pickers and incorporating orgies of fights; I don't know why they gave it to me. Another was *Million Dollar Baby,* with Priscilla Lane.

But that is the machinery of Hollywood. They don't care about proper directorial casting. "We have a film coming up, this guy's being paid, he's under contract, let him do it!" If it's objected that he may never have done that kind of picture they reply: "Never mind, he'll do it somehow."

Happy-Go-Lucky, which I made on loan-out at Paramount, started out as a punishment for me because I had turned down a film at Warners and was on suspension. Buddy de Sylva, then head of Paramount and before that a greatly successful Broadway musical writer, had seen the Priscilla Lane comedy and thought I was just the right man for *Happy-Go-Lucky,* although I'd never done a musical. It starred Betty Hutton and Rudy Vallee, for that time a big-name cast.

Norman Panama and Melvin Frank wrote the book. When I read the first draft script I went to Buddy de Sylva and said: "Mr de Sylva, take me off this film. It's all slapstick and I don't want to do slapstick."

"Wait till we get the second version," he said. "It will eliminate all that."

When I received the second version it proved to be worse. "Mr de Sylva," I said, "you told me you would change all that and it's still full of slapstick."

"That isn't slapstick, Curt," he said. "That's hokum." With that he dismissed me.

I made the film, it was fun, and it went over beautifully.

Then came a film more after my own heart, *Devotion,* the story of the Brontë sisters. This is the kind of film I like to do. I'd always been interested in the Brontës and was more than satisfied with the casting of Olivia de Havilland and Ida Lupino respectively as Charlotte and Emily; the third sister, played by Nancy Coleman, wasn't very important.

We also had Arthur Kennedy playing their brother

Branwell. This was his first really important part and he was stunningly good. It was the best performance in the film.

By that time, I'd attained a position at Warners where I sat regularly with the writers and worked out sequences. That is how the dream episode of Death on the moors as a horseman enveloping one of the sisters in his black cloak was conceived. It was done in a studio and not on an actual location because it is almost impossible—at least it was in those days—to make a sequence outdoors where you have a trick shot of a horseman with a black cape on a black horse, riding towards a person and enveloping that person in a death-like shroud. To do this out in the open you have to have considerable help from the lamps and reflectors and from the trick department. I remember we worked very long to get this done smoothly.

Also, to have done it on the moors we would have had to go to England. The war was on, and that made it additionally difficult. Besides—and later I was to suffer very much from this—it hadn't yet caught on in Hollywood that, if you have an appropriate subject, it pays to go out on actual location. In the nineteen-fifties I made a film set in Damascus on the Columbia backlot, and it looked like it: it lost all its veracity and all its colour.

Devotion was followed by one of my favourite films: *My Reputation*, with Barbara Stanwyck. It was a comedy-romance, with George Brent as the leading man. It was fun, mostly because Barbara is a real pal, a real trouper. You can pour water over her head or put a hot-foot on her and she takes it and laughs. The crew likes her, everybody likes her.

For the ski-ing scenes, we had a second unit shoot ski locations. Then we built a little hill with false snow on it. When Brent came down the hill to a stop, we rear-projected the snow scenes until it looked as if he was in the middle of a snowfall; yet it was all done indoors. Max Steiner wrote a charming score for the film, one of his less pompous scores.

My Reputation started my career on a new tack, because Miss Bette Davis saw it. She was then the queen of the Warner lot, and had her own company within the Warner organization. She was in Georgia or somewhere alone on vacation and sent back the order that I would have to direct her next picture, which was *A Stolen Life*. Despite what she claims in her autobiography, she did *not* produce the picture, although it was made by her production company; I'll face her any day on that. It had, in fact, no official producer. I was stuck with both ends of the thing, with producing and directing—which I don't like, because it's too much unnecessary bother.

It started out with a tremendous clash between Davis and me on the first running of her wardrobe tests. The tests were all done by her favourite designer. We all sat in a little projection-room, about twenty people, looking at those wardrobe rushes.

I hardly knew Miss Davis at that time, and I thought one test was more horrible than the other. She always exclaimed: "Isn't it beautiful?" And everybody would chorus: "Oh, it's gorgeous."

At the third costume I said carefully: "Now, Miss Davis, don't you think these things are a little theatrical?"

To which she replied: "Let's cut this 'theatrical' talk. Nobody can ever say that things connected with me are 'theatrical'." And she orated throughout the auditorium.

I thereupon became hot under the collar and saying "Goodbye, Miss Davis", I got up and walked out.

"Where are you going?" she asked.

"I'm going home," I said.

"What do you mean?" she called after me.

"You don't need a director," I said. "You need a yes-man, Miss Davis, and I'm not cut out to be a yes-man."

"I didn't mean it," she then said. "Come back, now, and tell me why you don't like the costumes."

So I told her. "I think you're right," she said, and from that moment on we were close friends. She has her own opinions, but an intelligent actress has a right to her opinions, if she's willing to argue them out and debate them with her director, and is not too stubborn. There were some scenes where she'd say, "Let's try it both ways."

Although *A Stolen Life* was set in New England, all the location work was done north of here at Pebble Beach, near Carmel and Monterey; nothing was done in New England, which the locations closely resembled. Most of the film, however, was shot on studio stages.

The story involved a pair of twins, and we were very anxious to achieve a completely new breakthrough in the screen handling of double exposure. Generally, with twins, one is in one-half or one-quarter of the screen and the other is in another, and they talk to each other that way.

But we did entirely new things. We actually had them pass each other, shaking hands, helping each other on with coats, even lighting each other's cigarettes. We only used a double very occasionally in over-the-shoulder shots; otherwise never.

I've forgotten how we did all that now, but I do know that when Warners made a similar film a few years ago with Miss Davis, called *Dead Ringer*, they sat all day long in front of *A Stolen Life*, studying it. They even called me in to advise them.

The climactic storm sequence was staged in the studio tank. It was very difficult and Bette almost drowned in it. In these tank scenes, you see, we have a boat with wires underneath it to control it and jiggle it around wherever you want it. Well, in this tremendous tank we had chutes coming down and waves coming up, and one of them was supposed to swish her overboard. She should have come up immediately but she went down and didn't come up. I was horrified because I realized that she had been caught in one of the wires.

We had what probably today would be called frogmen standing by who instantly dived in and pulled her out. A tank like that normally contains fifteen to seventeen feet of water, quite enough to drown in. I don't know whether she could swim or not, but, like a trouper, she took it all.

While Bette and I wanted Glenn Ford for the male lead, Jack Warner was dead against him, even barring him from the lot. So we smuggled him in through a back door and did secret tests which we later showed to Jack Warner, who then accepted him.

It's not true that Bette had anything to do with the lighting of her closeups. I saw to it that she didn't assume any authority that didn't belong to her, which was often quite a struggle. I would never have an actor tell me where to put my camera or anything like that. Once a director lets an actor interfere, he is lost. That's why I could never work with Sinatra or Marlon Brando. It would be out of the question because these guys assume rights and attitudes which properly belong to the director. Let them direct themselves, if they know how.

Compared with Bette Davis, Joan Crawford, whom I subsequently directed in *Possessed*, was as easy to work with as can be. She was naturally a little subdued because she was the studio's second-ranking star, Bette being Number One. She threw her handbag at me several times when, having just done a picture with Bette, I called her "Bette" by mistake.

The chief difference between Crawford and Davis is that, while Bette is an *actress* through and through, Joan is more a very talented *motion-picture star*. That means that, while she is just as professional, she is also simpler.

Granted, she's not as versatile as Bette. If Bette has an emotional scene she tackles it completely consciously and when you say "Cut" she might ask, "Do you think that was a little too much this or a little too much that?"

But, when Crawford plays an emotional scene, you have to wait twenty minutes until she comes out of it after you have said "Cut", because she is still crying or laughing or whatever; she's still going.

Conflict, which came from a Robert Siodmak story, was my first film with Humphrey Bogart, and it started exactly like my first film with Bette—with a row.

I was saying something to Bogart and interrupted myself to say something else to the cameraman. When I turned back, I found that Bogie, offended, had retired to his dressing-room in a rage to console himself with a bottle of whisky.

When I went in, he was boiling mad; he came right up close to me, pointing his finger in my face. "Mr. Bogart," I said, "I assure you I am unaware of having done anything to offend you." Suddenly he took me in his arms and literally embraced me, even though I do think he'd had quite a bit of whisky by then, and after that we were friends.

My first film made outside Warner Brothers was *High Wall* at Metro-Goldwyn-Mayer in 1948. I'd originally chosen Warner over MGM—having had offers from both studios on arrival from Europe—because it was less "tricky" to work in. Also, their pictures' greater realism, compared with the other studios' concentration on fantasy and schmaltz, appealed to me.

MGM was like a big, big opera-house, where you had to please this star and that prima donna. Warners had only one prima donna, Jack Warner. If you had him on your side, or if he said Yes, that was it: you knew that you could go ahead with whatever you wanted to do. Once you had a decision, that decision stuck.

Technically, Warners was a good studio. It had good

cameramen, sound people and art directors and some very good stars. They included Bette and Joan and Jimmy Cagney and Bogart and a host of splendid supporting players who all—and this was their advantage over the other studios—were disciplined. That was a bunch of star actors the like of which can no longer be found nowadays. They were there at nine o'clock sharp ready to shoot, they worked until six or seven in the evening, and there were no bones about it: you *worked* there.

Stars at other studios were already beginning to rebel, saying, "What the hell! I'll come at eleven o'clock, or if I don't feel like it, I won't come at all."

That sort of thing didn't exist at Warners. It was a studio run with an iron fist, and it was good. I long for those days when, if you had a rebellious actor, you just said, "O.K., let's get Jack on the phone." And Jack—except in Bette's case—always took the side of the director. He'd say: "You are the captain, you run the ship. The authority is yours. I hold you responsible for the actors' coming in on time and everything else."

In the case of Bette it was a little different. When Warner heard that Bette wanted to see him, he turned white because he knew he was in for trouble. She'd sweep regally into the room and give him a tough time. But there were also occasions when she listened to reason.

Warners was thus a really well-run studio, although I had a few difficult personal experiences there which I'd rather not go into. I was on suspension two or three times for turning down stories they wanted me to do. Going without an income for three months didn't particularly worry me because I never paid too much attention to money, and I knew that in a major studio like Warner Brothers an appropriate story would turn up sooner or later.

Films in those days, the nineteen-forties, derived their "dense", "crowded" visual texture, their extraordinary rich surface look, largely from the fact that most of them were in black-and-white and not in colour. Also, today's wide screen systems like CinemaScope and Todd-AO diffuse the image. I think the conventional, square 35mm ratio was ideal. Nowadays the image is not as *concentrated* as it was then; directors and cameramen have to cope with a vast expanse of space on either side of people photographed at close quarters, and they don't know what to do with it.

That critic's pejorative word "glossy" to describe the typical forties film is quite wrong.

However, to return to 1948 and *High Wall*: having served my seven years' contract of "peonage" at Warners, I made the film—a mystery story starring Robert Taylor— not caring very much about money or things like that, and it turned out quite nicely.

So did *Payment on Demand* a few years later at RKO. That had some very fascinating flashback effects using negatives and transparent sets, incorporating a technical innovation of my own invention. Frankly, I cannot understand why it hasn't been used since.

It was all a play with light. In part of it, Bette Davis had to play a thirteen-year-old girl, and I had her sort of impressionistically in the middle ground of the set. When we reverted to the past—the cameraman was the late Leo Tover—the foreground became dark, the background lit up and the walls disappeared, because the walls were actually transparent. But you couldn't discern that when they were illuminated for foreground action; they were like screens. As soon as you took the light off them and moved into the background, the walls vanished.

The film was originally to have been called *The Story of a Divorce,* and I wish we had kept that title. Davis was lovely in it, and so was Jane Cowl, who died very shortly afterwards; this was her last picture. Her scenes with the gigolo were very touchingly played, I thought.

At RKO I also did one of my favourite pictures, *The Blue Veil*. Jane Wyman, the star, got stacks of awards for it. Norman Corwin wrote the script, which was actually a remake of a French film with Gabrielle Morlay, *La Maternelle*. I had seen it, but we did our version quite differently.

The producer was Jerry Wald. I made a number of films with Jerry, including his first, *Juke Girl,* which wasn't very interesting. *Possessed* and *Miss Sadie Thompson* were his productions, too. With the exception of *The Blue Veil,* all the films he did at RKO were flops.

He was a really creative producer. Perhaps his greatest single contribution was his enthusiasm. Ninety per cent of the time he was wrong, but the remaining ten per cent, or sometimes five per cent, was *good*. He shot out ideas like bullets. Most of the time you were pained by them because he often had very bad taste, but out of a hundred suggestions, you could sometimes maybe use three, and they were fine.

He never resented it if you said: "But that's crap, Jerry." "All right," he'd answer. "How about this then?" And he'd always come up with something new. I liked him a lot and we had a wonderful time together.

His influence on scripts stemmed mainly from his enthusiasm. "Fellows," he'd say to the writers, "tell me what you've done today ... well, that's fine ... but couldn't we just ...?" Once the script was written, however, and provided he had a good director and a good editor, he left you pretty much alone—although I do remember that, when I was on location in Hawaii for *Miss Sadie Thompson*, he bombarded me with stacks of cablegrams from Los Angeles every day. I threw most of them away.

When he talked to you, it was like listening to a young man. He was a big, heavy guy, but bubbling over with enthusiasm. I think the way he lived was suicidal, and I told him so many times. After a day at the studio he'd go home and watch a movie through dinner, and then another movie. I was often at his house while he took notes after seeing a film. He had this tremendous wall of files in his study, containing hundreds of possible motion-picture subjects all indexed and cross-referenced. Fantastic. He was an unusual man.

I must honestly say, though, that he did not contribute anything significant to the finished work in *The Blue Veil*.

Lately I've been associated with the Westinghouse organization and the producer Jack Skirball in a scheme to do nine pictures in two years. I won't be directing them all, only as many as I can. Westinghouse will later have the North American and Canadian television rights, leaving the rest of the world to the producer and me.

These features, made in Europe for about $500,000 each, would cost about $800,000 or $900,000 if made here. This gives me a certain freedom, because I know that we'll always get back $500,000 and the finance people won't lose a penny. I won't be shaking in my boots saying, "My God, I have three or four million dollars at stake here. I hope the film will recoup it." That sort of thing ruins a lot of directors. This way I have no worries.

Our first picture under this arrangement was made in Hungary in collaboration with the Hungarian State Studio. Based on the widely acclaimed book *The Widow Maker* by Mrs Ladïslaus Bus-Fekete, wife of the famous playwright, it concerns a macabre but real event that occurred in a remote Hungarian village in World War I. Here the women, their husbands away fighting, became completely demoralized and took Russian prisoner-of-war farm-labourers as lovers. In a period of sixteen to eighteen months they poisoned forty of them; men disappeared *en masse*. Everybody knew about it but found nothing wrong with it. Afterwards six or eight women were hanged and other went to gaol.

This story has unfortunate parallels with the present-day general breakdown in moral fibre everywhere. Killing has become an accepted thing. The story shows that, once you let the reins of restraint go, everything goes.

What I like about moviemaking are small touches like, for example, the calm way in which the villain played by Herbert Marshall in *High Wall* casually flicks someone to their death down a lift-shaft with his cane, or the scene in *Payment on Demand* when the husband played by Barry Sullivan comes home, has to dress for dinner, puts on his tux and just unconcernedly says—after twenty-five years of marriage—"I'd like a divorce," as if he might say, "Please give me my tie."

These are the joys of making pictures, these little moments.

George Cukor

Animated, darting eyes behind lightweight bifocals; a protruding lower jaw enclosing irregular gold-inlaid teeth; a manner tense and excitable, giving off nervous energy like a shower of sparks: George Cukor's is not the sort of company one can readily relax in. Yet his supercharged dynamism affords a clue to why he has stayed at the top of the Hollywood directorial heap while many of his contemporaries have long since lapsed into retirement. He has a rare faculty for keeping emotionally and intellectually abreast of the times while, at the same time, sufficiently detached from them to draw profitably on his vast reserves of theatrical and motion-picture experience guiding some of the century's most volatile and luminous acting talents. Garbo and Garland, Barrymore and Bergman, Hepburn, Harlow, and Holliday: from all he has drawn performances of star quality, iridescent and glowing with an inexplicable magic. Not an easy man to talk to, he discusses the past with obvious reluctance; what counts for him is always the current picture and the one after that. Thus the interview starts not at the beginning of his film career, with his arrival in Hollywood as a dialogue director in the infancy of the sound era, nor even with his work on such films as Lewis Milestone's All Quiet on the Western Front *or Ernst Lubitsch's* One Hour with You; *we skip, too, his directorial triumphs of the early nineteen-thirties, such as* Dinner at Eight, Little Women *and* David Copperfield, *and start somewhat arbitrarily, perhaps—with* Camille *in the middle of the decade. So brilliantly crowded a career, and limited time, necessitate some such compromise. But Cukor's personality, bright, sophisticated and yet strangely unsure of itself, does nevertheless come through quite strongly.*

At the time we did *Camille* [1937] Robert Taylor was an up-and-coming young star; he wasn't all that inexperienced. Armand is historically a terrible part. I never quite knew why: perhaps because it was usually played by middle-aged men. As a result he seemed stupid doing the things he did. When you get someone really young playing Armand, you understand him; he becomes appealing, with a kind of real youthful passion; whereas if he were thirty-eight years old you'd think, "Oh, you ass, why do you do that?" So that very crudity, that intensity of young passion made Robert Taylor an extremely good Armand. He lacked maybe some of the style, but he was very handsome and did remarkably well in the role.

He worked in very harmoniously with Garbo. She saw to that—although, like all silent-picture people, she liked to tell herself stories about the character she was playing in order to preserve the illusion. It's a very curious thing; they involve themselves more deeply in their parts that way, it becomes less artificial. As a result, she was rather distant with him and he, a very nice young man, was rather hurt.

"You know," she told me, "I do that so I can always tell myself stories about the character I'm playing, whereas if I got to know him too well it would only confuse the images I've been making of myself as *La dame aux Camélias*, and of Armand."

She didn't improvise, except maybe plastically: she spoke every "if", "and", and "but". When people utter the word "improvise" it's rather like waving a red flag in front of me because I think improvisation is a lot of crap. Everything must come from the text, must touch the actor's imagination. You may enrich a performance, deepen it, by taking the text and developing the characterization in rehearsals; that's what rehearsals are for.

Improvisation, on the other hand, means something taken from the top of your head. Acting should *appear* improvised, but, truth to tell, it is really deeply felt: not thought out in a foxy way, but thought out through your talent and felt through your talent.

I've never had a really gifted, magical actor go into long explanations and long theories and long intellectualizing about the acting process. For example, Spencer Tracy used to tell you, "Well, I certainly learned those lines, spoke those eight pages down to every 'if', 'and', and 'but'; I knew every word." That's all he would tell you. Now there was a great deal else that went on with him, but he wasn't telling it to you. That would have taken the magic out of it somehow, to have chewed it all over beforehand.

I think the creative process in acting involves thinking about it, using your brains and your emotions and whatever creative talent you have. When you say "improvisation" it's as though you said of Artur Rubinstein: "Didn't he do that well?—he improvised." Well, I don't think he does that. I'm sure Rubinstein discovers new things every time he plays a familiar piece, he does it with freshness, but they're always the same notes. I believe in discipline, in other words.

As for preplanning my pictures in the way that Hitchcock is said to preplan his—well, I don't quite know what he does. Although he says he does preplan, I'm sure there are all kinds of things he finds out in production. You can sketch the shots (as he's said to do) up to a certain point. He's a master of it, but I'm sure something is left for that moment when he actually does it on the set.

I start from the text, and, of course, I have a general idea about how the film should go. The things that happen on the set enrich it or change it or surprise me a little. I might perhaps plan a *sequence* in detail, but I always watch the actors and discover things; I don't plan every tiny movement.

It all depends on the point of departure. I don't think you can hem people in. Here the three of us are sitting down, and we could have planned to sit this way. But no one could plan that I put my hand up like this, or that you put your hand up like that. Those are things that "happen", and I'm sure that they must happen in Hitchcock's case. I've never seen him work, but his pictures are very clever and adroit and full of talent. However, I'm sure they involve more than just mechanical planning; that would be too simple.

I saw *The Women* the other day for the first time since it was done in 1939, and there *was* a bit of improvisation there. I am one of the few directors who cannot write brilliant dialogue, and there was a scene toward the end of the picture when everything was going wrong for the Mary Boland character: she'd found out her cowboy husband had been untrue to her, and she was sort of luxuriating in her tragedy, with the women standing around sympathizing.

She was lying outstretched on a chaise-longue being the heroine. The line was "The publicity! The publicity!" All through she'd been using French phrases. Then suddenly she got up—she did it with such wit—and exclaimed: "*La publicité! La publicité!*" in mock-tragic tones. That was pure improvisation.

When I'm asked if I recall any more amusing anecdotes about the making of the film, it has a paralysing effect; my mind goes absolutely blank. Quite frankly I don't remember that sort of thing unless it's funny. But I do recall that, just before Paulette Goddard and Rosalind Russell were due to have their on-camera fight—women are much tougher, prepared to put up with much more than men are—they were saying to each other, "Now kick me, be sure to kick me hard!" And they really did roll around there as if they meant it.

Often when you work for a number of consecutive days among the same group of people, especially in this business, some are bound to become a little testy or cranky. But on *The Women* they were all rather a jolly bunch. There was a little bit of incidental rivalry among them, because each had her clothes fitted separately, and they'd see each other in them for the first time on the set. They'd then give each other quick little appraising glances, as if to say, "How does *she* look?" But there wasn't really much of that.

I enjoyed making *The Philadelphia Story*, too, very much. It was marvellous material, an enormous success on the stage. Katharine Hepburn was quite wonderful in it.

I've found very often that when you transfer a stage play to the screen—especially with the people who've played it—you have the problem of trying to retain its spontaneity. This problem bothered Rex Harrison a great deal in *My Fair Lady*; he'd never played anything on the screen that he'd previously done on the stage. Fortunately, there'd been a three-year interval, and the trick was to catch it with an absolute freshness.

In the back of their minds the actors know where the true values of the piece lie. Katharine Hepburn certainly did in *The Philadelphia Story*, which she'd played for a long time in the theatre. Sometimes I deliberately threw her off. If she played an unimportant scene laughingly, I'd say to her: "I think this should be played rather seriously." I did that because I knew that the *values* would all be there, but I also wanted it to have freshness.

Similarly with Judy Holliday in *Born Yesterday*: she was used to saying a certain line on the stage and getting an enormous laugh. She said it on the movie set and, although they were amused, the crew obviously couldn't laugh. That kind of threw her a little, so we made them all cluster round her and laugh when she rehearsed it. That reassured her. Then when we did it again they *didn't* laugh, but she knew that it was funny because she'd previously heard the laughs. That's how you do it so that it's quite fresh.

Although it's been said that there were thirteen or fourteen scriptwriters contributing to *A Woman's Face*, that is simply not true. As I remember, there was only one, Donald Ogden Stewart; he was the only person I worked with, his was the script we shot. Christopher Isherwood and others may have been involved before I came on to the project. I might even have read their scripts, but we didn't use them.

Conrad Veidt, who played the villain Torsten Barring, was absolutely charming to work with, not at all like the parts he usually assumed. He always looked like the wickedest man in the world, yet he was really very gay and funny. I'd be awful with him and say, "No, no, let's not have any of that UFA acting." Everybody liked him very much. He would do everything with a great gusto. I remember we had hysterics when, whipping a pair of mechanical horses, the poor thing fell between the two of them.

He had a great sense of humour. I kept a dog on the set which I'd named Connie, after Constance Collier, the actress. And Conrad Veidt would exclaim: "I find it *so* insulting that he brings this wretched mongrel on the set ..." But he was really tickled by it.

Albert Bassermann, the venerable German actor who played Torsten Barring's uncle, did not speak one word of English. He learned his entire part phonetically. He knew, really, what it was all about, but I would have to explain things to him in my wretched German. He would read it aloud first in English, and if his inflection was sometimes wrong I'd correct him; and his ear was so impeccable that he would get the correct inflection immediately. He did not speak English in real life. Nor did Anna Magnani when I first worked with her—although, of course, they often know more than they say they do.

In the first half of the picture, when Joan Crawford played a facially scarred criminal, I thought she displayed great gifts. It wasn't difficult to extract that standard of performance out of her. I think you have to touch her imagination. She's a very accomplished actress and she realized that the part was "twisted". Right before every scene, in fact, she'd try to "twist" herself mentally.

The whole thing built up to a courtroom scene in which she finally told the story of her life. (I'm the hero of this anecdote.) When we did it I told her: "We've all been waiting for this revelation. Will you just say it absolutely as though you were reciting the multiplication table—'I was a girl, I was nearly burned to death,' etc." The situation was so strong that it had a great deal of style when she played it that way.

Joan Crawford was very easy to work with, very sensitive. Actresses have to trust you, to trust your judgement, and have your confidence; you give them confidence, too. You do it differently with every actress. If you call upon their resources in an appropriate way, they respond equally appropriately.

Naturally we ran the original Swedish version of *A Woman's Face*,[1] starring Ingrid Bergman, and took everything out of it that was any good, even while changing it a little: the unwrapping of the bandages, for instance. A great deal of the other stuff was invented.

I'm a great believer in that. I believe that, if you adapt a play for the screen, there's no point in trying to make it "cinematic" just because you're doing a film. Or if you do a novel, you must very often try to grasp its essence, why it's good, and keep that.

On the other hand, you mustn't try to slick it up too much. People often say to me: "The first part of your film version of *David Copperfield* is better than the second." To which I reply: "Well, the first *volume* of *David Copperfield* is better than the second."

Similarly, *Little Women* has a rather awkward construction: the hero is introduced in the last quarter of the picture, the little girl seems to die twice. There's no point in slicking that up, because in doing so you lose some of the vitality. But you have to know why you're doing it:

[1] *En Kvinnas Ansikte* (1938).

the main aim should be to preserve the strength of the story.

Some of the more bravura bits in *A Woman's Face*—such as the opening when Crawford is led through the corridors, the final sleigh chase, and the sequence of the overhead suspension car—were the inventions of the writer, of the producer Victor Saville, and I should think of me too.

Saville was extremely clever technically. He'd been a director and knew all about everything. That scene of the tram going over the valley with the waterfall in the background was a marvellous job. The special effects man, Buddy Gillespie, and his people did it. They'd had a second unit shoot backgrounds somewhere, and then we shot on the stage with plates. For the final sequence, showing Veidt's body washed down the river, they made a miniature artificial waterfall out of the sand with such virtuosity that when it was blown up you believed it really existed.

I didn't like *Two-Faced Woman* very much. We really had no script and it was just disasterville; the film didn't work at all. Garbo wasn't very happy about it either. It was the final film she did under her Metro contract, and when it was over she asked to be released. Louis B. Mayer was lost in admiration over the splendid way she behaved about it.

People often say glibly that the failure of *Two-Faced Woman* finished Garbo's career. That's a grotesque oversimplification. If only life were tied up in such neat packages! It certainly threw her, but I think what really happened was that she just gave up; she didn't want to go on.

However, she did attempt to make a picture after that in Italy. That experience rather threw her too, mainly because she'd never worked anywhere other than at Metro since she was very young. Against my advice—she asked me to direct it but I declined—they planned to do something of Balzac's, *La Duchesse de Langeais*. It struck me as being a very old-fashioned story and I begged her not to do it. When she arrived in Italy, they weren't prepared for her and she was just piffled around. That episode, coupled with the failure of *Two-Faced Woman*, depressed her terribly, and she hasn't attempted to do another film since.

I did enjoy making *Keeper of the Flame*. I thought the

first part of the picture was bang-up—there was less to this than meets the eye—and then it sort of went to pot. The early scenes had enormous intensity, but toward the end—what with fires, suicide, and insanity—the story just pooped out. That was the real trouble. I find that if the situation holds, the thing will play all right, but in this case it didn't.

Making so much of it indoors was the fashion at the time at Metro. I don't know why we did it that way. I suppose I wasn't wilful enough to do it differently; I let myself be persuaded. Yet, to your eye, the mock studio exteriors look awfully good. There were just a couple of scenes—such as the one between Spencer Tracy and the boy—where it did appear very artificial after we'd put it together, although it looked all right when we shot it.

Some critics have purported to see the influence of Orson Welles's *Citizen Kane* in *Keeper of the Flame,* but there were no conscious echoes of it in the picture. The resemblances were just an accident. There was something in the air; it was simply a result of the prevailing political climate.

In those days at Metro, a great deal of prehistory of which one was often unaware happened on each picture before one became associated with it. Thus, for all I know, Hedy Lamarr may have been considered for the Ingrid Bergman part in *Gaslight,* as she claims in her autobiography, but by the time I came to it there was no talk of Hedy Lamarr and they cast Miss Bergman shortly after.

The film had three writers: John Balderston, Walter Reisch, and John van Druten. I worked only with the last two; Balderston I think was on it before my day. Reisch is a marvellous, very inventive screen constructionist, while van Druten was a very good playwright and dialogue man. They were very sympathetic and entered into a real collaboration. They worked out the plot's suspense elements together but Reisch, whose *forte* is telling a story visually, did not write any dialogue; that was mostly van Druten's.

Ingrid Bergman had no difficulty in grasping the character of Paula Alquist's essential frailty, but she would complain, "Oh, I look so *healthy.*" However, I think healthy people *can* be frightened. In fact, very often it's perhaps more moving.

Although Ingrid and I became fast friends, she was at

first rather put off by one aspect of my working technique. Between setups I try to compensate for the absence of an audience, and the special tone and excitement that an audience can lend a performance, by going in and talking to the actors about all sorts of things. I'm really not quite sure what I say, but it's just to keep them stimulated, on edge. They can't maintain their involvement constantly at fever pitch, particularly when the cameramen have to reload. So sometimes I tell them "It's almost right," and go in and chat with them between setups.

When I did this with Ingrid, she'd look at me with those cool Swedish eyes and say, "You've already told me that. I'm not stupid, I remember it." So I thought: "Oh dear, well, well, well, I mustn't say that." Then, when I wanted to say something, I thought: "I'd better not." And then: "Oh, the hell with this. That's the way I work and she may as well get used to it." She did, and we became good friends.

I think *Gaslight* owed its tingle of excitement to that technique of mine. It was helped, too, by Charles Boyer's unorthodox style in the role of Paula Alquist's tormentor, Gregory Anton; he had a kind of line, a manner of implacable coldness, and he kept that up all the time.

Bergman's clothes were very good. In one scene she looked like Queen Alexandra, and was particularly elegant and charming when she went to the Tower of London. The film's sets were exceptionally beautiful and a lot of the decoration—for which we had the advice of Paul Huldschinsky, a refugee who had been very rich in Germany and who had enormous taste—was modelled on *Punch* and du Maurier drawings of the period. That gave us a great deal of the proper late-Victorian atmosphere, as well as an interesting visual quality.

This was Angela Lansbury's very first picture. She'd been recommended to me by John van Druten who, knowing we were looking for a girl to play the part of Nancy, the corrupt Cockney maid, informed me that Moyna MacGill and her children—of whom Angela was one, then aged about sixteen or seventeen—were here as refugees from wartime England and working in Bullock's Wilshire department store, packing parcels for the pre-Christmas season.

Angela was accordingly sent up and I made a test with her. She'd had no movie experience at all. Yet the moment she stepped on the stage she was an absolute professional: she had this sullen mouth, and assumed the look of a thoroughly "bad lot" girl.

She did what I thought was an awfully good test, but then they decided she wasn't sexy enough. I remember calling her and saying: "Now you may not get this job, Miss Lansbury, but I think you're a very gifted girl and you may go far."

Anyhow, she did get the job, and from the day she started she was so completely professional and authoritative that she absolutely *was* that girl Nancy. She could also sing and dance and was altogether enormously gifted. Then immediately after *Gaslight* she appeared for a friend of mine, Albert Lewin, in *The Picture of Dorian Gray*, playing a terribly difficult part, that could have been saccharine, so touchingly and affectingly that it was never for a moment ridiculous.

Winged Victory, which I did soon after *Gaslight*, was a little far afield, but it interested me. I went around to all the training commands watching air force trainees being tested. That sort of thing was very much in the air then; it was wartime, and there was great patriotic fervour everywhere. I thought the story was rather hokey-pokey, but Moss Hart had written it to order, and it must be viewed in the context of its time. Technically, although the material was somewhat out of my line, I didn't find the film hard to handle.

While I was shooting *Winged Victory* at Twentieth Century-Fox, the studio head, Darryl Zanuck, suggested I take a look at a girl he had under contract, whom he'd seen performing with other people in a nightclub, and let him know whether I thought she was any good or not. The girl came in, made-up and rather nervous, and read for me. "Can you do this all the time?" I asked her. "Yes," she said, "I think so."

That girl was Judy Holliday. She played a perfectly serious part in *Winged Victory*, did a couple of more small movie roles, and then went to New York to do *Kiss Them for Me*. When she came back to Hollywood several years later, it was as a comedienne.

My first collaboration with the scriptwriting husband-and-wife team of Ruth Gordon and Garson Kanin was on *A Double Life*. In it, Ronald Colman as a demented actor had to play a number of scenes from *Othello*. While I don't think he was as great an Othello as Sir

Laurence Olivier is on the stage, I still thought it was a respectable try. We obviously did the best we could. Olivier's Othello is of course absolutely thrilling, but I thought Colman looked wonderful and he spoke some of the lines very movingly. I'm sorry some of the critics objected at the time; I don't know why they did. I wonder what the hell makes them such great experts on *Othello* anyway.

The comedies I subsequently did with the Kanins were much better. They were bang-up, marvellous scripts, and a lot of what seems like comic invention was actually written into them, including shots and things like that.

What a wonderful cast we had in *Adam's Rib*! There was so much invention in it, and we had this glorious ensemble playing with Hepburn and Tracy.

Garson and Kanin reminded me recently, when he and Ruth and I were all together, of a memorable occasion involving Spencer Tracy. Pointing to a corner in the room of my house, he said: "That's where I witnessed the greatest single piece of acting I ever saw in my life." Apparently—I don't remember the occasion—we'd had a reading there of *Pat and Mike*, just a run-through of the text. Spencer put his glasses on—we thought he would simply read the words—but suddenly he departed and instead there appeared in his place this crude prize-fighting manager of *Pat and Mike*. There was no sign of the Spencer Tracy we'd just seen there a minute before. It was absolutely magical, Garson said: there Spencer was, and suddenly someone else appeared.

For *Adam's Rib*, which was partly about a murderess, I went and attended a murder trial here. Katharine Hepburn played a judge in it, and in New York we went to all kinds of trials where judges sometimes allowed her to sit on the bench.

The same thing happened on *The Marrying Kind*. I went to a domestic relations court and it was fascinating, because then you really understand what a judge's function is, and it's not the way it's usually played in movies. Even though *Adam's Rib* was a comedy and *The Marrying Kind* was serious, I came away with a real understanding of what judges and the whole court staff were trying to do, although naturally I'd known beforehand that it wasn't just a question of a man banging a gavel and saying, "Silence in court!"

Thus I find that one always goes back to the source of

things, and you're often amazed at how this makes them appear fresh. I'm terribly familiar with Washington and I was born and grew up in New York, but when you look at these places for the purposes of making a picture they become quite new, a whole new world. It's very interesting, this kind of research.

I don't think *The Marrying Kind* was as successful as some of the other pictures I did with the Kanins, but I still liked it very much. Aldo Ray was remarkable in it, and the early scenes we shot in Central Park and Times Square had, I thought, a kind of fun and fantasy quality.

I saw it again quite recently, and one thing that struck me about it was that it all seemed so frightfully antiseptic. These two married people are going to bed, and it's practically their wedding night. She's in one bed, and far away he's in the other bed. Then he gets up—he's a postal clerk—and gets into a dressing-gown and comes over and kisses her, with both his feet safely on the ground.

At the time we had all sorts of codes, and it didn't strike me as being particularly odd. Now, of course, it's gone quite the other way, and people—any place, any time—are always jumping into bed, and putting their hands up under each other's clothes when there's no occasion for it. But *The Marrying Kind* must be viewed in the context of its period. People probably did behave much more that way than they do now, so we were more or less representing—via the Production Code—what did in fact happen.

Ruth Gordon based her screenplay for *The Actress* on her own autobiographical play, *Years Ago*. She was accordingly very much involved with the film's art direction, and the sets—including interiors—were exact copies of her family's old house in Wollaston, Massachusetts. They were technically quite difficult to cope with, and we just had to crowd everything in. The picture probably seems more real for that reason.

Before production began, we went up to Wollaston, went through the actual house, through the Mellons Food Company where her father had worked, and through the whole town. We picked out things that no screenwriter could possibly have invented: a small kitchen with eight doors in it, and all the little details—a cupboard, a cellar—that in reality are so interesting.

Somebody told her that the lady who'd lived next door was still there, and Ruth, dressed in a mink coat, rang the bell. When this lady opened a screen door and peered at her, Ruth said: "Mrs So-and-So, dear, it's Ruth Jones." This was 1952, and Ruth had left there I think in 1917, calling herself Jones (her name was Ruth Gordon Jones). The poor woman was quite startled!

The story of what happened to *A Star is Born* is rather sad. We previewed it and it went wonderfully. I thought it was too long and asked that Moss Hart, the screenwriter, and I be allowed to sweat out some footage. But everybody had gone to Europe and alas the cut pieces were lost. I never saw it all the way through in its cut form.

The version cut by Moss Hart and me was the original release version, shown complete with great, ravishing, enormous success. After the initial release the studio found that its length restricted the number of daily showings, so they cut it further, and I think disastrously.

They cut wonderful, wonderful scenes. There was a most charming scene where James Mason proposed to Judy Garland on a soundstage. There were some wonderful scenes on the way to the preview, where she got sick and went behind an oil well and threw up, and others downtown at Bunker Hill, where he visited her in this terrible apartment house she lived in. All these cuts interfered with the development of the love story and reduced the impact of their relationship. So much was lost that I felt it was a great pity. Bosley Crowther wrote an article about it called "A Star is Shorn".

Also, that huge fifteen-minute "Born in a Trunk" number threw everything out of kilter. The studio thought they should have it, so in it went. It was in fact too long. I didn't direct it; I don't know who did.

James Mason's performance as Norman Maine was terribly good, very moving, but I don't think it was the equal of Garland's. I thought she was absolutely staggering.

The film's opening première scene was a mixture of all kinds of things. We'd shot some long shots of Grauman's Chinese at the opening of *The Robe* and then we reproduced it down at the Shrine Auditorium, so that it was a *mélange* of both, and you could never tell where one began and the other took over.

A Star is Born was done in the early days of Cinema-Scope, which we used rather boldly. We never went on location at all, except maybe for one shot. The final beach-house scene was all done in process; there was really no such building.

I think what makes the film alive is the fact that I always have a wind-tunnel on the stage: not a fan, because a fan makes a noise and the sound man always wants it cut down. A wind-tunnel, on the other hand, keeps the air constantly circulating and gives the atmosphere a lift.

We were going to make *Bhowani Junction*, based on John Masters's novel, in India, but they wouldn't let us do it there. We made it in Pakistan instead, where we received every co-operation. Later we did some of the interiors in London, reproducing the exteriors we'd shot in Pakistan, and they matched perfectly. That Sikh wedding ceremony we used in the film was authentic, photographed in an actual temple, and the train wreck—which was all the work of the art director, Gene Allen—was done in a London depot using an upside-down train.

Unfortunately the story went wrong in *Bhowani Junction*. The audience simply thought—whatever the failure was—that the character played by Ava Gardner was rather sluttish to go abruptly from one man to another whereas, truth to tell, in the book she wasn't.

The film also suffered from some rather stupid and prudish cuts—for example, a scene where Ava Gardner used her lover's toothbrush disappeared, together with several other erotic scenes, which horrified people at the time (1955), but which if done later with, say, Jeanne Moreau would probably be considered absolute masterpieces.

All that stuff is awfully easy to do, I think. In fact, during some of our very amorous scenes, Ava giggled so much that we were all in hysterics. Those supposedly passionate sequences just become comic after a while. But the film had an atmosphere and Ava herself was charming. She's a real movie queen, really exciting; lovely looking, too, with marvellous legs. When *she* crosses the screen, you're bound to follow her.

I thoroughly enjoyed making *Les Girls* with that adorable girl Kay Kendall. It was very jolly. In a stylized way, I think we managed to capture the essence of Paris without using any genuine Parisian shots—although later, against my better judgment, I let them put in a couple of long shots of the real city. Gene Allen and I had been all through the city gathering material for the rooms and apartments to be used in the film: it was he who very carefully put together the Cézanne-like arrangements of bread and wine on tables, and things like that.

Certainly one or two things went wrong, such as the technicians' passion for using a lot of coloured lights which we don't use any more. Apart from that, I thought *Les Girls* was impeccable in a colour way. It irked me terribly when the London critics, after the film's Royal Command Performance showing, said they thought it looked like tomato ketchup.

"You've got a hell of a nerve," I thought. "You're just poor cornball provincial people, you critics, you just don't know what the hell you're talking about."

I was particularly annoyed over that because, since *A Star is Born*, I've had two brilliant people helping me on the design of all my pictures: the late George Hoyningen-Huene and Gene Allen. We worked together as a team; where one stops and the other starts, I don't know.

When I brought Hoyningen-Huene to the screen he'd been for years the most distinguished photographer on *Vogue* and *Harper's Bazaar*. He was a friend of mine, living in Paris, and had done a great many books. He was shooting a documentary movie at the time, and, as *A Star is Born* was my first colour picture, I thought he would be ideally suited to assist me on its colour problems, since he knew all there is to know on that. Since then he's profoundly affected all my films. He was nominally the colour coordinator but he touched every department with his enormous taste and knowledge.

Gene Allen was a sketch artist on *A Star is Born*. I thought his sketches for that film disclosed a lot of talent, and we've been working together ever since. His contribution has changed from that of art director, because he later took on writing and editing and producing; he also shoots second unit. He's with me constantly. On *My Fair Lady* he did art direction, and he did script work on *The Chapman Report*.

The last picture—*The Chapman Report*—had some very extraordinary and revealing scenes of the women in it, subjects in a suburban sex survey, being interviewed. They had a kind of candour and purity I'd never seen. The sum total of the picture—this is the cop-out—was all hocus-pocus, but the interviews with these women were fascinating.

The costume designer, Orry-Kelly, was very clever about their clothes. One woman wore white all the way through, another wore black, and you weren't aware of it. All the girls in it were attractive. Glynis Johns and the boy, Ty Hardin, were funny, Shelley Winters was touching at times, and Jane Fonda was very pretty.

But the most striking performance was Claire Bloom's. The character she played was a depraved nymphomaniac, and I wanted somebody for the part without any vulgarity whatever. Claire had never done that type of role before, and she was marvellous: such a "bad lot", and so driven by her impulses, that as a result it became—*I* think— terribly moving. I think it had a kind of tragic pathos.

The scene where she was subjected to a mass rape by a group of jazz musicians was cut like mad in many places. That scene was absolutely marvellous. The high point occurred when she began to enjoy it. The censor jumped on us with both feet. Today, of course, you could do it much more candidly. The picture was ahead of its time in that respect.

The first preview of *The Chapman Report* at San Francisco was quite fascinating because the audience understood it and it went over great. Then the studio stepped in and cut it, and by the time most audiences saw it the film had been drastically altered for the worse.

With *My Fair Lady* it was quite different. People say, "Oh, it's just a photographed stage piece." But it isn't. When you have these absolutely marvellous theatre scenes, and you know people can play them, there's no point in trying to tear the thing apart, to make "cinema" out of it. You retain as much as you can and try to do it with a kind of fluidity.

Although it was originally planned to do one sequence— a pubcrawl—in London, this finally didn't seem necessary, not only because there were no suitable pubs in London to crawl in, but also because by the time the picture was finished all the numbers had been accounted for. Rex Harrison's charming rendition of "I've Grown Accustomed to Her Face" was done right there on the set in Hollywood. The whole thing wasn't realistic, it was a kind of stylized London.

The differences between me and Cecil Beaton to which he refers in his book *Fair Lady* were not on details of interpretation but on methods of work. He irritated me. I don't think he knows how to work in concert, and he would be doing still pictures when we should have been rehearsing. When I got annoyed at his holding up production—especially since he was an old friend—I think he got rather hoity-toity. That's what the disagreement was really about.

You often work on many things which fall into abeyance and to which you periodically return. One such subject is *The Spiritualist,* the story of Florrie Cook and Sir William Crookes. I think that's a fascinating set of circumstances and I'd still love to do it.

It's a rather tricky subject. The trouble is that there's no story as such. It's a situation rather than a story; you have to invent a climax for it. Walter Reisch did a treatment, and it didn't quite work. I don't think either of us has licked it. There is a way of doing it—there's a way of doing everything—but we haven't yet found the key to it.

Sir William Crookes, a respectable man of science, offered to test the sincerity of Florrie Cook, a teenaged "medium" who claimed to be able to materialize the spirit of a dead young girl named Katie King. "This is not a fraud," he declared. "I saw the apparition of the girl." As a result of that, Florrie Cook became a well-known spiritualist. It later transpired that Crookes, a forty-year-old father of nine, was in love with her, and all sorts of strange things went on. It's funny, in a kind of ghoulish Victorian way.

I think Florrie Cook was a deliberate deceiver and that amongst so-called spiritualists of that time there was a great deal of hocus-pocus, which took different forms. Crookes at forty was still very naïve, and she was a minx. The characters are all so marvellous: the man she eventually married, for instance, a sea captain. One never knew if he was her collaborator. She was up to everything.

I don't really know who I want in the Florrie Cook part. It should be a young "bad lot" girl. I think the film could be done without offending any relatives or descendants of the participants who may still be living; it's all such old stuff.

After my new film *Justine* I'd like to do Arthur Schnitzler's *Casanova's Homecoming,* featuring Rex Harrison. This is Casanova at the age of fifty-six, on his uppers, trying to get back to Venice. It's a comedy, quite unlike *La Ronde,* of the episodes involving Casanova before and after his Venetian reappearance.

I was unfamiliar with the Schnitzler novella but I'd read, of course, quite a bit about Casanova. Then, as I began reading more deeply, I discovered the interesting fact that his celebrated *Memoirs* were first published twenty-seven years after his death, in an inaccurate German translation, although he'd written them in French. The original French text was first published in France as recently as 1961.

The English playwright John Mortimer has been working on a treatment of *Casanova's Homecoming* for some time. My colleague Gene Allen will produce it.

It's true that I've been involved with a number of films which I didn't finish, which were abandoned, or were completed by other people. *Gone With the Wind* was not the first of those; there were a great many others. I'd prepared it for a year, made all the preliminary tests, and shot for a month. I believe all the stuff I shot is still in the picture. As I remember, it included the opening scene on the steps of Tara, the bazaar, and the scene where Vivien Leigh came downstairs and slapped Butterfly McQueen.

At the end of a month I was removed from the film; I was never really quite sure why. Yet I still remained great friends with David Selznick.

I chose not to do *The Razor's Edge*. Maugham wrote a wonderful script but we couldn't cast it. Then I had to go back to Metro, and while I was there doing another picture, Tyrone Power got out of the services and they cast him in it as Larry Darrell. I wasn't available at that time, and, besides, they weren't using Maugham's script; so I never did the film. All I did on it were tests with a boy called John Russell.

We shot about seven weeks on *Something's Got to Give*, Marilyn Monroe's last, unfinished picture. That was a terribly sad occasion, because she arrived on the set looking absolutely lovely and then found she had frightful difficulty in concentrating.

I used to tell her: "You do it so easily, you're so accomplished", and as she'd perform some straightforward action like walking down a path I'd say: "Oh, that's great, perfectly simple."

But she'd reply: "Oh, no, I've lost it", and her inability to concentrate got worse. At the end she couldn't do anything and was quite incapable of sustained mental effort. What the reason for that was, I don't know.

I'm not being affected when I say I don't really remember the other films on which I've only been partially involved. It's honestly of that little importance to me. I just didn't finish them. I thought in most cases they were wrong, and I've sometimes suffered the slings and arrows of indignity because of them.

I consider all these vicissitudes are only bad if you let them affect you, if you let them throw you. One has to roll with the punch and not let it injure one's morale, because really that's all one has, isn't it?

John Frankenheimer

In John Frankenheimer's powerful film Seconds, a man gets a second chance at life by recapturing his youth through the use of plastic surgery. He goes to California, where the organization which has made him over has supplied a ritzy beach-house at Malibu, complete with kidney-shaped swimming pool and spectacular views of the Pacific; there, and on his private beach, he discovers a brief moment of happiness. Startlingly, Frankenheimer's house turns out to be the same one: he lent it to Paramount for the shooting in return for some paid-for additions to the structure.

You reach it along the curving road that sweeps through Santa Monica, past giant toppling sandhills, crested by tall palms that strut across the skyline as regularly as sentries. On the left are the one-storey timber shacks, the low-lying seafood restaurants and seedy electric signs that have been seen as the background to chases or high-powered dramatic clashes in a thousand films. Beyond them lies the Pacific, almost always as drably blue-grey as the Atlantic. The waves seem flat this summer, and the carved golden bodies of the surfriders are hunched pessimistically over their boards, rocking up and down in barely perceptible swell. Few birds fly, and even here the sky is smeared with smog.

Frankenheimer's house is hidden by a tall, rather formal gateway, like the entrance to an Italian villa. A short path leads up to a stern-looking door, but inside everything has a massive informality: huge pink chairs in patterned cotton, a great table loaded with books in higgledy-piggledy piles, a solid-looking clutter of figures. To the left is the cool, secluded studio-room where Antiochus

Wilson, artist hero of Seconds, *painted his rather indifferent works.*

We look out, during the conversation, at the Pacific, stone grey under a driving wind and sudden bursts of rain. The noises off are, as always in Hollywood, deafening, even in this remote house: the shriek and jangle of ambulances and fire-engines, the incessant zooming of jets, the crash of surf, and the shrill cries of sea-birds. The phone often punctuates the conversation: a casting director in London, discussing problems connected with Frankenheimer's new film, The Fixer.

Frankenheimer himself is handsome, large-boned, dark-haired; he looks older than his thirty-seven years. He is extremely tense, keyed up over and over again during the interview almost to breaking-point. His eyes dilate at moments of stress, and he sometimes trembles. His casual clothes, slacks and T-shirt, slippers, have, as usual in California, nothing whatever to do with relaxation.

He speaks quickly, softly and nervously, and has a sharp feeling for the absurdities of human behaviour. His sense of humour is very sophisticated, but never malicious or cutting, Hollywood-style. His films all deal with important themes, and he doesn't know how to be trivial: in The Young Stranger *and* All Fall Down *with the agonies of growing up; in* The Manchurian Candidate *and* Seven Days in May *with the dangers of extremism in politics; in* Seconds *with the futility of pursuing the illusion that youth is everything. In an increasingly impersonal and mechanical industry he has held out for the personal statement, for a young and committed cinema. He is an artist in a world of carpenters, and one wishes him well.*

I came from a well-to-do family, never rich, not poor either. I went to private schools then to the Los Alamo Catholic Military Academy, on Long Island. From there I went to Williams College in Williamstown, Massachusetts. When I got out of Williams, I got married; I had done a lot of acting in Williams while I was there, followed by two years of summer stock, and when I got out of college I wanted to continue acting. I wasn't doing too well, and my parents had violently disagreed with my choice of profession. I kept getting damned things in the mail from my father about "the average actor's yearly income is $700". Things like that. The poor man had a terrible choice to make because my second occupation was a racing-driver. I wanted to do that too, because I did compete in some midget races while I was in college, and I imagined I could make a very good career of it. Being nineteen at the time, the thought of death never bothered me. You know, as Thomas Wolfe says, "You're twenty-one and you will never die", and I wasn't going to die either.

I decided on acting, just getting a few bit parts on television at first. But luckily for my survival, around that time I got a reserve commission in the Air Force. It was during the Korean conflict, and they called me in as Second Lieutenant. I made three hundred dollars a month, which was a hell of a lot more than I'd been making; my wife had been supporting me. She was a schoolteacher. Once I was in the Air Force, they assigned me to the Mail-Room in the Pentagon, which is a horrible, horrible place to be.

The boredom was so great that I read almost everything that came through there, and I read a directive that said they were forming a motion-picture squadron in Burbank, California, and you did not have to go through channels to apply to join it, which is really quite way out for the American military. So I immediately applied, and lied my tail off about how experienced I was with cameras and so on, and mentioned I had acting experience, and kind of *elaborated* my career generally. Before I knew it, I was assigned.

When I got to Burbank, I went clear out of my mind. I had never *seen* a movie camera. Here I was at the old Lockheed Air Terminal and I found that *everybody* had lied, none of the assignees knew *anything* about movies whatsoever, and our commanding officer used to be in the grip department at Warner Brothers!

It turned out they had two cameras and four hundred men. So the first thing the commanding officer says to me is, "Look, you've got to take this crew and shoot a film!" So I said, "On what subject?" And he said, "On anything, you've just got to keep them busy!" So my first job was taking this group of derelict air force men out to do the film and the only thing that was close enough was an asphalt plant. My first production was on how to make asphalt! It was the first time I had ever looked through a movie camera in my life! I ended up letting the whole crew go—they didn't know anything, and didn't want to know—and I shot the film myself. And I kept on making movies, all of which I'm sure must be somewhere in the archives of the Pentagon, including one on registered Hereford cattle. Now, the only cow I'd ever seen was from a moving car on a parkway when I was moving from one place to another, because I was brought up in New York City. While I was doing this film on registered cattle, a fellow named Harvey Howard had a thing going whereby you'd hire one of these registered cattle. It would be fertilized by his bull, and you would then be able to sell the offspring.

The guy had a weekly television show in Los Angeles, which he called the Harvey Howard Western Roundup, which was really Harvey Howard trying to sell people into buying his cattle. He had several fly-by-night producers doing the show, then he had a violent fight with them and fired them. One day I was there and I saw two of these guys in dark suits driving away. He came up to me and he said, "Kid, do you write?" And, of course, the only thing I wrote were letters. "I certainly do!" And he said, "I just fired my producer-writers, and I need somebody to write my show. Will you do it?" And I said, "I certainly will. How much will you pay me?" "Forty dollars a week." So I wrote twenty-four Harvey Howard Western Roundups.

We were finally taken off the air by the FCC because they said that you were allowed six minutes of commercial in a sixty-minute show. And we had fifty-four minutes of commercial. To write the Roundups I would look in the encyclopaedia and put in various things about cows. Harvey Howard used to bring his cows over to the studio, mind you, defecating all over the place, these huge things—a registered Hereford bull, my God, in a room no bigger than my living-room! And one director of this show only had two cameras, and there was a choice of cutting to Harvey or the cow and since both looked exactly the same it was difficult to tell the difference. So he, in anticipation of doing this weekly horror, would get stone drunk, out of his mind! And as a result, in my second lieutenant's uniform, *I* would direct the show! I added some singers to the show, and Howard wouldn't pay professionals, so we used amateurs—until the picket line started to form outside the studio.

After that show was taken off by the FCC, I was sent to do one legitimate film for the Air Force on an aerial gunnery meet in Yuma, Arizona, and that turned out to be a disaster. It came time for me to get out. But in the meantime I would take the camera and I would go out on weekends and shoot the hell out of stuff. I did films on everything—the desert, the freeway, I'd stand out there at rush hour and shoot the horrible congestions and accidents, and over them I'd have a sweet, dulcet voice reading the California Chamber of Commerce's spiel about how great the freeway system is.

I decided now to get into the film business. But the idea of going into a Hollywood type of film appalled me, because I knew what the system was: you had to be fifty years old to direct. I also knew it was almost impossible to get a job. So I thought it would be a good idea to try television first.

I banged around a lot and got offered a job as a parking-lot attendant from NBC and a mail-clerk from CBS; I was told there were Ph.D's in the studio mailrooms. Finally I got a job offered to me as a scenic supervisor at ABC, which would mean I had to check that a sufficient number of nails were being hammered. I had one hundred and fifty dollars left, and the last thing I wanted to do was to ask my father for anything. So I went back to New York, where I had a lot of friends I'd acted with who were now in production jobs in television, and they were all terribly glad to see me until they knew what I was there for, which was to get a job. I got the nicest turndowns you ever saw. And finally I went back to CBS, where I didn't know anybody. I got in to see the guy who hired assistant directors. He believed in me, and he called me three weeks later. In the meantime I'd done anything to stay alive: extra jobs, waiter in a restaurant, just to have enough money to eat. The CBS man called and said "We can give you a job for eight weeks temporarily, as an assistant director." That was in 1953, and it all worked beautifully from there.

I was Sidney Lumet's assistant on a programme called "You Are There". It was a dramatization of historical events with CBS newscasters actually "interviewing" the people of the past—Washington, Napoleon, and so on. Then I started studying with Sandy Meisner, to learn something about what I had luckily fallen into.

I watched every bit of television I could possibly watch. I went to see every film I could possibly see, and I was in museums and art galleries all the time, and what really has influenced me most is the work of painters and photographers. As far as perspective is concerned, Gauguin has taught me more than any book could, and he was influenced by Japanese painters in his turn; Japanese painters taught me about perspective. You look at Kurosawa's films, with the long lenses he uses, and you can learn more from him than from anybody. Among photographers, I learned most from Robert Frank, Ernst Haas, Eisenstadt, and Werner Bischof. I learned from these men that every rule, so far as composition was concerned, was made to be broken. You read Eisenstein's film books and they're fine, but what you don't read is that you can break the rules, if you want to.

Hitchcock influenced me deeply as well. Any American director who says he isn't influenced by him is out of his mind. René Clement was a very great influence also. And, of course, Welles: from the photographic point of view he made just about the perfect film in *Citizen Kane*. The only problem with it is you really don't care about anybody in it. And I suppose that really violates the whole concept of drama, which is that you have to have somebody you can really care about. And here's a clinical approach to the whole thing, just a bisection of it. That's why you can look at the film again and again. Because it's what he wanted it to be, just a technical exercise.

Getting back to television, I enjoyed being assistant director; an assistant director in television was completely different from an assistant director in the movies, a very creative job. You set up shots for the director, as a cameraman does in film; I was very young, twenty-four years old, and I didn't want to be a director. I was making a base salary of one hundred and twenty dollars a week, plus overtime which came to about one hundred and eighty dollars a week, plus being paid under the table by directors for doing their shows, which came to about two hundred and fifty dollars, plus doing about three commercials a week for the shows, bringing me up to about three hundred and fifty a week. I was unmarried in New York and I didn't want to change that. I worked a five-day week and had the days off I wanted, which were Wednesday and Thursday; on Friday night I was the fellow who directed the remotes for Ed Murrow on *Person to Person*, so I would get to go to all kinds of places, and then I'd come back the same night, still on penalty time from the union, and do a rehearsal of *You Are There*. I'd do that show on Sunday. Then on Monday and Tuesday I'd do a show called *Danger*.

At that time television directors were being paid next to nothing, so I was glad not to be one of them. They were also being fired left and right. There were only three places to go, you could run out of networks very quickly if you slipped. From CBS to ABC to NBC and that was it. Now *Danger*—very aptly titled—was the show they would put all the directors on they were going to can. Just to give a final test of their ability—if they failed there, they were *out*. I was put on the show to try and help these bums, to try and get these damn things on the air. And of course they would know that they were on the verge of being fired, and they'd be very tense before the rehearsal ever started, and they'd give me these ridiculous sums of money to help them keep their jobs. I didn't want their money, but they insisted on it. And, no matter what I did, I couldn't help them keep their jobs, because they were just *terrible*.

After about fourteen directors in a year, I was very upset about the whole thing. One night I was planning to go out with a girl whom I later married, and I was wearing the first 150-dollar suit I'd ever worn. The director came on, the video flashed, and the director suddenly panicked and said, "Take two!" in a shrill voice. Of course, camera two happened to be pointed right at the control-booth, and there we were, coast to coast! And I said, "No! Take one!" and so the technical director did that, and the director stood up and screamed "Take anything, save me, *save me!*" And proceeded to vomit all over me! On the air! The production assistant had been a prize-fighter and stood up and decked the director with one blow. They carried him out, and with vomit all over me I did the show.

The vomit-all-over-me was kind of symbolic of what had been going on during the whole past year, and I walked into the vice-president of CBS and quit.

Then the V.P. offered me a chance to be director. So I proceeded to do a hundred and twenty-five live TV shows. I did *Climax* on the west coast with the producer Martin Manuelis, and we won the "Emmy" with it three times. I had got going.

Then we went on to "Playhouse 90". Of these, the best were *The Comedian*, with Mickey Rooney, adapted by

Rod Serling from an Ernest Lehman story; *Days of Wine and Roses*, from a story about alcoholism; Faulkner's *Old Man* and Hemingway's *The Fifth Column*; and a show I did on tape in Arizona with Lee Marvin, *The American*.

My average week was a seven-day one—I couldn't do that now, but I was young then. We rehearsed for two and a half weeks, and then three or four days on camera. First day, you block it out with your cameras; the second day, you have a very rough run-through; the third day would be dress rehearsal and then, finally, air. The tensions were tremendous then. And you'd also be working on your other scripts at night—meetings with writers about a script you were going to do in another month. It enabled me to work with so many different actors and writers, and I could be my own cameraman—nobody told me where to put the camera. The pressure of live TV was very good for me. And in "Playhouse 90" you could develop a character, you could improvise. It was all very creative; I had colleagues like Ralph Nelson, George Roy Hill, Franklin Schaffner, Delbert Mann, Sidney Lumet, and Arthur Penn, and we all got along fine. We'd discuss each other's problems.

TV shows in those days often starred "B" Hollywood names, and sometimes you'd find that very hard to cope with: some of these people were just taking jobs so they could get back into the movies, and their agents would connive with CBS to get them a job, and then they would be terrified of the fact of going on live. But despite the disadvantages it was easier to do creative work then. I just don't know how, today, they can make an hour-long show in five days, and I can't see a new crop of directors coming from TV today: if you're doing a thing quickly, it doesn't necessarily mean that you're doing it well.

Then I came to my first film feature. I had done an original on *Climax* called *Deal a Blow* written by Robert Dozier, who was Bill Dozier's son. It was an account of him and his father when he was a boy. We used Jimmy MacArthur, the son of Helen Hayes, in the TV show; it was the first thing he had ever done. When Bill Dozier became head of RKO he decided that one of the things he would like to do was this film, and his son also wrote the screenplay. It didn't involve much work: it was just a question of dramatizing the things the TV show hinted at. A great deal went wrong with the film. First, I was a new

director and the production department tried to in-
timidate me by saying, "You have only twenty-five days."
I had a producer who wanted to be a director, and we
didn't get along at all. I had a cameraman who had been
under contract to Metro-Goldwyn-Mayer for twenty-five
years, so that everything I wanted to do he said you
couldn't do it. I was afraid to repeat the TV show, and
realized I had to do it differently, but I didn't do it any
better; in fact the whole film was a very constipated
effort.

The crew I had was just awful, a typical American crew
who couldn't have cared less. They gave me open hostility. At a quarter of six suddenly you'd hear, "Fight night,
tonight", that kind of thing, and you'd be trying to get a
scene! I was so tense I would drink a bottle of Amphergal
a day; my stomach was just a wreck, trying to finish this
thing in twenty-five days. Finally I said to the cameraman,
"Look, I want this shot, I want the depth of focus across
the boy to the man coming in the door", and he said "It
can't be done." I said, "We're going to do it." Well, he
took half a day to light it. On a twenty-five day picture
you can't afford that time for one shot. So in the end I
wound up doing it his way.

The tension kept building up. I'm a very shy man. I
can't work in an atmosphere of hostility, and I felt that
crew didn't like me at all, or the movie. I mean there were
remarks like, "Trying to make an 'A' movie on a 'C'
budget." And "Let's face it, what we're making is a 'C'."
Out of that came what I think people have referred to as
my temperament. I swore I was never going to put myself
through anything like that again as long as I lived. And I
was going to have a film my way or I wasn't going to do
it at all. Of course, it's different now: if anyone doesn't do
what I like, they're out, fired. I don't care who it is, even if
it's the lead actor; I have to have complete control. And I
didn't on *The Young Stranger*. It's a *lousy* movie. RKO
cut it, and I thought, "Who has to take that kind of
crap?"

I went back to television and didn't make another
movie until 1960. I didn't want to. But finally the TV live
work stopped, and I didn't have a bloody dime. Then
David O. Selznick adopted me. He helped me work on the
script of *Tender is the Night*, which I was going to do for
him; but unfortunately he abandoned the project. He

taught me all I needed to know about film-making, right down to the most complex technical details.

Then I got a real break: Harold Hecht gave me the script of Evan Hunter's *A Matter of Conviction,* and the idea was that Burt Lancaster would appear in it: a story of hoodlums in New York, to be retitled *The Young Savages.* It was a bad script, but I could see something in it; it was set in New York, and I knew all the locations: I lived only five blocks from the area in which the movie was set. Luckily, Hecht let me throw out the script and rewrite the whole thing with J. P. Miller, who had done *Days of Wine and Roses* with me. I had a fight with Hecht over casting, but I won, except for the Dina Merrill part: I didn't want her, but the producer wanted to put in a rock-'n-roll singer as one of the leading juvenile delinquents, and to get rid of him I had to have her; we traded. I didn't think she could hurt the picture too much, but she did.

The boys were great, were real. Selznick and I cut the picture together. It came out quite well.

Then came *Birdman of Alcatraz.* I'd always wanted to do it—for "Playhouse 90" originally. And I had it in my hands at one stage. Then the Prison Bureau came to CBS, and said, "If you do this, you will never get any co-operation again from us, for anything." Well, having done the film, I'm very glad I didn't attempt to do it on live TV. With the problem of getting those birds to act, it could have been one of the great disasters of all time.

I knew that Hecht-Hill-Lancaster owned the rights to *Birdman.* While I was in the midst of *The Young Savages,* I had asked if I could do it and they were very non-committal, chiefly because I did not get along well with Burt. We fought. I just wasn't going to do what he said, that's all. He tried to direct all his films, and he and I had already fought on *Savages.* Hecht would come in screaming, "God, how can you do this, you're working with a big Hollywood star!" And I'd say, "Either I'm directing the film, or he is. After all, I'm not trying to act in it am I?" So they finally decided against me for *Birdman,* and hired an English director named Charles Crichton. I learned about this at the same time I was finishing *Savages* and I was in the midst of terrible domestic problems, so terrible I couldn't come to California for the *Savages* preview later on. I'd have to fly out under an assumed name because if I arrived under my own I'd be served process papers as soon as I arrived. When I got to California I was surprised to find Harold Hecht very warm and friendly—he hadn't been before. While we were driving into Los Angeles he said, "Look, I want you to direct *Birdman of Alcatraz*. We've been shooting for three weeks and we're very unhappy with what's happened." I said, "Thanks very much, but Jesus Christ, Harold, it's very tough after somebody has started the picture, and cast it." "Burt wants you very much", he said.

I had a long talk with Burt and we decided I *would* direct. I looked at the film that had been shot and it was no good, but I knew the property so well there was very little I needed to do to prepare it. The only thing I disagreed with totally was the set that they had. It should have been shot in a real penitentiary. They said, "We can't get one; the prison authorities won't co-operate." So I said, "That's a lot of crap; we could find an abandoned one." But that was a battle I didn't win.

I did win practically everything else. The script was a hundred and eighty pages, and we went ahead and shot it as it stood. In the film version, he finds the bird within eighteen minutes. In the script, the bird did not show up for an hour and ten minutes! We shot it, as I've said, as written. When I'd finished it, it was four hours and ten minutes long! I said, "You can't cut it. You have to *rewrite* it. You just have to trim the whole of the first seventy minutes down to eighteen; you have to have a totally new concept."

So Burt went ahead and did *Judgement at Nuremburg*, and we closed the picture down. The writer, the late Guy Trosper, and I rewrote the beginning. I went back and reshot it, and came out with the movie I wanted. Burt and I then became very good friends. We've since worked together on *Seven Days in May,* and *The Train,* and gotten along beautifully.

Birdman was a terribly difficult film to make. If it had been in colour I don't think we could ever have done it, because there is just no such thing as a trained bird. You've got to use a hungry bird. We used canaries in some scenes, and you can't train *them* at all. At other times we used sparrows—about fifty for one bird. Ray Berwick is a bird-trainer and he would work with a bird, but once you got the lights and the camera and the crew around, the bird would be petrified, and we had to sit there until it felt like doing it. It was torture, it really was. And it was like being in prison because we had a netting, a wire mesh constructed over the set, so the bird couldn't fly out. We were all trapped; it was a very claustrophobic movie.

All Fall Down came next. I had read James Leo Herlihy's novel about a young man growing up, liked it very much, and had always wanted to work with William Inge; this seemed an ideal subject for him to adapt. John Houseman, the producer, had done one of my TV shows, and he called me and said: "I've got a three-picture contract with MGM. You can do any one of three properties you want." So I chose *All Fall Down*. I loved making that movie; it was a very happy time for me. In a love scene we had a lake and swans: I wanted it to be almost a parody of idyllic love as the boy, Clinton, would have imagined it. In the novel, the whole story is told from Clinton's point of view, and the one fault of the film is that it isn't totally from his point of view, as it should have been. It is the story of a man's emergence from boyhood, the difficulty of becoming a man. The loss of innocence was a theme that fascinated me. Warren Beatty, the star, was very insecure, having only done two films, one of which, *The Roman Spring of Mrs. Stone,* he knew was no good. He was terribly worried about his career, his image as a star and so on, but he was never difficult at all, and Warren and I are quite good friends. He's a talented actor, and he was good in the film, but he wasn't up to the last scene, when he is left behind by the younger brother, and you see that he's no longer the hero he had been imagined to be.

I would have preferred to make the whole picture on location at Key West. The picture didn't do too well at the box-office, but about two years later they made the same movie and called it *Hud,* and that did very well.

After *All Fall Down,* I made *The Manchurian Candidate.* George Axelrod and I had wanted to work together for some years, because we had been friends, and before we did *Birdman* we bought *The Manchurian Candidate* together. We had started to work on *Breakfast at Tiffany's* together, and worked a great deal on the script in 1959. But Audrey Hepburn didn't want me; she wouldn't work with me because she hadn't heard of me and didn't know anything about me, and they had to replace me. I never shot a foot of it. *The Manchurian Candidate* varied a good deal from the original, yet I think it kept the essence of the book. George and I realized we had a problem: the film had no third act. In the book, Marco orders the executions of the mother and father. Now, you can't do a film that advocates killing people. We couldn't get around it, until we hit on the idea that he doesn't know what Raymond is up to.

The preview was hysterical (that was the last picture I ever previewed: previews makes me so nervous I can't think of anything; I'm sitting there like a rock). It took place in San Francisco, and the audience reaction was fantastic. In the foyer a man came up to me and said, "Did you have anything to do with this movie?" I said, "Yes". And he said, "The goddamned Commies are never going to let you release it. This really shows 'em what they are." I walked round the other side of the table and this other guy said, "Did you have anything to do with this movie?" "Yes". And he said, "Those right-wing bastards are never going to let you release it." So I brought the two guys together and introduced them. The last thing I saw they were having a heated argument in the lobby.

At one stage we were going to be picketed by both the American Legion and the Communist party at the same time, which we tried to encourage of course; after all, the whole point of the film was the absurdity of any type of extremism, left wing or right.

Then came *Seven Days in May*. I was out of work after *The Manchurian Candidate* because I had had such fun creating my own material that I never wanted to go back to something somebody handed you. Besides, they weren't handing me the scripts I wanted. I fired my agents also because they suggested I do the Edith Piaf story with Natalie Wood. It would have been the end of me. Now, I was very active in the American Civil Liberties Union and we were going to do a television show, and we all got together in the office of Edward Lewis, the TV producer. But we never did do it, and later Lewis rang me and said he had just read the galleys of *Seven Days*.

I read the galleys, and hired Rod Serling to do the script. I loved the anti-MacArthur, anti-McCarthy theme. It was at a time when the military was very strong in this country and, God knows, they're strong now, too, but this was just after Kennedy got in, after eight years of Eisenhower, which was pretty tough to take. Those were the days of General Walker and so on. I think that, even though we are involved in this ridiculous thing in Vietnam, the temper of the country has swung the other way; but then things were bad. President Kennedy wanted *Seven Days in May* made. Pierre Salinger conveyed this to us. The Pentagon didn't want it done. Kennedy said that when we wanted to shoot at the White House he would conveniently go to Hyannis Port that weekend.

The studio worried a good deal about the subject matter. But there was nothing they could do about it because we came in with such a strong package, and paid for it with our own money. I had to borrow money from the bank for that. We had Kirk Douglas, Burt Lancaster, Rod Serling, Edward Lewis, and the number one best-seller in the country, and there was nothing they could do to us. We had total, final control.

Kirk Douglas was very jealous of Lancaster; he felt he was playing a secondary role to Lancaster, which indeed he was. I told him before he went in he would be. He wanted to be Burt Lancaster. He's wanted to be Burt Lancaster all his life. In the end it came to sitting down with Douglas and saying "Look, you punk, if you don't like it, get the hell out and stop playing it like a Western hero. Jiggs Casey, no matter how you look at it, is kind of a despicable human being; he does rat on his friend."

Seconds had a theme that fascinates me: the old American bullshit about having to be young, the whole myth that financial security is happiness—you could keep going for half an hour about what *Seconds* really means. There's the point that there are lots of people going to psychoanalysts, trying to get away from what they are. You are what you are, and you live with yourself, and that's what life is all about. This man couldn't, and ended up with an appalling situation on his hands. I thought the film had a terribly important and powerful statement to make.

The novel was sent to us in galleys—to Eddie Lewis and myself. Lewis Carlino wrote the script with us. I didn't know how to cast the central role of the man who goes back for a second chance at life. You see, in the novel, you believed that the same man went through plastic surgery, but there was this problem: the confrontation with his wife. What surgery could they do to prevent the wife from recognizing him?

We had to get around that problem. We also had the problem that the film demanded extreme closeups of the actor as both Arthur Hamilton, the New York banker, and Antiochus Wilson, the West Coast painter. I had originally intended to have Sir Laurence Olivier in the part, playing both roles, but I couldn't get the film financed with Olivier; his box-office pull wasn't strong enough. Paramount was upset, anyway, about having to do it at all, and Olivier just wasn't what they wanted.

And finally I thought, if you've got to go through all this horseshit of operations and so on, what would you want to come out looking like? Marlon Brando? He turned it down, so I went to Rock. And he said, "I can't do it. I'm not that good an actor to be able to make the transformation." So I said, "What would happen if you just played the second part?" "O.K.," he said, "fine." And I suddenly realized that this was the way to do the movie, that the same actor couldn't play both roles anyway. Of course, there were endless problems in using two actors: John Randolph, who played the older man, was right-handed, and Rock's left-handed; their hairlines were different, and so on.

In many ways I adored the movie, but we always knew we had a weakness in the second act, which was why he didn't adjust to life in California. The wine-crushing scene that symbolized his release and showed how he got rid of his inhibitions wasn't meant to look like an orgy. It was just that, in the English and American versions, they made me cut so much that it came out looking that way. In reality, it's the cleanest thing in the world! These people, most of whom are terribly attractive, take off their clothes and get into a vat stark naked and stamp the grapes. And it really is an exhilarating experience. I did it—with some inhibition. I had to get in that goddamned vat when we were shooting that thing. I had a camera, and I wore a bathing-suit, but they pulled it off immediately. No one gets an erection in the vat! You wouldn't believe it! And they have a kind of a rule, no hard-ons in the vat!

Usually they had the ceremony in October, and we wanted to shoot it in August, so we had to bring the grapes in specially from New Mexico, so they had two wine festivals that year! And they just wanted a new vat from us, that's all. Finally, we had to do some retakes, so we went back to the real one in October. The old Chinese photographer, James Wong Howe, wouldn't get into the vat. He was out there impeccably dressed and we were trying to figure out ways to get him in, but he said, "I won't get in, I won't get in the vat!"

The Train was something I would never do again. I did it to pay off a favour to a friend. Burt Lancaster was doing one of those bail-out pictures of his to pay the debts on his Hecht-Hill-Lancaster company. He and the first director didn't see eye to eye and Burt called me after three days shooting and asked me to come over to France and do it. I said no, but he finally persuaded me. And I wanted to get out of this country, too; I wanted to work abroad. He sent the script to me at the Los Angeles Airport. If I'd been a pilot, I'd have turned the plane round and landed it. It was the worst script I'd ever read, two hundred and forty pages long. It made no sense, and they didn't get the train out till very late. I made them shut the picture down for three weeks while I brought in some new writers, and we took a hotel room and rewrote the whole damn' thing. I would shoot the railyard scenes while we were rewriting.

We never really finished the script because of problems with its construction, not until we had to close the picture again in December because of weather. But the film came out well, and I *loved* working in Europe. I got tired of living in Saranwrap, which one does in Hollywood, and I wanted to get out and see what the world was like. I live out of the company town atmosphere here anyway, at the beach, and I'm not a person who feels any compulsion to go to Beverly Hills dinner parties. What the French crew perhaps lack in efficiency they make up in interest; if you get to the rushes the entire crew is there. I don't want to knock American crews, but they *are* very conservative. And there are no young people in Hollywood. They have cinema schools here and you wonder why the kids go to them, because they can't get a job in Hollywood. It's like getting a degree in something you can't work in.

My next picture in Europe was *Grand Prix*. We had several rewrites on it. The actors really drove, there was no process work. I ignored the problems of Cinerama. The other Cinerama films I saw had been done with an anamorphic lens, but I used a spherical lens for super-Panavision. The lenses are much smaller and you have a good deal of height, while with the others you have no height whatsoever. I used an anamorphic process in my next picture, *The Extraordinary Seaman,* an anti-war comedy, and it was *murder.*

My latest movie, from Bernard Malamud's *The Fixer,* is very exciting. The story of a man who will not give up, like *Birdman.* And then *The Gipsy Moths,* about three men who defy conformity.

Above all, I look forward to working in Europe. Bergman, Losey, these are the men. And I want to be part of it all.

Alfred Hitchcock

In the middle of the Universal-MCA lot, a little bit of England: a small white cottage, and inside a grandfather clock, antique furniture, two barking terriers, and the ritual of morning tea. Hitchcock, short and plump, his figure hugged by an immaculate coffee-coloured suit, is still, for all his years in California, very much a Londoner. His eyes, small and brown and extraordinarily penetrating, have a way of seeming to concentrate into their gaze all the power of his personality. To be on the receiving end of his displeasure, one reflects, would be a most uncomfortable position. Today, however, he exudes charm, but even more than charm he gives off an overpowering air of authority, and when he speaks of something that passionately interests him, his voice takes on an urgency, an enthusiasm, that is electrifying. The interview, punctuated by the ticking and chiming of the grandfather clock and by the scratching and yapping of the dogs outside the room, suggests that, second only to making films, the Master of Suspense most enjoys discussing them, for he is a marvellous talker, and his pleasure in talking communicates itself to us forcefully.

I first came to the U.S. in June 1938 to sign a contract with David O. Selznick. There had been American approaches in previous years by Universal and Sam Goldwyn, but I was always under contract to either Gaumont-British or ABC in England. In those days I was called England's "ace" director, and it was through David Selznick's brother, the agent Myron Selznick, with whom I'd been acquainted over many years, that I received an offer from David Selznick to come out to Hollywood and

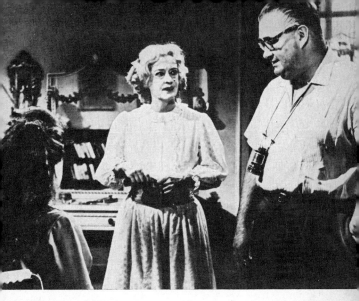

Joan Crawford (*back to camera*), Bette Davis and Robert Aldrich on the set of Aldrich's *Whatever Happened to Baby Jane?*

Bette Davis, Jack Warner and Joan Crawford.

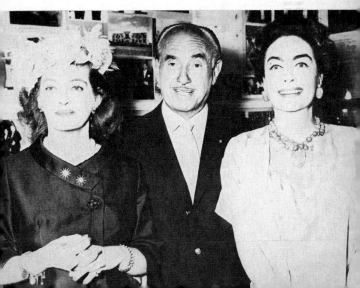

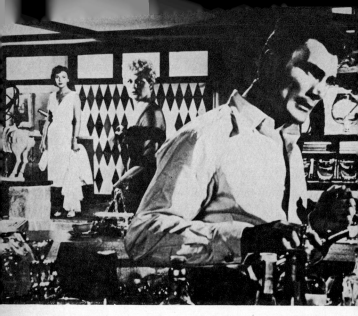

Ida Lupino, Shelley Winters and Jack Palance in Aldrich's film of Clifford Odets' *The Big Knife*.

Bette Davis in Aldrich's *Hush . . . Hush, Sweet Charlotte*.

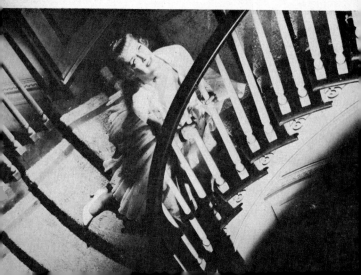

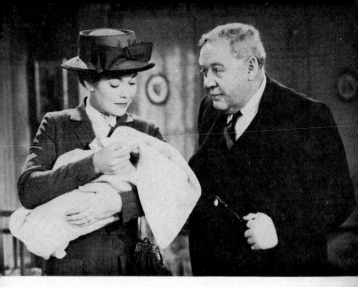

Jane Wyman and Charles Laughton in Bernhardt's *The Blue Veil*.

Curtis Bernhardt.

Bette Davis in Bernhardt's
A Stolen Life.

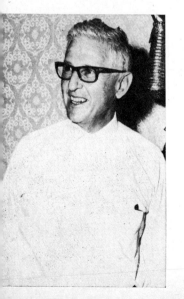

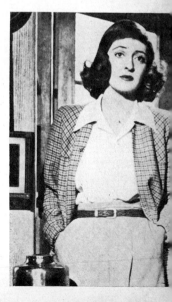

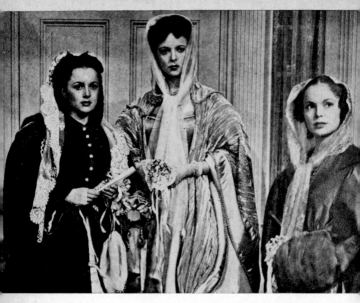

Olivia de Haviland as Charlotte, Ida Lupino as Emily and Nancy Coleman as Anne in Bernhardt's film about the Brontë sisters.

Audrey Totter and Robert Taylor in Bernhardt's *High Wall*.

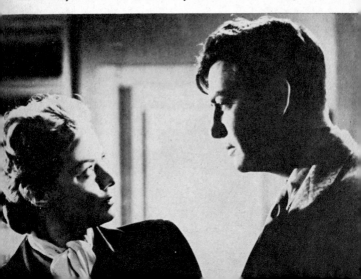

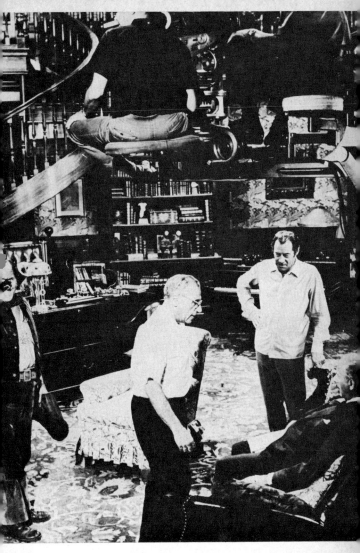

Stanley Holloway, director George Cukor, Rex Harrison and
Wilfrid Hyde-White on the set of *My Fair Lady*.

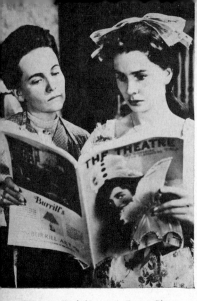

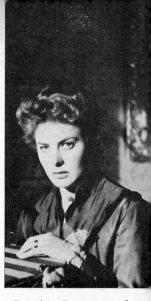

Teresa Wright and Jean Sim-
mons in Cukor's *The Actress*.

Ingrid Bergman in
Cukor's *Gaslight*.

Joan Crawford, Rosalind Russell, Norma Shearer and Joan
Fontaine in Cukor's *The Women*.

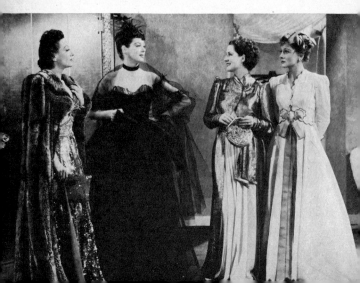

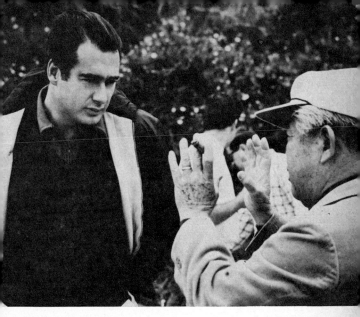

Director John Frankenheimer and chief cinematographer James Wong Howe during the filming of *Seconds*.

Karl Malden, Angela Lansbury and Brandon de Wilde in Frankenheimer's *All Fall Down*.

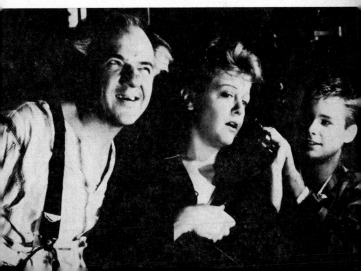

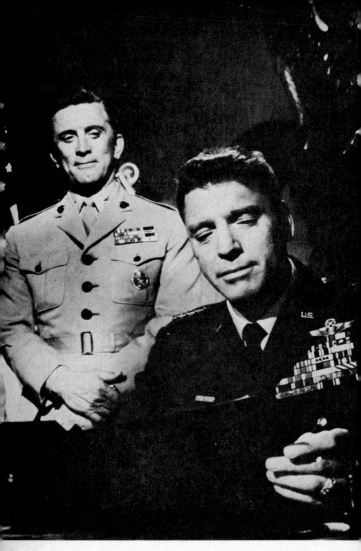

Kirk Douglas and Burt Lancaster in Frankenheimer's *Seven Days in May.*

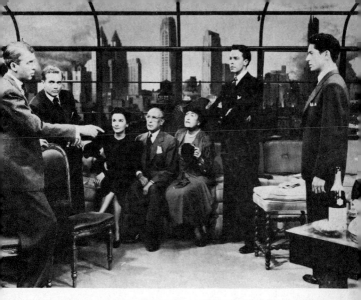

James Stewart, Douglas Dick, Joan Tetzel, Cedric Hardwicke, Constance Collier, John Dall and Farley Granger in Alfred Hitchcock's *Rope*.

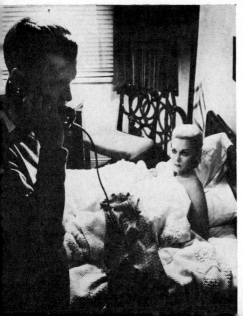

James Stewart and Kim Novak in Hitchcock's *Vertigo*.

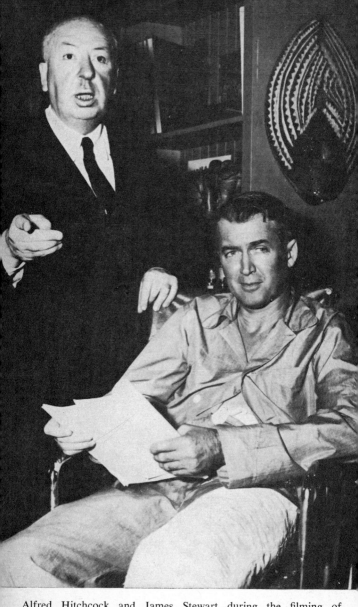
Alfred Hitchcock and James Stewart during the filming of *Rear Window.*

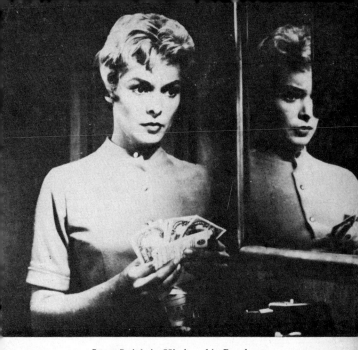

Janet Leigh in Hitchcock's *Psycho*.

"Tippi" Hedren in Hitchcock's *The Birds*.

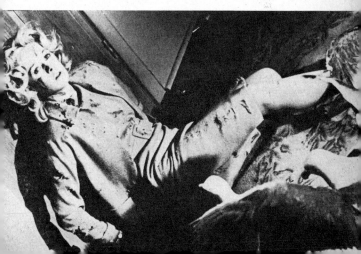

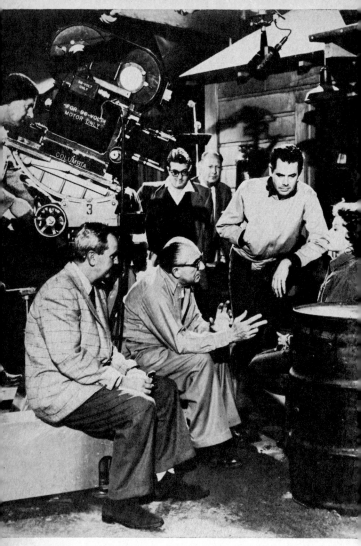

Fritz Lang (*center seated*) on the set of *Human Desire* with Glenn Ford and Gloria Grahame.

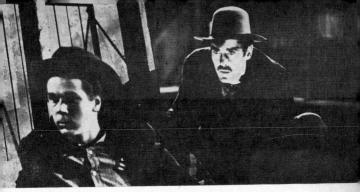

Jackie Cooper and Henry Fonda in Lang's *The Return of Frank James.*

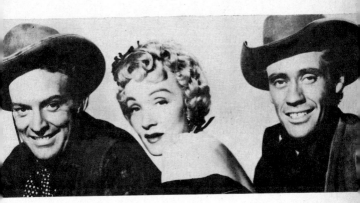

Arthur Kennedy, Marlene Dietrich and Mel Ferrer in Lang's *Rancho Notorious.*

Robert Ryan and Marilyn Monroe in Lang's *Clash by Night.*

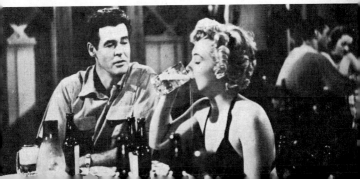

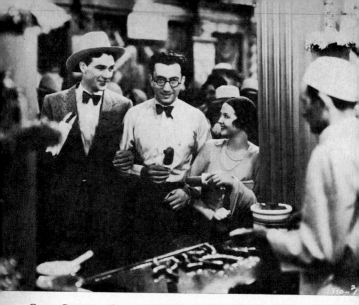

Gary Cooper, director Rouben Mamoulian and Sylvia Sidney making *City Streets*.

Myrna Loy in Mamoulian's *Love Me Tonight*.

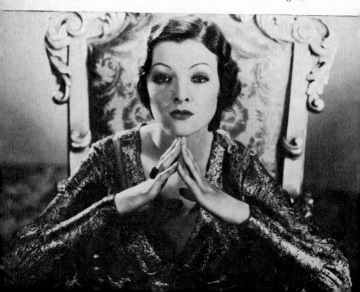

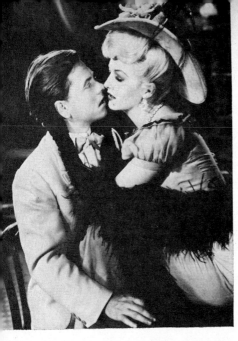

Mickey Rooney and Marilyn Maxwell in Mamoulian's *Summer Holiday*.

Tyrone Power, J. Carroll Naish and John Carradine in Mamoulian's *Blood and Sand*.

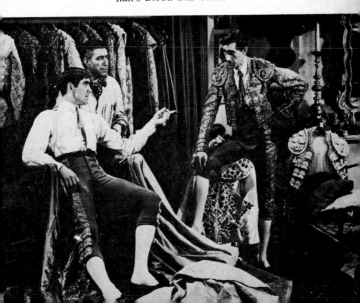

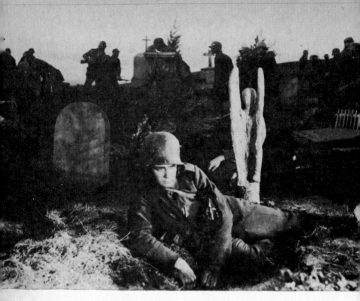

Lew Ayres in Milestone's *All Quiet on the Western Front*.

Lewis Milestone (seated on crane) during the making of *All Quiet on the Western Front*.

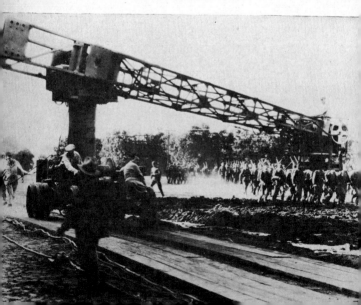

do the story of the *Titanic*: that was the original intention. The offer came while I was shooting *The Lady Vanishes* and Selznick was very pleased with his buy, because the following year I received the New York Critics' Award for best direction for *The Lady Vanishes*. Just before I left England—where I'd returned after signing the contract—I got a message saying that he would like to change from the *Titanic* to *Rebecca*. So when I arrived here to start work in April 1939 it was on *Rebecca*.

Selznick had just made *Gone with the Wind* and he had a very strong theory that a best-seller should be adhered to, because readers had their favourite scenes and if you left any of them out they would be disappointed. He accordingly followed the book of *Rebecca* fairly closely, sometimes I felt *too* closely. I felt that one would like to have got more movement into it, rather than have many static scenes. It was a novel, whichever way you look at it, and the plot had certain holes.

One of the main holes in the *Rebecca* plot is this: here is a man whose wife is dead. She's a paragon, and in the middle of your story she is washed up in a boat. But he had already identified his dead wife some time before. So, on the same night that he killed his wife, by some good fortune another woman was washed up on the shore several miles away. Nobody ever realizes this, it's obscured by the general overall interest in the surface story.

The ironic thing about *Rebecca* is that it was an English picture, in effect. The only two—shall I call them foreigners—were Robert Sherwood, who did the main work on the script, and Selznick. Although Joan Fontaine was our first choice for the female lead, I had to go through the *motions* of testing every woman in town, because Selznick wanted to do the same publicity that he had done for Scarlett O'Hara. So I was testing all these women—Loretta Young, Vivien Leigh even, Anne Baxter, Anita Louise, a whole lot of them, some of them totally unsuitable—although I'd already made up my mind that Fontaine was the best.

I got on very well with Selznick. He once made the remark—and it's a very scary remark if you ponder its meaning—that I was the only director he'd ever trust a picture with. The significance of that remark is that it was the *producer* who would employ the director and take him off if he didn't like him and put another one on, just as they used to do with cameramen. Selznick did that on two occasions: he swapped George Cukor for Victor Fleming after two weeks on *Gone with the Wind,* and when Ingrid Bergman made her first Hollywood picture, *Intermezzo,* he replaced the original cameraman, Harry Stradling, with someone else. Stradling had had a big reputation in Europe although he was an American cameraman—he'd done films like *La Kermesse Heroique*—and being taken off this picture was such a shock to him that he was missing for nearly a week. They found him out on one of the gambling-ships off Santa Monica. In this town it was nothing to be taken off, but in Europe it would be considered almost professional death.

Working with Walter Wanger on *Foreign Correspondent* was different from working with Selznick. The book he had, Vincent Sheean's *Personal History,* was ridiculous as the basis of a film. So we started from scratch on a brand new idea. As always, I preplanned the picture in detail. I have such a strong sense of the visual that I can see a film beforehand from beginning to end. It's almost a "must" to me to make it first on paper, just as a composer can compose music on paper. When I hear of a man shooting a film off the cuff, making it up as he goes along, I think it's like a composer composing a symphony before a full orchestra. I like to improvise in an office, not on a stage in front of a hundred technicians.

The windmill episode in *Foreign Correspondent* was a notion of mine based on a particular approach I have to settings. I'm a great believer in that; if you have a setting, it should be dramatized, and be indigenous to the whole picture, not just a background. For example, in *North by Northwest,* I had Cary Grant trapped in an auction gallery. How is he going to get out? Not by hiding and running, but by bidding for things in a crazy way, causing him to be thrown out by the police and thus escape. In the same picture, I was barred from using Mount Rushmore properly—they said I was "making fun of the Shrine of Democracy", or something. They wouldn't let me use action over the faces of the presidents. We had to work *between* the faces, and any fighting or struggling had to be on the mountainside out of view of the four heads, which was ridiculous because I wanted to have Cary Grant slide down Lincoln's nose and then hide from his enemies in the nostril, and then while he's in the nostril have a sneezing fit. That way you can spur your background into something that *functions* for you.

Years ago I made a film of Somerset Maugham's *Ashenden*, with John Gielgud and Madeleine Carroll, *Secret Agent*. I said to myself, "I'm going to Switzerland. What have they got there? Lakes, alps, chocolate factories—we'll work all those in." So in *Foreign Correspondent*, set partly in Holland, I asked myself, "Now what is there in Holland that I can dramatize?" Tulips? There was no colour in those days, so no tulips. Windmills? Naturally. And how did I use them? I had one mill going the wrong way while Joel McCrea's hat blew the other way; then he realized it was a sign for an aeroplane to land.

I'd like to describe the staging of the final plane crash carefully. The first principle is, in order to have an audience participate, treat it subjectively, keep it inside the plane, make it *feel* what it's like to be in a plane that's being attacked. So it becomes subjective—all the attack is seen through the windows. You only became *ob*jective when the plane actually crashed into the water. Now, I had one shot in this sequence that was never questioned, no one asked how it was done. It was a shot shooting over the shoulders of the pilot and the co-pilot, and beyond them the glass front of the cockpit, diving towards the ocean. And in this shot the camera never moved from behind the two men, the plane hit the water, smashed the front of the glass and enveloped the two men with water and drowned them, without a cut, and nobody ever asked, "Were you all drowned in that shot? How was it done?"

Well, it was done this way: I had a trick pilot—a man called Paul Mantz, he died recently—go up over the Pacific and do some nose dives with the camera stuck out on the front of the plane and pull out of the dive at the last minute, so that the plane was practically touching the water. He did two or three of those. Then we brought those films back. When you looked at them on the screen you felt you were diving towards the water, and at the last moment you came out of the dive.

Now I built the cockpit in the studio with the glass front and the two men in it, and on a screen, back-projected, I had the dive towards the ocean. So it was a combination of the screen with the dive on it and the cockpit in the front. But nobody asked: How did the water come in and envelop the people? I had the screens made of rice paper, without any seams, twelve feet wide by eight feet high, and behind the screens two dump tanks with 2,700 gallons of water in each, and a chute pointing at the screen. So, at the crucial moment, when I felt we were just about to touch the water, I pressed a button and let the whole of that 5,400 gallons go: it tore through the screen in such a volume that you never saw the screen go, and the whole cockpit was filled with water, all in the one shot.

To achieve that shot of the people apparently drowning in the cabin we had a tank, and lowered the set with the people in it into the tank, so you got the effect of the water coming up. We had the ceiling made of paper so their heads went through the paper; we cut just before the paper ceiling broke. Herbert Marshall presented a special problem because he only had one leg. So we built a chest-high tub for him, photographed him in the water, and just skimmed over the top of that tub; but he was dry underneath.

Suspicion suffered from a compromised ending because the star, Cary Grant, obviously cannot be a murderer. The original ending had the wife dying from a poisoned glass of milk given her by her homicidal husband. Of course it was impossible to use that in the film, but I did have an ending whereby the wife now knows that she's married to a murderer who's going to kill her, so she writes a letter to her mother saying. "I don't want to live any more, I'm in love with him, he's going to kill me, but I think society should be protected." She writes the letter, seals it, puts it beside the bed, and when he brings up the fatal glass of milk she says, "Would you post that letter for me?" So she drinks the milk and dies. Then you fade out and fade in again on one shot: Cary Grant walking down the street whistling very cheerfully and popping the letter in the box. But I couldn't use that ending either.

Dorothy Parker wrote a couple of amusing lines for my next picture, *Saboteur,* which I think rather escaped a lot of people. Our hero and heroine are on the run and get a lift with some freaks on a circus train. The midget is having a row with the thin man, who's terribly tall, and the thin man says to the midget. "If you were two inches taller I'd knock you down", which is a typical Dorothy Parker line. Her other line involved a pair of Siamese twins who come out of the end of their bunk sort of half-asleep, not speaking to each other. They're communicating through a third person, and one of them says to the third person, "I wish you'd tell her to do something about her insomnia; I've done nothing but toss and turn all night."

The villain's fall from the Statue of Liberty in the final sequence was done by a double-printing matte process. We have the man in closeup against black velvet in a kind of swinging chair, all covered in black, with only the man visible. The camera, at first close to him, is suddenly whipped up to the ceiling of the studio. When you see it on the screen you get the opposite effect, and that's printed in by matte. Of course, to have had the total involvement of the audience it should have been the hero who was in danger, not the villain, but the story demanded it otherwise.

Shadow of a Doubt is one of my favourite pictures. It started as a nine-page original by a man called Gordon McDonell. His wife happened to be Selznick's story-editor in those days. I was being loaned out by Selznick, and we met in the "Brown Derby" in Beverly Hills, where she told me her husband had this idea for a story. I suggested she go and type it out. She did and we bought it. Then I invited Thornton Wilder to come out and do the script because, as the author of *Our Town*, he was the best available example of a writer of Americana. We used to talk in the morning and he'd write in the afternoon. He didn't work in continuity either, he jumped around.

Before he arrived we'd already selected Santa Rosa, California, as our location. We stayed in the town and studied it before any script was written, and constantly used local citizens in the cast. I found the little girl who played Teresa Wright's sister looking in a store window, brought her down here, tested her, and put her in the picture. This was wartime, and very few films of that type had been shot on real locations. They mostly used studio back-lots, so going into a real town and shooting it all there made quite a big difference.

The opening scenes of Uncle Charlie on the run from his hotel room were shot in Newark, New Jersey, before Joseph Cotten had been cast. I shot them three times—there were only about four setups—using three different men: tall, medium, and short. So when Cotten was cast I used the shots with the tall man.

Lifeboat was a back-projection picture from beginning to end. There again I adopted the principle—as in the aeroplane in *Foreign Correspondent*—of never going outside the boat, keeping the camera inside all the time, except for one shot: I couldn't photograph a becalmed sea from inside the boat, and that's the only shot in the whole picture that's shot objectively, outside. We did the storm in tanks using back-projected film of stormy sea taken off the Californian coast. I remember that, when Tallulah Bankhead took her first dump-tanks, which involved about 100,000 gallons of water coming in at once, she got a round of applause from the crew for surviving it.

The picture was my idea, a kind of microcosm of the war. I sent it to both Hemingway and Steinbeck. Steinbeck accepted and wrote the whole thing. I never even heard from Hemingway, although I knew him. The film drew many complaints. Dorothy Thompson, who saw it and gave it ten days to get out of town, went after it terribly. So did Crowther of the *New York Times*. The main complaint was that I'd shown the Nazi in ascendancy over the rest of the people. But that was ridiculous because, after all, he *was* a submarine commander, he'd be the man who'd be more proficient at handling a boat than anyone else. It also showed that they were all at sixes and sevens with each other, and, to get rid of his man, they had to combine. Irrespective of whether Henry Hull was a Fascist or John Hodiak a Communist, they had to get together.

Spellbound started as a book I bought for Selznick called *The House of Dr Edwardes*, written by a two-man team who published under the name of Francis Beeding. One was a man called Hilary St. George Saunders who I think became librarian in the House of Commons or something, and the other was a man named Palmer. Originally set in England, the story was about a crazy patient being taken to an asylum who overcomes the doctor and turns up as the doctor himself. The book went in for Black Mass and all kinds of things, so Ben Hecht and I just took that one idea and worked out a whole new story.

I wanted to open the film with two men in a train dining-car: one was the doctor and the other was the patient. One of them sees a fly crawling over the tablecloth. He catches it, tears its wings off and puts it back again. But what I couldn't decide was: who would have done that, the patient or the doctor? So I never used that idea.

I brought in Salvador Dali to do the dream sequences, not for publicity purposes—as Selznick thought—but because I wanted to have dreams photographed vividly. Until then, movie dreams were always blurred, always double exposures, and misty; and dreams are not like that, they're very, very vivid. What I wanted out of Dali was that long perspective, that hard, clear, solid look; I wanted his sequences to be shot in the open air in bright sunlight, so they would have to stop the lens down to make it really hard in contrast. But they wouldn't do that. Dali wanted all kinds of crazy things. He wanted Ingrid Bergman covered in ants at one point. He was really a kook.

I also used Ingrid Bergman in my next picture, *Notorious*. There's a whole story about that film. In any spy story you have to say to yourself, What are the spies after? Now in Kipling's day they were the plans of the fort. Later, they were the plans of the aeroplane engine as in *The Thirty-Nine Steps*. We always called this thing the "MacGuffin" because actually, when you come down to it, it doesn't matter what the spies are after. The characters on the screen worry about what they're after, but the audience don't care because they only care about the safety of the hero or heroine.

People would ask, "Where do you get the word 'MacGuffin'?" And I'd tell them the following tale: Two men are sitting opposite each other in an English train. One asks the other: "Excuse me, what's that on the luggage-rack over your head?" "Oh, that—that's a MacGuffin." "What's a MacGuffin?" "Oh, it's an apparatus for trapping lions in the Scottish Highlands." "But there *are* no lions in the Scottish Highlands." "Well," comes the reply, "then that's no MacGuffin."

In the *Notorious* story, you had Ingrid Bergman sent down to South America to ingratiate herself with a group of German friends of her father who's just gone to gaol, and Cary Grant was the FBI man who goes down to be her contact. The question was: What are the Nazis up to? What does she have to find out? I remember Ben Hecht and I tried to figure out all kinds of MacGuffins. At one point we even had the escaped crew of the *Graf Spee* drilling and training a German army to take over the Argentine.

Finally it got so wild that—being a connoisseur of wine—I came up with the idea of uranium in wine bottles. When I mentioned this to Selznick he said, "What uranium?" I said, "It's Uranium 235." "What's that?" he said. I said, "It's the stuff they're going to make the atom bomb from." "What atom bomb?" "David," I said, "everybody knows about this. The Germans are trying to make heavy water in Norway: this is what it's for." He said, "I think this is the craziest thing on which to base a picture." "All right," I said. "If you don't like uranium let's make it industrial diamonds, anything you like— jewellery—I don't care."

He couldn't understand. A lot of people make the same mistake when it comes to thriller stories. They seem to think—especially in America, less in England—that this is the most important item. It isn't. It's the *least* important. As I said before, it's important to the characters but not to the audience. Eventually Selznick sold the whole project—half-finished script, Ingrid Bergman, Cary Grant, myself—to RKO for $800,000 and fifty per cent of the profits.

Ben Hecht finished the script—after Clifford Odets tried and failed—and we went to see Dr Millikan of Cal Tech, a leading local scientist, to find out more about Uranium 235. We walked into his office with its impressive bust of Einstein, and I said, "Dr Millikan, how big would an atom bomb be?" Mind you, he was right in the middle of the top secret Manhattan Project! "Do you want to get arrested?" he asked. "Do you want to get *me* arrested?" Then he corrected himself; he'd spoken too soon, and spent an hour telling us how impossible the whole thing was.

I understand that I was watched by the FBI for three months afterwards. And the only information I'd ever had was from a man called Russell Maloney on the *New Yorker* who told me, "There's a place down in New Mexico where men go in and are never allowed out again, it's so secret." I guessed it was the atom bomb. So I made the picture—a year before Hiroshima! After the war, coming back from Europe on the *Elizabeth*, I met a partner of Hal Wallis—Joe Hazen—who said, "By the way, I've often wanted to ask you: how did you get on to that atom bomb thing all that time ahead?" I told him, and he said, "When that script was submitted to us we thought it was the goddamnedest thing on which to base a picture." "You made the same mistake as Selznick," I said. "You thought the story was about Uranium 235.

Well, it wasn't. It was a love story." "Well," he said, "we know it now."

About a year later, Selznick gave a cocktail party down in Malibu. I vividly remember the moment when I was talking to Clare Boothe Luce and he called me away and said, "You ought to go over to Germany, your name's become very big there since *Spellbound* and *Notorious*. Those Germans are very clever: now that uranium is out of date they made it narcotics." He was telling me the very same thing I'd been telling him all those years before, and if he hadn't made the error of thinking the public wouldn't go for stories about uranium he could have had a hundred per cent of the profits because the picture cost two million dollars and grossed eight million; that would be equivalent to about twenty million today.

I was lucky to get Leopoldine Konstantin, a newcomer to films, to play Claude Rains's mother in *Notorious*. Your big problem in casting is to avoid familiar faces. The best casting man is the novelist: his principals are always new, unfamiliar. I've always believed in having unfamiliar supporting players even if your stars are known. I learned that lesson years and years ago while watching a Metro picture, called *Trader Horn*, at a London press show. It all took place in the African jungle. They had Harry Carey as the lead and two brand-new people, Duncan Rinaldo and Edwina Booth, as the boy and girl. Everything was fine until the moment towards the end when Carey went up to the counter of a trading-post and there—in the middle of the jungle—up popped C. Aubrey Smith. I've never heard an audience laugh so much. And one's always learning that lesson: that's why I went to such trouble to import actors from Germany, for *Torn Curtain*, who'd never been seen before. Otherwise the whole thing would have been spoiled.

For *The Paradine Case* we had a pile of scripts two feet high. My wife, Alma Reville, did the first one, based on the novel entirely, because Selznick wanted a script for budget purposes. He wrote the final shooting-script himself. That was his great ambition—to be a writer—and I think he should have stuck to producing, the thing that he was most proficient at.

He also cast the picture, to my mind unsatisfactorily. Alida Valli as Mrs Paradine wasn't really what I wanted. She was too impassive and didn't know her English too well, which is a tremendous handicap to an actress. The part was originally offered to Greta Garbo, who turned it down immediately because Robert Hichens described this woman as "working in a barber's shop in Stockholm": he'd based it on her. She was also infuriated at being offered the part of a murderess.

Gregory Peck wasn't really an English lawyer either. It should have been an Englishman, someone like Ronald Colman or Olivier, if they could have got him. Here again you're casting for star value and not for proper casting. But the biggest casting mistake of all was Louis Jourdan, a pretty-pretty boy. It should have been a man like Robert Newton, because the whole point about the lawyer falling in love with the murderess was to realize the degradation of falling for a woman who'd had as one of her lovers a manure-smelling groom. He should have had to sit face to face with a coarse, horny-handed slob, and look and say: "I've sunk low enough to become infatuated with a woman who will even sleep with *this*." And of course it was all lost because Selznick had signed up this pretty-pretty boy.

I had one shot in that picture of Charles Coburn and Gregory Peck walking through Lincoln's Inn in London towards the camera, with the camera in front of them. They turn into a house, close the front door, come up the stairs, turn the corner, go along the top landing into an office and continue the scene in the office—all in one shot without a cut, and shot in Hollywood and not in Lincoln's Inn.

This is how it was done: I had a background shot made in London of where they would have walked, had it turn into a doorway and then stop. Then I had them shoot about two or three hundred feet of the stationary setup as through we were in a doorway. We put that on a screen outside the door of a set, which consisted of the door, some stairs, an upper landing and so forth. A big crane started at the bottom of the stairs at the front door. The screen showed the background, then the turn, then it came to a stop. The two men were walking on a treadmill in front of the door, but the camera was clear of the door and shot right through it on to the screen only. When the men appeared to turn and come in—they'd been on a treadmill all the time—the effect of the turn was on the back of the screen, not on them. They then came off the treadmill into the set, closed the door and cut off the screen, and the crane took them up the stairs. But Selznick never used the shot.

On *Rope*, we followed Patrick Hamilton's play fairly closely, except that we had Arthur Laurents to polish the dialogue because the locale was changed from England to New York. The New York background was a complete model and it took up more space than the set itself because you had to see it from all angles. It was semicircular. We had moving clouds of spun glass that were part of a plan—Cloud Number 1, 2, 3, 4, 5, etc. Some were hanging, some standing. We kept moving those every reel. The play covered a hundred and five minutes—from 7.15 p.m. to 9.0 p.m.—and so did the film. The apartment set was actual size, with a special floor for the camera and no ceiling. The camera movements and everything were all worked out in advance.

I think the two principals did quite a good job. There was one very interesting sidelight: as you know, we always have to dub sounds in afterwards because they conflict with the dialogue, and there's a scene where Farley Granger's playing the piano, for which we used Poulenc's *Perpetuum Mobile*. Of course, he wasn't that proficient on the piano so his hand was straying all over the place. After the film was finished, one of the men at Warners' music department had to study his fingers and then rewrite the music according to where his fingers went, so that, when it was ultimately played, it correctly matched his fingers.

I can't work well with mystery or thriller writers because I can do all that stuff myself. I'd rather work with writers who *don't* normally do thrillers so that I can get an extra contribution. That was Raymond Chandler's trouble on *Strangers on a Train*. He'd say to me, "What shall we do here?" And I'd say, "Why don't we do this?" "If *you* can think it out," he'd say, "what do you want *me* for?" Czenzi Ormonde, who did the picture's dialogue, was one of Ben Hecht's writers. He was like a chess player in those days, playing five scripts at once.

About two-thirds of it was based on Patricia Highsmith's novel. I've always liked stories involving trains because trains are movement. Unfortunately they're not so romantic now. We've lost the steam engine, and the diesel locomotive is a very dull affair to look at. There's nothing exciting even up front. At least in the steam trains they did open that door and shovel in the coal and all that. Now that's all gone.

I still perspire when I think of the little man crawling

underneath the carousel at the end of the picture because he actually did go under the machine. It couldn't be faked because it was a forward movement. The final collapse of the carousel, however, was done with a miniature against a background of live people. We put the miniature in front of a screen, and on the screen were the live people. Then, when we'd got that, we put it on a screen again and put live people in front of the screen, so you had a kind of sandwich: live people behind the carousel, the carousel miniature, live people in front.

The tennis match was done partly out at Southport, California, and partly from long shots done during the Davis Cup matches. I remember asking them would they mind moving that Davis Cup out of the way, please? And for our purposes they did.

I Confess was based on an idea by Louis Verneuil. It didn't really come off because the public as a whole couldn't believe that a man will sacrifice his life for the secrets of the confessional. Protestants won't understand that, or Moslems, or Buddhists. The dream sequence, Anne Baxter coming down a circular staircase in slow motion with her dress floating around her, was the sort of thing they do a lot today, but of course I've pioneered much of that.

I found Montgomery Clift—like all Method actors— very difficult. You can't get them to look the way you want when you want to cut. The actor must conform if you have some pre-cut ideas, and sometimes you cut for certain subjective effects. If you're using an actor who says, "I don't know whether I feel like it", you're up against a problem, and that was the problem with Clift.

Many people make the mistake of thinking that motion pictures are all galloping horses and racing cars. I think you can make a cinematic scene in a telephone-booth because you have so much detail to cut to. You're using the language of the camera. I use subjective treatment like that all the time. It's not practised enough. The most clear example of a purely cinematic subjective treatment in my own work is *Rear Window*. Here you have a man in one room, in one position, looking out on a courtyard: you show his closeup, what he sees, how he reacts. And he discovers a whole murder.

The idea for *Rear Window* came from a short story by William Irish. It didn't have any woman in it or anything like that. The challenge it posed was to have one man in a confined space and that's why it became such a cinematic picture. I tried to be stylistically consistent, to stay away from the people he was observing until he got out his camera with the long lens. The set had to be pre-lit because it was such a tremendous job. We had thirty-one apartments, twelve of them fully furnished. The people moving around in them had microphones on, which you couldn't see at that distance, through which they received instructions. It was a sort of walkie-talkie effect.

One of my favourite pictures is *The Trouble with Harry*, and it's the only losing picture I've had since 1952. I suppose it flopped because it had no well-known stars on which it could be sold. Shirley MacLaine, whose first film this was, had been understudying in the musical *Pyjama Game*. Hal Wallis had her under contract and I saw a test of her he'd made. I found the story in a small English novel and changed the setting to Vermont in autumn, because I wanted to counterpoint its macabre elements with beautifully coloured scenery.

Vertigo came from a story by Boileau and Narcejac, the same two men who wrote *Diabolique*. I changed its locale to San Francisco but, more important than that, I revealed its main secret in the middle of the picture. This wasn't a calculated risk because, when you save a twist like that for the end, you wonder how the audience are going to react to the middle part of the story.

One girl is dead and the James Stewart character has had a nervous breakdown. Then he discovers a brunette girl who resembles the dead woman. You're really starting a new story and asking yourself: What are the audience saying now? "Oh, he's found another girl. She looks like the dead one so he wants to make her over." By revealing the truth you give the audience two more things to think about: What will Stewart say when he finds out it's the same woman? Will the girl submit to the making-over? We can understand her objections. Previously we wouldn't understand her objections. Had I saved everything till the end the audience would have been more or less impatient with Stewart making over the girl.

That's why I always try to avoid last-minute revelations. In the case of *Psycho*, it's an *explanation*, not a dénouement, an explanation of *how* this boy came to be that way. The film is really over. By telling people all, you give them more suspense. That's the big difference between suspense and surprise: in surprise you have maybe ten seconds of shock; in suspense you have all the time you want because you've given the audience all the information. It's my old analogy of the bomb: the bomb is under this table, goes off, gives the audience ten seconds of shock. Tell them five minutes beforehand that it's going to go off, and there you have suspense. Big difference. That's why whodunits are not successful to me. It's an intellectual exercise. There's no emotion in a whodunit. They're wondering whether it's the butler or whoever. But give them all the information at the beginning and they'll say: "How are they going to find out that it's him?" They've a more intellectual kind of excitement going for them.

North by Northwest grew out of an idea I had for doing a story called *The Wreck of the Mary Deare*, having tried to lick *The Mystery of the Marie Celeste* many years before. MGM owned *The Wreck of the Mary Deare*, so I sat down with Ernest Lehman—he was under contract to Metro—and, after about a month, we gave up. But I still owed Metro a picture. Now it so happened that a New York journalist had given me an idea about an ordinary businessman being mistaken for a decoy spy. I took that and, with Ernie Lehman, worked up the whole thing. It took about a year to write.

The crop-dusting scene, staged out near Bakersfield here, was an example of avoiding the cliché. In ordinary circumstances, if they're going to put a man on the spot, they make him stand under a street lamp on a corner at night. The cobbles are washed by the recent rain. A black cat slithers along the wall. Somebody peers from behind a curtain. A black limousine goes by and—boom, boom, boom!—that's the cliché.

So I said: I won't do it that way. I'll make it in bright sunshine, without a tree or a house in sight. Thus the audience are worked up much more: they know the man's put on the spot, but they're mystified as to where it's going to come from. I had him waiting and waiting. Then a car pulled up, a man got out, approached our hero and said, "That's funny." "What is?" "There's a crop-duster over there dusting a place where there are no crops." And with that he hops a bus and is off. Sure enough the plane then dives on our hero (Cary Grant) and attacks him: no cliché.

James Mason was the heavy, but I didn't just want him

behaving villainously. I wanted him to be polite, but not so polite that he wasn't sufficiently menacing. So I divided the character into three: gave him a secretary who *looked* menacing and a third man who was brutal.

Psycho all came from Robert Bloch's book. The scriptwriter, Joseph Stefano—a radio writer, he'd been recommended to me by my agents, MCA—contributed dialogue mostly, no ideas. The shower-room stabbing sequence took seven days to shoot, although it was only forty-five seconds long on the screen. I did it with heads of Janet Leigh, a nude—a girl in full figure—and the woman doing the stabbing. I shot a lot of the nude in slow motion because I had to have her breast covered by an arm at the crucial moment; it was speeded up for the final film. There were actually seventy-eight cuts, seventy-eight little pieces of film, used in those forty-five seconds. The prop department made me a very nice pink rubber torso filled with tubed blood which shot out whenever you stabbed it, but I didn't use it.

The picture took about thirty-six days to make, including retakes. I used my TV film unit because of speed and because I wanted to make it for a price. I only slowed up when I came to something cinematic, like the shower scene. You could never have shot that under TV conditions—seven days' work for forty-five seconds' screen time! TV work is nine minutes *a day*. Unfortunately, feature film-makers are attuned to a minute and a half a day. There are very few feature cameramen—unless they're *passé* or semi-retired—who'll bother with TV.

The Birds posed so many problems that I didn't even bother bringing them up before we started the picture. I did not say, "Can you do this? Can you do that?" The scenes were written in and we had to discover how to do it afterwards. We trained 3,200 birds all told: gulls, crows, ravens, individual ones, groups. The whole thing was a matter of double-printing.

The shower of birds down the chimney was real. We rented so many finches. The trouble was that we had to keep them flying by the use of air hoses (of course we had the Society for the Prevention of Cruelty to Animals on the set) because by nature they went to perch, they wouldn't fly around, they were domestic birds. Then we printed them. Then we put a lot in a glass cage and let them fly around against a plain background and printed it on top of the real ones. So we had a double lot of birds: those in the room around the people and those in the glass cage.

The final scene of the birds' going out was done with about sixteen exposures on one piece of film. One little tiny section was shot down a road with five hundred ducks painted grey. Foreground birds were printed over. That was a tremendously complicated job. It's done by optical printer; a man from Disney was in charge of it. It's quadruple-treble printing. It's by far the most difficult single shot I've ever done, but nobody will ever know.

Nor does anyone apparently wonder about the "bird's eye view" shot over the gasoline station, asking, "Where was that shot from? A balloon?" The seaside was up at Bodega Bay. The other side of the road was on the studio back-lot, because there were only meadows opposite at Bodega Bay. We created the town on a matte. We did it by putting the camera on a high hill shooting down to a new parking-lot they were building. We put in the blazing car, etc., and all the rest was left blank. Then the matte artist painted in the whole scene and we fitted the two pieces together. In other words, on his painting the live parts looking down are black. On our side you can see the live part, but all the rest, all his part, is painted black. Then you put the two together.

Now the travelling matte system is a means of printing one thing over another without ghosting. In order to do that you must have a silhouette. Let me describe how it was done in the old days. Say I wanted to do two men talking on the corner of Fifth Avenue. Normally we'd do that in Hollywood with a back projection: Fifth Avenue on the screen and the two men in front. But supposing we are making this film in the summer and we want snow on Fifth Avenue. We aren't going to release it until January. In those circumstances we photograph the two men against a white backing (I'm talking about a black-and-white film). We put that film aside and wait until about November or December when the first snows fall and then we photograph the background independently.

What do we have now? We have a background of Fifth Avenue with snow and two men shot last July against a white backing. You have to superimpose one over the other without ghosting. In other words, if we printed the two together you'd see through the men, as happened in the old days when you could take two snaps on the same film.

So we take the positive, the print of the two men against the white, and overdevelop it to such a degree that the two men become silhouettes. That is called a travelling matte. Then we put raw, unexposed film in the printing-machine. Against that we put the negative of Fifth Avenue and against that the silhouette of the two men. Now you print that.

As the printing light goes through, it's printing Fifth Avenue blocked off by the two men. If we were to print that at that moment, we'd have two white figures, two white silhouettes against Fifth Avenue. But you don't print it. You rewind your first film, the raw film, take away the negative of Fifth Avenue—you've finished with that—and take away the black silhouettes of the two men. Now you put in the *negative* of the two men which was shot against a white background. On the negative it's now black, and you can see through the two men. So you put it through again so that the unexposed portion—the two men—is now printed in its proper place.

That's how we made *The Birds*, except that we made our silhouette at the same time as we made our colour shot. Our colour shot is done against a yellow background, and in the camera is a prism. The prism will take the straight colour negative and at right angles it will take a second image on black-and-white film through a red filter, turning that image into a silhouette. The red filter, the prism, is what we call a split beam: it takes the thing twice, once straight through and once at right angles. The right-angled one is on ordinary black-and-white film, not on colour film. The reason the background's yellow is the same as fog light's yellow: it's the lowest band in the spectrum of colour and comes out black. It's the one colour that won't photograph, this yellow light, called sodium light.

So in that shot I described before—the one from above—I wanted the gulls to descend. We went out here to a high cliff, put some food behind the camera and gulls came immediately. Then we took the food and threw it down to a beach below the cliff, whereupon the gulls went down for the food away from the camera and down to the beach.

When the film was brought back to the studio we had gulls going down towards a beach against surf, sand, and the side of a cliff. It took two women three months to copy each gull on a plain board and a silhouette on another board, frame by frame. They had a method whereby they transferred the thing almost like a lantern slide on to a card, and they merely had to paint over the actual birds themselves. Then they would take that and make a silhouette as well. When they made their film, we had live gulls against a plain background, each one drawn separately, and *that* was printed over the other matte shot. And people thought we shot it from a balloon or a helicopter!

Similarly, in the birds' attack on the children, we shot the children in a real place running down the street, and then in the studio, against a plain background, we shot the birds flying from one perch to another, about thirty feet apart. We made a silhouette of that against a yellow background and printed it over the shot of the children, and then the real birds over that.

The bird pecking "Tippi" Hedren's head was done by the same method. We let a bird dive against a plain background, and doubleprinted it over a shot of "Tippi" against the sea to coincide with the moment when we sent a squirt of air through a tube placed in her hair, which shot up as if the bird had actually pecked her.

The basic theme of *Marnie* was a fetish of a man wanting to go to bed with a thief, like going to bed with a coloured woman or a Chinese girl. But I don't think it came off, quite apart from the fact that Sean Connery wasn't really a Philadelphian. Even Hunter did two scripts ahead of Jay Presson Allen's, but they didn't work. It was a hard thing to lick. I think there was too much talk in it, it wasn't cinematic enough. Jay Presson Allen, the wife of Lewis Allen, producer of Truffaut's *Fahrenheit 451*, had been recommended to me by Hume Cronyn.

When I'm asked how I feel about Truffaut and other French critics describing me as a metaphysician and so on, I can only say that it's very nice. Some of it makes sense to me—Truffaut's comment for example that I'm one of the few people who know how to use the medium—but all these "philosophical" theories hold no water at all.

After Leon Uris's *Topaz*, a spy story, my next film is rather similar to *Suspicion* in its genre. It's a study of a psychopathic killer of three women, with the audience as it were inside the killer's mind. He has an ordinary life, he's charming and attracts women, but the moment it comes to the sexual act, of course, he loses his head and kills. You see him get acquainted with the first girl and eventually murder her. You're shocked by this, but you know the second murder is coming. The question is when and where, and will the girl get out of it? So you give her narrow escapes until she's finally done in. The third girl is a police decoy, but running terrible risks. She's aged about twenty-two or twenty-three and the character is based on a girl who took part recently in the Richardson torture-gang case in London.

When the case was over, the judge asked the Scotland Yard chief who'd been in charge of it to line up in front of the dock all the officers and detectives—there were about eight or ten—engaged on it: this was after sentences had been passed and the prisoners had been taken away. And, while thanking them for their services, he noticed among them a young blonde girl of twenty-two. When he asked her why she'd been chosen for the case she said, "Well I suppose it's because I'm rather proficient at judo", adding that she had been assigned to many "awkward" tasks: we know what that can mean. She'd been in the force since she was nineteen and had told her family she was on plain clothes duty!

I'd been contemplating for a long time making John Buchan's *The Three Hostages*, but I let it go because I don't think that you can put hypnotism over on the screen. The public can't appreciate it. It's like putting an illusionist in front of them. I don't believe people can feel or sense it. It's something outside their experience. Also, your central situation is that Hannay—the same character as in *Thirty-Nine Steps*—has to *pretend* to be hypnotized. Now, this is awfully hard to make the public understand. But I do love the scene where Hannay, pretending to be hypnotized, is told to go on his knees like a dog and bring an ashtray back in his teeth: I think it would be hilarious.

I'm still keeping *Mary Rose* on ice. I regard that as almost a science fiction subject. I think it can be put over, not only as a sentimental Barrie story, but also as an illustration of the proposition—in which I believe—that a person can be atomically disembodied, made to disappear and then be reassembled. I think there will come a time in the future when either we will be disembodied, taken apart by someone or be able to do it ourselves, and transfer ourselves that way to another place and come together there again.

The story I've always wanted to do is the big city from

dawn till dusk, or from dawn till the following dawn. It's a tremendous task. The main problem is getting a plot that will encompass all the back stage of a city, what makes it work. Would it be a chase? What takes you to all these different urban places?

Fritz Lang

The chauffeured limousine—supplied by courtesy of Universal Pictures—sweeps past some of the world's most opulent private homes, lush and handsome in the Californian afternoon sun, depositing us finally at Fritz Lang's house atop Summit Ridge Drive, beside a canyon so redolent of the Australian bush that—apart from the built-up surroundings—we might almost be in New South Wales. At the door to greet us is Lily Latté, the director's devoted secretary, who has been with him for more than thirty years. Possessor of an agreeable sardonic sense of humour, she promptly conducts us to the living-room where Lang, a barrel-chested septuagenarian dressed in a casual open-necked sports shirt and slacks, makes us run through our proposed list of questions prior to the actual taping, which occurs to the accompaniment of full-throated outdoor birdsong. His presence is awesome: here is someone who has seen and experienced it all, Berlin's Golden Age in the twenties and Hollywood's in the thirties and forties; and their passing has not left him embittered—as it well might—but serene and detached, contemplating their folly and grandeur with a super-sophistication that manifests itself in a simplicity and directness quite devoid of affectation or pretence. "The last of the dinosaurs" is how he half-mockingly describes himself, and the image is apt: for giants such as Fritz Lang have long vanished from the motion picture scene, and we shall probably never see his like again.

By birth I am Austrian, not German. But I liked pre-Hitler Germany very much and I liked the German language, so I was very hurt that such a thing as Nazism could happen. When, in 1933, the then Minister of Propaganda, Joseph Goebbels, offered me the leadership of the German film industry, I left the country that same evening and did not return until 1958, on my way back from India.

From that moment I never spoke German again. I spent nine months in Paris and made a film there for French Fox from Ferenc Molnar's play *Liliom*, starring Charles Boyer.

Then David O. Selznick brought me over to the United States on an MGM contract. He was on a talent-hunting European trip, and in those days it was the fashion for Hollywood producers or studio-heads visiting Europe to come back with some—I say it in all humility—famous man. That's how Selznick found me.

I'm quite sure now that I made many initial mistakes here and I know what they were. I spent a whole year at MGM without being given a picture, and when the year was up they said, "Goodbye, Mr Lang."

That wasn't unique. There was a very famous story about a writer—I forget his name—under contract to the studio head, Irving Thalberg. The writer was eager to work, but Thalberg never summoned him. Every time he tried to see Thalberg the latter was always too busy and said he'd call. However, the writer still drew his weekly cheque. This went on for months, until the writer finally said, "To hell with this, to hell with the cheque", and, locking the door of his office, he went to Europe for three months without telling anyone. At the end of that time, his conscience made him come back, and under his door he found all his weekly cheques for the previous three months: when Thalberg did get around to calling him a couple of days later, no one knew he had ever been away!

During some of the time that no pictures were offering, I lived with the Navajo Indians on their reservation, meeting traders and sharing their existence. That was an extremely interesting experience. I did it because I'd always been interested in the Red Indians and wanted to know as much about this country as possible. At the same time I acquired my lousy English by reading American newspapers and, most of all, by reading funny papers.

Eventually I approached Louis B. Mayer's right-hand man, Eddie Mannix, saying, "Look, Eddie, you can't do this to me. I came here willing to work and with a considerable European reputation. If I'm not given anything to do, my reputation will suffer." Eddie Mannix realized I had a genuine grievance, and that's how I came to do my first American film, *Fury*.

Fury was a film based upon a three-page or four-page long story by the writer, Norman Krasna. He and I spent the time and worked as long as we wanted to on the script, and when it was finished I had ample time to prepare the picture. Later, conditions were not quite so favourable; schedules gradually became tighter, much more so than they had been at UFA in Germany. For example, I shot a silent film called *Spionen* (*Spies*) in about a hundred days, while here I've never had more than forty-two or forty-five days in which to shoot a film.

I found the whole procedure of shooting a picture quite different from Europe. In Europe, for instance, I didn't have to halt filming after five hours so that extras or the crew could eat. I'd dismiss, say, *half* the crew, and the cameraman and I would continue working in the studio with a sandwich or something; then, when the half-crew came back from their meal, we'd send out the other half. Naturally, I made lots of mistakes here in the beginning, and learned how to do things the hard way.

Louis B. Mayer interfered only once on *Fury*, and for a very peculiar reason. In the picture I had a scene showing a group of Negroes—an old man, a very beautiful buxom girl, and a young Negro with two children—sitting in a dilapidated Ford car in the South listening on the radio to a transcription of a lynching trial. As the state attorney spoke about the high incidence of lynchings in the U.S. each year, I had the old Negro just nod his head silently without a word. Mayer had this scene, and others like it, removed because at that time I think even he was convinced that Negroes should be shown only as bootblacks, or carhops, or menials of some description. Otherwise I was allowed complete freedom.

The only other time I struck the Negro problem in one of my films was in a picture I don't particularly like: *The House by the River*, with Louis Hayward. It opens on a very hot summer day. Hayward's wife is out of town, and on the staircase of his house he encounters a coloured maid, just coming out of the bath. He tries to kiss her and she fights him. During their fight—which is quite friendly, not sexy or anything, almost joking—he looks out of a big french window and sees a female neighbour, a woman who likes to chat and gossip. He's so afraid that she might talk about his attempt to kiss the girl—who's yelling "Leave me alone!" etc.—that he puts his hand over her mouth. She struggles and he struggles and finally he strangles her. The Hays Office would not permit me to make this a coloured girl; she had to be white.

After I finished *Fury*, nobody at MGM believed that it was any good. A reporter, who has since died, asked them one day: "What kind of a picture are you previewing today?" "Oh," they said, "a lousy picture. Don't watch it, it is by that German son of a bitch, Lang." But he knew of my European reputation and insisted on seeing it. And, contrary to the expectations of the people at MGM, the picture turned out a tremendous success. I received national prizes for it, but wasn't given another job at MGM for nearly twenty years.

My next assignment after *Fury* was *You Only Live Once* with the independent producer, Walter Wanger. The script, based on a story by Gene Towne and remotely suggested by the exploits of Bonnie Parker and Clyde Barrow, was almost finished, but I worked on it as I'd been used to doing in Europe. I think a director should always work on a script. I knew I would have Henry Fonda, who'd recently made a very successful motion-picture début, as the leading man, and for his co-star I brought over Sylvia Sidney, whom I'd used in *Fury*. The other parts were filled by General Casting.

I think there is one thread running through all my pictures: the fight against Destiny, or Fate, or whatever you want to call it; this has maybe something to do with my so-called philosophy of life. In *You Only Live Once*, it is the fight of a three-time loser against something which is stronger than he is.

In those days, there were still certain strange taboos in the moive industry. For example, I wanted to have a kind of ironic touch when Fonda and Sidney flee from the law and she goes and buys him some cigarettes, which ultimately provide the means for his betrayal. I wanted her to buy Lucky Strike cigarettes to stress the irony of the bad luck they bring him. But that was forbidden because it constituted advertising.[1]

---

[1] The situation has since altered radically the other way. (Authors' Note.)

I can't explain why I used the sound of bull-frogs' croaking over one of the love scenes in *You Only Live Once*, any more than I can explain the use of rain against the window in a similar scene in *Fury*. There are certain things you cannot explain. Very often people ask me, "How did you do it?" or, "Why did you do it?" Well, those things make a director. It is a little more than instinct, it is something you cannot analyse but which you know will "hit".

You Only Live Once was a success. But Walter Wanger had prominently displayed in his office a portrait of Mussolini. Now if I am anything I am an anti-Fascist, and I didn't like the whole setup. Meanwhile, in New York, I'd become friends with Katharine ("Kit") Cornell, then the first lady of the American stage. Despite my friends' warnings not to write anything for her because she would never consent to make a picture—and she never did—I still went ahead and wrote a long, unfilmed scenario for her; I was very green and inexperienced in American ways. It was a panoramic story, stretching from the First World War almost till 1936; I've forgotten the details.

Simultaneously, I met a man who had a lot of influence at Paramount. Afterwards he went into politics and became, I think, U.S. ambassador to Spain. He, Kit and I were very close and at his suggestion I went to Paramount to produce and direct just one film, *You and Me*.

I don't think *You and Me* is a good picture. It was—I think deservedly—my first real flop. I made it probably a little under the influence of my friend Bertolt Brecht, who had created a style in the theatre which he called *Lehrstück*, meaning a play that teaches you something. And I wanted to make a didactic picture teaching the audience that crime doesn't pay—which is a lie, because crime pays very well. The message was spelled out at the end by Sylvia Sidney on a blackboard to a classroom of crooks.

Kurt Weill had nothing to do just then. You may think whatever you like of him—some people said he could only write in one key—but he was good. He and I worked together, and he composed introductory music for certain sequences. For one scene, in which a bunch of crooks sit together around a table on Christmas Eve and indulge a sentimental nostalgia for prison—which is, of course, stupid—I wanted to have not music but only sound effects: people hitting the table, or one glass against another, etc.

But then Weill left me in the lurch by going to New York where he had an offer to work with the Spewacks. The music score for *You and Me* was finished by Boris Morros, a Russian who was then the head of Paramount's music department, and as a result it was no longer truly Kurt Weill.

For a while, after finishing *You and Me* I was out of work. Then a producer at Twentieth Century-Fox, the late Kenneth Macgowan, offered me a picture called *The Return of Frank James,* a sequel to the Tyrone Power vehicle, *Jesse James.* That was the first of my three Westerns, the other two being *Western Union* and *Rancho Notorious,* and I thoroughly enjoyed doing it.

I found some new locations for it which no one had ever used before; they were north from here, near the Sierra Nevada. The same thing happened on *Western Union,* for which I found in Utah a very isolated spot—since used often by movie companies—where there were *real* red and blue mountains. *Frank James* was my first colour picture, which made it an additionally enjoyable experience, and Fox's technical facilities were really wonderful.

That was the great difference between Europe and America: Hollywood's mechanical superiority. In Europe, for example, we didn't know what a crane was. We had quite different lights. I remember that on "*M*" I wanted to have a camera follow someone down a staircase, but we had no way of doing it. So we took a chassis—four wheels with ball-bearings—and in front of it we put a very long two-by-four, and at the end of the two-by-four we put the camera, and that was our crane.

Most of *Frank James* was imaginary, not historical, except for certain minor things like a contemporary song about the James brothers and how Jesse was killed. My contribution extended also to the script, although in a minor capacity; for *Western Union* I wrote much more. That was based on a Zane Grey novel which Darrel F. Zanuck had bought, but we practically ignored the book.

The film, in fact, was almost entirely imaginary and fictitious, not based on actual episodes at all—although it purported to deal with the laying of telegraph-wires from Omaha to Salt Lake City in the eighteen-sixties. We depicted the engineer, for instance, as a married man with children, whereas he was really a bachelor.

The only true incident we used was when the linesmen went down into nearby valleys looking for timber for their wire-posts after some buffaloes, plagued by itchy ticks, had rubbed themselves against the existing posts and dislodged them.

I shot *Western Union* in two months—longer than it took them to lay the actual line—and after its release I received a letter from the Old Timers' Club of Flagstaff, Arizona, saying: "We have never before seen the old West more accurately depicted in a motion picture than in your *Western Union*. How is this possible for a foreign-born director?"

While I was naturally tickled pink by this letter, it was based on a misconception, on these old peoples' idealization of the West as reflected in the film. The real West was certainly quite different, as I knew from stories which had been told me and from certain things I'd seen.

Zanuck had liked *The Return of Frank James* so much that, when John Ford turned down a script, it was offered to me through the producer of *Frank James,* Kenneth Macgowan. I read it, had some more work done on it, and then made it as *Man Hunt;* it was based by the screenwriter Dudley Nichols on Geoffrey Household's novel *Rogue Male.* That was my first picture with Joan Bennett.

I made it deliberately "Germanic" in style, which was rather funny because this was just before America entered World War II, and Zanuck had told me, "Fritz, don't show too many swastikas; we don't like them in this country." But you cannot make an anti-Nazi picture—and for me it was primarily an anti-Nazi picture—without showing swastikas. So I shot it the way I wanted it, only to have many things changed by the studio. The scene showing Hitler at Berchtesgaden was done with an actor, and a mask over the camera lens to simulate a telescope.

I then became interested in doing *Confirm or Deny* because the original script incorporated reports we'd heard about Hitler's attempt to cross the Channel to England. But the final script eliminated all that and consequently it didn't interest me much any more.

I also wanted it to contain echoes of my last German picture, *The Last Will of Dr Mabuse,* which I'd used as a political weapon against the Nazis. In *The Last Will of Dr*

Mabuse, I'd put all the Nazi slogans and catchcries into the mouth of an insane criminal. The Nazis said for example: "We must destroy the average citizen's self-created belief in the authorities, and when everything has broken down we will build on the ruins of the old order our Thousand-Year Reich." So I had my insane criminal propose a "Thousand-Year Era of Crime" as a mockery of this doctrine.

In *Confirm or Deny* I wanted to do something similar but I couldn't convince Zanuck or anybody, and I thought the whole thing as the studio envisaged it was very phony. Fortunately, after I'd been shooting the picture for about four or five days I had a gall-bladder attack. Now, contrary to European practice, you cannot change an actor in Hollywood because he's already on film, it costs a lot of money to replace him and reshoot his scenes. But you can easily change the director. If a director is sick for maybe two days and he's in very good standing with the company, they might get another director as a temporary replacement to shoot certain scenes in order to save time and money.

My case was different, however. I was delighted that I was unable to shoot, and told a very good friend, who acted as a go-between between all the shooting companies and Zanuck, that my doctors had put me out of action for three or four days or a week. So when he came one day shortly after and told me that Zanuck had taken me off the picture, I couldn't have been more pleased.

My next project was to have been a musical with Rita Hayworth. I would like to have done it very much because—apart from *You and Me*—I'd never done a musical and had many new ideas about the genre which I thought extremely interesting. But Zanuck, who liked my work very much, said, "Fritz, I have something much better for you." And he assigned me to *Moontide*, starring Jean Gabin.

Gabin hated the picture, probably with justification. I didn't like it either, but when you're under contract you often have to do things you don't like. Audiences usually have a very false notion of a director: even a director has to live, he cannot afford to be put on a lay-off.

Anyway, I started to shoot *Moontide* and was very unhappy about the whole thing. Originally it had been planned to make the film on location on the quay at San Pedro. But the war interfered: it became a strategic area, the whole vicinity was mined, and it was impossible to do the film there. So Zanuck decided to do it entirely in the studio, although it was set mostly on the high seas. They accordingly built an artificial indoor quay on the Fox lot and stuck blue backdrops all around it, and I was even less happy with the project than before.

Gabin's dissatisfaction grew, too. He was very good in other types of part, but he couldn't persuade the producer to change the script, because the producer was a tyro and insisted on shooting the script Zanuck had handed him. Then something personal occurred between Gabin and me and he told Zanuck he could no longer work with me. I was very happy indeed when Zanuck then took me off the picture.

I'd no sooner read about the assassination of Reinhard Heydrich, the Nazi *Gauleiter* of Czechoslovakia in World War II, than I immediately thought it would make a great picture. At that time the German playwright, Bertolt Brecht, was living in America. I liked him very much—he was never a Communist Party member, incidentally—and was very glad to have been instrumental in bringing him over here by putting up certain guarantees and complying with other formalities, the details of which I've forgotten.

I used to meet him quite frequently, and when I put up to him the idea of working on a picture about the assassination of Heydrich, he readily agreed. It was such an obvious motion-picture theme that we had a story outline written within a day, and shortly afterwards I concluded a deal with an independent outfit to make the film.

However, we had a problem with Brecht, who didn't speak English at all and wanted to write his contribution in German, because he was, after all, a professional German writer. He'd always written in German wherever he was—in Denmark, France or the U.S.—and always looked forward to the time when he could go back to Germany. I, on the other hand, *never* wanted to go back; besides, I had meantime become an American citizen.

I felt his attitude was perfectly justifiable and so we found a bilingual collaborator for him. But to my distress he quarrelled with this man, who claimed sole screenwriting credit for himself. The whole matter came up for arbitration before the Screen Writers Guild, and at the hearing—attended by both Brecht and his rival—the composer Hanns Eisler and I appeared as witnesses for Brecht.

Despite our testimony, they withheld screenplay credit from him, and for a very peculiar reason. "Mr Brecht" they said, "is going back to Europe eventually and thus doesn't need a screen credit, whereas the other writer does need credit."

In the circumstances the most I could do for Brecht was to give him joint credit with myself for the story idea and its construction. I think it was all rather unfair to him, because the picture contained certain scenes which no one but Brecht could have written.

For example, there was a scene in which the Czech professor, played by Walter Brennan, instructed his daughter in the ways of clandestine anti-Nazi resistance, drawing on examples illustrated by letters of the alphabet; and when he came to the letter "G" he declared: "And this stands for Gestapo!" Another scene involved the professor, visited in a Gestapo prison by his daughter, dictating a last letter to his son for her to memorize. Both these scenes were so typical of Brecht, as indeed was the whole film, its entire construction.

I was extremely pleased with the performance of Hans von Twardowski as Heydrich. I'd known him in Germany—he'd acted in a picture of mine called *Spies*—and he was unemployed here at the time. I was less happy about the casting of the girl,[1] but I couldn't help that, despite the fact that I fought as hard as I could over it with the independent producer who wanted her in the picture.

Alexander Granach I loved; he was my choice; and Brennan's unorthodox casting—he usually played cowboy types and deputies and that kind of thing—was my doing, too. In my opinion, he was extremely good as the Czech professor.

I shot the film in, I think, the former Chaplin studio, where I built one or two street corners in an attempt to reproduce Prague. By some lucky accident, I managed to get hold of actual shots of the city—I remember particularly a clock with mechanical figures walking around it as it struck the hour, a death's-head skeleton, and others—and, by cutting these into the picture, I gave it great authenticity.

Although I don't know Graham Greene personally, he is one of my favourite writers, and I wanted very much to make a film from his "entertainment" novel, *The Ministry*

[1] Anna Lee.

of Fear. Accordingly, I instructed my agent to try to buy it for me, but he declared it was impossible because Paramount, who were also interested in the book, were outbidding us.

Then I went to New York, and one day received a cable from my agent containing an offer to make *The Ministry of Fear* for Paramount. I jumped at it, but made a big mistake by not specifying in my contract that I wanted to be able to work on the script; I took it for granted, after all the years I'd been accustomed to working on scripts, that my agent would have seen to it that the contract contained some such clause.

When I came back here, I found someone in charge of the film who'd never made a picture before and who'd been a trombone player in a band or something. On top of that, I was handed a script which had practically none of the quality of the Graham Greene book.

When I wanted to have changes made in it, the writer resented it deeply. Then, when I wanted to step out of the project, my agent told me I was contractually obliged to complete it. So I finished the picture to the best of my ability.

While I don't care for *The Ministry of Fear* as a whole, there are still some things in it that I like: the séance, for instance, in which Hillary Brooke was very good, and the performances of Marjorie Reynolds and Dan Duryea. He was excellent, I thought, in the scissor-stabbing scene, which was my own invention and not in the book. I liked, too, the performance of the English actor Percy Waram as the police inspector.

The script for my next film, *The Woman in the Window,* was written by Nunnally Johnson and based on a story by J. H. Wallis called *Once off Guard.* They changed the title because they thought the word "guard" sounded too much like "God".

I had known Nunnally since the days we both worked at Twentieth Century-Fox in the early nineteen-forties. We didn't get along too well then because he had notions of becoming a director himself, and wrote articles attacking other directors, which he was later forced to retract.

However, I liked the script for *The Woman in the Window* very much. There was only one thing wrong with it: all the male parts in it were written for old men, not only Edward G. Robinson's and the man who kept Joan Bennett, but also the part ultimately played by Dan

Duryea. I'd liked Duryea's handling of the scene with the scissors in *The Ministry of Fear* so much that I was able to persuade the studio to let me bring him in; that was the only way I could introduce someone relatively youthful into the male cast.

Various things appealed to me in the story, but I took the liberty of changing the ending with such a corny old trick that it seemed almost new: I had the whole thing turn out to be a dream. I did it by having the main characters in the story revealed as employees of the club—the hat-check man, the porter, etc.—in which Robinson falls asleep. Having won the fight about Duryea, I had little difficulty in convincing the studio about this also.

"Look," I argued, "the whole story is not so heavy and serious that you can afford to have three deaths. Your audience will say, 'So what?' Robinson kills one man in self-defence with a pair of scissors, Duryea is killed"—I think—"by the police, and Robinson commits suicide. If the picture ends there it will be an anti-climax."

In the opening scene we'd had Eddie Robinson contemplating a portrait of a girl in a shop-window near his club. Then a girl strongly resembling the one in the portrait accosts him; he goes home intending to sleep with her, and the story unfolds from there.

At the end of the picture, after we've revealed that everything is a dream, and Robinson has seen Duryea as the club's hat-check boy and the murdered man as the porter, he contemplates the portrait again; and suddenly another girl, mirrored in the window-pane, materializes and asks him. "You wanna come with me?" Robinson takes one look at her and runs away exclaiming, "No!"

Thus I was able to end the film with a laugh. That, coupled with the feeling of relief engendered in the audience by the revelation that it was all a dream, was a major reason, I think, for the success of *The Woman in the Window*. Both these things were strokes of luck for which I was not one hundred per cent responsible.

Some reviewers attacked the "dream" ending, but that didn't worry me. I don't care about reviews, and I think my reasons are valid ones. Motion pictures are and have been the content of my life, everything. You conceive a picture, you write it yourself or help to write it; that is the initial creative process. Then comes the actual direction, in which my crew and I work for months, very seriously, doing the best we can; that is the second stage of creation. Finally comes the cutting process, in which I always have the main say; that's the third time you create something.

At last you give the finished picture to the audience and along comes a reviewer who has to meet a morning edition dead-line. In addition, perhaps his wife is betraying him or maybe he has haemorrhoids or something. In any case he cannot write an honest review and, good or bad, favourable or unfavourable, I cannot accept it. That's why I don't give a damn about reviews.

After I'd done *The Woman in the Window*, David Selznick wanted me to make a picture for him to star Ingrid Bergman and to be written by Dore Schary, later head of production at MGM. I signed a contract with David, to make this picture, and we started to write it. But—as I found out later—Ingrid Bergman was fed up at that time and didn't want to make any more films here, especially not with David Selznick. So the whole thing came to nothing.

When that happened, Selznick wanted to pay me out for less than the amount specified in my contract. I protested, but my lawyer—a wonderful guy—urged me to make a generous gesture in the hope of winning Selznick around. "What kind of a gesture?" I asked. "Tell Selznick," he advised, "that you don't want anything at all."

I told Selznick that, whereupon he just said, "Thank you very much", and I didn't get a penny compensation for the entire four weeks I'd worked for him.

Meanwhile I had created my own company, Diana Productions, in partnership with Joan Bennett and others. I owned fifty-one per cent, she owned twenty-five per cent, and the rest was split up among various people. Walter Wanger was not one of them; he was retained under contract at $40,000 per picture.

In those days I worked a lot with the writer Dudley Nichols, whom I liked very much. (He's dead now—I'm the last of the dinosaurs.) I'd heard that Paramount, on the recommendation of Ernst Lubitsch, had bought the rights to the old Jean Renoir picture *La Chienne*, which I remembered having seen in 1932, and that no one knew what to do with the property.

I discussed it with Nichols, and we bought it very cheaply from Paramount. My idea was to transpose the story from Paris into a kind of similar American *milieu*, retaining the basic situation of the novel by Georges de la

Fouchardière. I wanted to set it in Greenwich Village in New York, and that's exactly what Dudley Nichols and I did, retitling it *Scarlet Street*.

Neither of us looked at the Renoir film again; not a single scene was copied, and in that sense it was really one hundred per cent Dudley Nichols's creation.

We devised a very unorthodox downbeat ending for the film, allowing Edward G. Robinson to evade legal punishment for murder. Now, a director is something very peculiar. He has a nose for something, he smells something; I cannot explain it otherwise. He's not bound by laws such as "upbeat endings are mandatory". If you believe in what you are doing, the audience will never let you down. I found that out long ago in Germany, when the audience sat on its hands in response to flashy display sequences I'd inserted just for effect. But that will never happen if you do something honestly, something in which you strongly believe.

And I did believe strongly in the ending for *Scarlet Street*, which occasioned my second fight with the Hays Office. My first one was over the ending of *Hangmen also Die*, when Hays had said to me. "You want me to approve a film in which every Czech is—by implication—shown as a liar?"

"What would you do," I retorted, "if you were living under Nazi occupation?"

I had to give in finally on *Hangmen also Die*, and now I clashed with him for the second time on *Scarlet Street*. Arguing with Hays's chief *aide*, Joseph Breen, I said: "Look, we're both Catholics. By being permitted to live, the Robinson character in *Scarlet Street* goes through hell. That's a much greater punishment than being imprisoned for homicide. After all, it was not a premeditated murder, it was a crime of passion. What if he does spend the rest of his life in gaol—so what? The greater punishment is surely to have him go legally free, his soul burdened by the knowledge of his deed, his mind constantly echoing with the words of the woman he loved proclaiming *her* love for the man he'd wrongly sent to death in his place ..." And I won my point.

In a certain sense this man, played by Robinson, was doomed from the start. It was yet another struggle against destiny, against Fate. The man, Christopher Cross, a humble clerk, tries to escape from himself and becomes a painter, like Henri Rousseau (*Le Douanier*) in Paris. The paintings in the film were done by a dear late friend of mine, a man called Decker. I discussed the effect I wanted with him: it was to be a kind of primitive style, a little *bourgeois,* but still with the qualities of the French painter Rousseau.

Decker was a very peculiar man. "I can paint like any other painter," he would complain, "but I still haven't found my own style." He was unquestionably an alcoholic, and the last time I saw him was with my secretary Miss Latté when he was in the Cedars of Lebanon Hospital suffering from cirrhosis of the liver. They'd given him about thirty-six blood transfusions, which didn't help at all. It was maybe twelve hours before he died. We talked, and I thought he could be saved, but he was past saving.

Then something very strange happened at the last memorial rites in his studio. In it was a framed painting of perhaps his best friend, John Barrymore. If I remember rightly, it showed Barrymore on his death-bed, and it always stood on a big easel. The room was very crowded and everybody present can testify to the truth of what I'm about to relate.

The last speaker had alluded to the dead man's friends, saying finally: "And now he has gone where he will rejoin his dear friend, John Barrymore." And at that moment— *crash!*—the picture of Barrymore fell from the easel onto the floor. I'll never forget it.

I received a lot of money from Warner Brothers for making *Cloak and Dagger* the following year, but that's not why I made it. I made it for one reason only, and that reason was nullified by studio cutting.

The picture ends now with Gary Cooper saving the professor, played by Vladimir Sokoloff, and boarding an aeroplane back to the U.S. But the original script was different. In it the professor is a sick man unable to walk; they have to help him escape, and he dies of a heart attack. The American and English secret service people, anxious to discover German plans, find a snapshot of the professor and his daughter in the dead man's pocket, and in the background they notice a certain peculiarly-formed mountain in Bavaria. The next thing we see is hundreds and hundreds of parachutists dropping down on what was called during the war Hitler's "Last Redoubt" in the Bavarian Alps, and among them is the American physicist, played by Gary Cooper.

Cooper's part was based on the late J. Robert Oppen-heimer, whom I had met and who had given me a certain insight into the experiments at Los Alamos and the first atom bomb.

Anyhow, Cooper and his fellow-parachutists come across camouflaged highways and big barbed-wire barri-ers, but not a single shot is fired, every pillbox is empty. Trained soldiers among them test the wire and find it is not charged with electricity. They keep going and finally come to a tremendous cave in a mountain. Walking in, they discover on the first floor traces on the ground of enormous machines that have recently been removed.

One of the generals in the party then remarks that they are probably too late, that those formerly in charge of the establishment are doubtless now in South America or somewhere like that. At that moment a sergeant enters announcing that on the second lower level they'd found— and this was historically correct—the bodies of sixty thou-sand dead slave workers. And that was the reason I made the picture.

Gary Cooper walks out of the cave knowing Germany is beaten, and outside is a paratrooper sitting in high grass and chewing on a stalk.

"Nice weather, isn't it, professor?" he asks. And Gary Cooper says, "Yes", adding: "This is the Year One of the atomic age, and God help us Americans if we think we can keep the secret of the atomic bomb for ourselves." End of film.

All that was cut out by Warner Brothers. Don't ask me why. The producer was Harry Warner's son-in-law and he offered no explanation. I couldn't do anything about it.

The Secret Beyond the Door was a very unfortunate adventure, made for my own company, Diana Produc-tions, immediately after *Cloak and Dagger*. If one thing goes wrong with a project, then everything goes wrong; and this one went wrong from the beginning.

I don't know whose fault it all was; probably much of it was mine. The cameraman was very bad, Joan Bennett wanted to divorce her husband—lots of things like that went wrong. The basic idea—the bodies in the various rooms—was good, but our solution, which involved talk-ing someone into a radical change of outlook, was too glib, too slick. It would be very nice if a mentally dis-turbed patient could talk with a psychiatrist for two hours and then be cured; but such things cannot be done so quickly. And that was a great mistake in this picture; besides, I never really wanted to do it anyway.

During the war Darryl F. Zanuck had wanted to make a film set in the Caribbean, but the picture never eventuated. Now, five years after the end of the war, he decided to do it in the Pacific instead. He was on excellent terms with the Filipino representative in the Senate or House of Representatives—I forget which—and so I headed a unit sent out to the Philippines to make *I Shall Return* (called in some parts of the world *American Guerrilla in the Philippines*).

The producer[1] was also the scriptwriter and he'd based his script on an obsolete book. Many of the things mentioned in the book no longer existed because of the war, and so we had to make considerable changes on location. We shot much of the film in Bataan with the help of the U.S. Navy: I remember the sunken battleships still reposing at the bottom of Manila harbour. It was an awkward time to be making a film because there were big clashes going on involving the Communist Hukbalahap forces.

I was very lucky in one respect, however. I was shooting some dancing scenes in the big park of a Filipino estate and needed just one or two more shots when the first downpour of the rainy season started, wetting everything. Just as everybody left off eating and drinking and laughing the sun suddenly broke through. I hastily had everything dried and got my missing shots. After that, the rain didn't bother me.

I had long wanted to make a film with Marlene Dietrich, who was a friend of mine, so when Howard Welsch, a producer at RKO, told me I could have her if I could supply a suitable script, I collaborated with an extremely good new writer, Daniel Taradash—the same man who later wrote twenty-four *From Here to Eternity* scripts for Harry Cohn—on a Western story which we called *Chuck-a-Luck*.

The original Chuck-a-Luck is a very famous game, a kind of vertical roulette played with a round turning wheel. I myself have seen it played in a Mexican border town. The story revolved around a cowboy trying to find the outlaw killer of his fiancée at a ranch called Chuck-a-Luck, and this was, I think, the first Western to use a ballad theme throughout to point up the narrative. Lewis

[1] Lamar Trotti.

Milestone had done it in a war picture[1], but mine was the first such Western. The song was a very good one, with the same title as the film: "Chuck-a-Luck."

When the picture was finished something happened about which I can smile today, although then I was furious. Howard Hughes had just bought RKO. None of us had met him. It was Christmas Eve, and in Hollywood on 24th December you officially work from 9 a.m. till 12 noon, but nobody really works. You may have certain things to shoot, and you shoot them, but after that you proceed to celebrate from one office to another, while everybody gets drunk.

So in the afternoon I went to the office of the man who ran the studio for Howard Hughes—he was also head of the Hughes Tool Company or some such thing. "Mr. Hughes liked your picture very much," he told me, "only he changed the title to *Rancho Notorious* because he thought no one would understand the meaning of *Chuck-a-Luck* in Europe."

"Is that so?" I said. "Well, I suppose they'll have no difficulty understanding *Rancho Notorious!*"

It was a stupid thing to do because the words "Chuck-a-Luck" are constantly repeated in the song, and the ranch at which the cowboy locates the killer of his fiancée was also called Chuck-a-Luck.

Howard Hughes's behaviour was altogether most peculiar. When the news came around that he'd bought RKO, all the big-shot producers who usually turned up for work at eleven o'clock or later were there at 9 a.m. awaiting the new boss, who never appeared. This went on for about a fortnight until they said, "Oh, the hell with it", and lapsed back into their old ways.

Then after several weeks Howard Hughes finally appeared. I'll never forget it. He had a large entourage and never spoke to *anyone*. He went through the whole studio, looked at every stage, every shop, and after two hours and twenty minutes all he said was, "Paint it". Then he walked out and was never seen again. I was told that he looked at the rushes of one of my subsequent RKO films, *Clash by Night,* every evening; they would mysteriously vanish from the cutting room and turn up again the following morning and no one was sure whether he had really seen them or not.

---

[1] *A Walk in the Sun.*

The collaboration with Marlene Dietrich on *Rancho Notorious* turned out less happily than I'd hoped. I had the foolish idea—foolish because it led to a lot of unpleasant fights with her—of wanting to give Marlene a new screen image. In the script I'd described the character she played as "an elderly dance-hall girl", and she came on looking younger in each scene.

She has learned, I think, very much from von Sternberg, who was a cameraman before he became a director. They had a long love affair about which I don't feel entitled to speak. You can buy von Sternberg's book, *Fun in a Chinese Laundry,* and find the lot there. She claims to have learned much from him. On *Rancho Notorious* she would suggest certain things saying von Sternberg had done it that way; but this was my picture, not his, and so I did it my way.

I'm very happy with the way my next film, *Clash by Night,* turned out. I was very fond of the project, and of the late Clifford Odets, author of the original stage play. It had been set on the East Coast in the early nineteen-thirties, but the producer, Jerry Wald, and the screenwriter, Norman Krasna, updated it and changed the locale to Monterey, California.

I had some wonderful actors: Bob Ryan, Paul Douglas, Barbara Stanwyck, and, of course, Marilyn Monroe. Poor Marilyn was a scared girl, scared of everything. God knows why she was so frightened. I'm quite convinced that she never wanted to die. She'd taken those damned sleeping-pills, and I was told that they found the telephone-receiver dangling from its hook, which probably meant that she wanted to call somebody for help but was too weak from the pills.

But working with Barbara Stanwyck was one of the greatest pleasures of my career. She's fantastic, unbelievable, and I liked her tremendously. When Marilyn missed her lines—which she did constantly—Barbara never said a word. I remember a particularly difficult scene between the two of them in which Barbara was hanging out some laundry and Marilyn had to say one or two lines. Although Marilyn missed her cue three or four times, all Barbara said was, "Let's try it again."

It was all rather distressing for Barbara and for us because we were all doing our best, and reporters would visit the set saying, "Who wants to talk to that old

Stanwyck dame? Who's that girl over there"—indicating Marilyn—"with the big tits?" That sort of thing made everyone very unhappy. Paul Douglas, in fact, hated Marilyn.

After finishing *Clash by Night* I suddenly stopped getting jobs. Howard Hughes's representative promised me heaven on earth but I got nothing. Wherever my agent went they said, "Yes, yes, we know Fritz Lang is a great director, but we just don't have anything that fits his special style."

Finally I discovered that I was on a blacklist, alleged to have been a Communist, which I never was; this was the height of the McCarthyist Red-baiting period here. My New York lawyer reported that some people in the American Legion had not actually accused me of subversive activities, had *not* said, "Hollywood, watch out, here is a Communist"; what they said was, "We have found Mr Lang's name on the stationery of certain pro-Communist organizations."

That could have been easily explained. One day, for example, while shooting *Scarlet Street*, I got a letter from a very famous actress asking for contributions to such-and-such an organization. I instructed my secretary to send them a hundred dollars and thought no more about it, until I suddenly found myself described as a sponsor on the letterhead of an organization later characterized as pro-Communist.

Thus my accusers, while not actually describing me as a Communist, nevertheless wanted producers to have me checked. Now you know producers: why should they check? They don't run a detective agency. It was much easier for them to say: "No more pictures for Lang—to hell with the son of a bitch."

As a result I was unemployed—in the "doghouse", as they say here—for a year and a half, until finally Harry Cohn obtained a job for me at Warner Brothers. The film was *The Blue Gardenia,* which I made in twenty days for a producer who was married to Billy Rose's sister in New York. It wasn't much, but I was very happy with Anne Baxter's performance in it. She's a very good actress.

Then I made two films at Harry Cohn's own studio, Columbia. I liked the first one, *The Big Heat,* very much. It was fun to do, shot mostly in the studio and on the Columbia ranch. Based on a story by the excellent crime-writer, William P. McGivern, it appealed to me because it combined yet another struggle against the forces of fate with a certain social criticism.

Those scenes in which Lee Marvin and Gloria Grahame have boiling coffee thrown in their faces were based on an impossibility: you cannot disfigure someone with boiling coffee, it would just heal. Alexander Scourby was very good as the crime boss, and there's a whole story about Gloria Grahame and the picture which I'd rather not discuss.

She starred also in the second picture I made under the Harry Cohn contract. It was called *Human Desire,* and was based on a very famous novel, Zola's *La Bête Humaine.* It was a great success in France, I don't know why. It certainly doesn't deserve it.

There is, as you know, vanity in every man. I did a very good job at MGM with *Fury* in 1936, but subsequently never landed another assignment there. So when, nearly twenty years after *Fury,* they offered to let me direct *Moonfleet,* I naturally said, "Yes".

In *Moonfleet* we tried to create a period film entirely in the studio; we shot everything there, even the exteriors. That was the first time I worked with CinemaScope, and I made a remark about it which has since become famous—or infamous, if you prefer. CinemaScope, I said, is a format for a funeral, or for snakes, but not for human beings: you have a closeup and on either side there's just superfluous space.

The producer, John Houseman, was very nice to begin with, approachable and friendly. Then things began to deteriorate: Stewart Granger, whom MGM had under contract, never knew his lines. We had a child actor, a little boy, who tried hard but just wasn't good enough. As a result, we fell further and further behind schedule.

I don't know what ending *you* saw, but my original ending had Granger deliberately deceiving the child in the little hut on the ocean shore, saying farewell, and then boarding the barge and sailing away. The boy stands by the window saying, "You will come back," but by then Granger is dead; we fade out as the boy stands there and waits. That was *my* ending.

Afterwards the studio substituted an ending in which Granger survives and returns to the old mansion, which is now his: does anyone care about that kind of thing?

Producers' cuts not only drastically reduced Viveca

Lindfors's part but rendered certain sequences almost unintelligible. The overturning of the coach, for instance: Granger hears the news of this diamond, disguises himself as an officer and goes to the well where the diamond is hidden; this was much more elaborate in the version I originally shot. They get the gem and flee, and then he comes back and saves the boy.

Then Granger makes a deal with the rich man played by George Sanders, and with Sanders's mistress[1]. Everybody tries to cheat each other and Granger, overcome by qualms of conscience for having wronged the kid, leaves the coach. A shooting affray follows, and as Sanders tries to stab him, Granger shoots; Sanders dies, the horses bolt, and the coach is destroyed.

Following *Moonfleet*, I made a successful picture for an independent producer, *While the City Sleeps,* a film I personally like very much. In one scene, Dana Andrews, as a crime reporter, is sitting alone, almost drunk—let's say he's tipsy—in a bar at night, when in comes Ida Lupino, a sob sister on the same paper, with instructions from her lover (George Sanders) to seduce Andrews because he wants to have Andrews on his side in an office power struggle.

She orders something fancy to drink—Pernod or something—and then takes a colour slide from her handbag and begins studying it. When Andrews asks her what she's looking at, she replies. "Oh, nothing, nothing." But you can sense that she's looking at a picture of herself naked; it was played wonderfully.

Andrews wants to see it, she won't let him, there's a bit of a struggle and the slide-viewer falls behind the bar. A bespectacled barkeeper pounces on it, takes one look at it, and registers disappointment: it's a closeup of a naked baby on a fur coat.

I thought the scene was very funny. My producer thought it stank and didn't want to have it in the picture. Now, in all my contracts I have a clause stipulating that a producer, or production company, can only cut a picture after it has been previewed. After five days, I finally persuaded the producer to allow the scene to remain in the film.

Then came the first preview. Naturally I'm sitting there sweating blood and tears, wondering how the audience

[1] Played by Joan Greenwood.

will react to my pet scene. To my great joy, they started to laugh and roar and applaud. The producer goes straight to my cutter and exclaims: "That son of a bitch Lang was right again! I'm going to preview this picture so often that I'll eventually find an audience that *doesn't* applaud the scene, and when I do, I'll cut it out." And that's the sort of thing you have to fight constantly in Hollywood.

No sooner had I finished *While the City Sleeps* than the same producer[1] offered me another picture. I agreed to do it provided I could make certain script changes. The producer promised that I could make whatever changes I liked, but owing to my agent's negligence, I had nothing to that effect in writing.

Once having signed a contract to do the film I found that I didn't in fact have the right to change anything. So I made the picture—*Beyond a Reasonable Doubt*—under duress. I hate it, but it was a great success. I don't know why.

I will tell you why I was opposed to *Beyond a Reasonable Doubt*. The story revolved around a scheme by a newspaper tycoon and his prospective son-in-law (played by Dana Andrews) to prove that circumstantial evidence is not enough to condemn someone to death.

Having already made a picture against capital punishment in *M*, I saw this as an opportunity to make another. But in the end it turns out that Andrews really has committed murder and is seeking his future father-in-law's help to escape trial. I cannot, I said, make an audience love Dana Andrews for one hour and thirty-eight minutes and then in the last two minutes reveal that he's really a son of a bitch and that the whole thing is just a joke. But thanks to my agent's mistake I was contractually bound to shoot the producer's original script.

He died soon afterwards of cancer, so he was probably already in pain, and it was a very disagreeable experience altogether. For example, he said: "Let's start with a scene showing a man being taken to the electric chair."

I knew San Quentin, had visited the death-chamber there, and had visited Sing Sing during the making of *Scarlet Street*. "Fine," I said. "Showing the reality of capital punishment is a very effective argument against it."

"Please make it as realistic as possible," the producer added.

[1] Bert E. Friedlob.

My argument against capital punishment is that the law forces some other man to commit murder. If he throws a switch or administers poison pills, he is responsible for the death of somebody else; so the State, trying to punish a murderer, makes another man commit murder. That is my main reason.

I accordingly shot the scene in question the way I myself had seen it: how they drag the man in, how he struggles and doesn't want to go, etc. It was very realistic. Now, every Hollywood set harbours a front-office spy, and the one on this particular set, who didn't know that I had talked the scene over very carefully with the producer, ran up to the front office crying that I was shooting something monstrous, horrible.

Front office calls the producer and what does the producer do? He denies everything, comes down to the set, and shouts at me: "How dare you shoot such stuff?" You have to have a scapegoat and the scapegoat is usually the director.

No wonder I was unhappy with the finished picture; and yet the producer still approached me with further offers, saying, "Let bygones be bygones." But by then—this was 1957 or 1958—I was really fed up with Hollywood. I'd seen too many people die here of heart attacks.

"I don't want to make any more films here," I told the man; "I don't want to die of a heart attack."

Then something very strange happened: I was sitting in Washington—where I had gone to spend the Christmas-New Year period—with a woman I loved very much when I suddenly received a telegram from my secretary announcing that a German producer, Arthur Brauner, wanted me to direct a remake of *The Indian Tomb*, a very successful German silent picture of the early nineteen-twenties.

The Indian Tomb was based on a book written by my former wife, Thea von Harbou, in 1920. It had been bought by a German producer named Joe May, and I was originally supposed to direct it. Mrs von Harbou and I—we were married later—collaborated on the script, which followed the then current fashion of envisioning a two-part film, each part of feature length and designed to be shown on successive evenings.

We gave the finished script to Joe May to read; with him were his wife, the silent star Mia May, who still lives here in Los Angeles (he's dead), and his daughter. In silent-films scripts each scene occupied a single page, the advantage being that you could interchange them, you didn't write the thing consecutively; you could interpolate new and/or better ideas as you went along.

Anyhow, the May family read each page in turn and were wildly enthusiastic. "Fantastic!" they chorused. "The greatest script we've ever read!" Mrs von Harbou and I naturally went home elated.

Three days later she brought me sad news. "Fritz," she said, "you cannot make the picture." When I asked why, she told me that Joe May—despite his name he wasn't English; he was a Viennese called Otto Mandl, and that was just his professional name—had declared he was unable to obtain for a young director, such as I then was, the amount of money necessary to make a big film like *The Indian Tomb*.

The fact was that he wanted it for himself. The result, a two-part film starring Conrad Veidt, was very successful indeed.

So when, nearly forty years later, I received Brauner's offer to make a new version of something I'd begun in the twenties, it was like the closing of a mystic circle, an illustration of the maxim that "everything comes to him who waits".

I got Brauner's telegram—which instructed me to be at a certain place in Europe on 2nd January 1958—on 30th December 1957. Despite the fact that my passport was in the bank in Los Angeles and it pained me to leave the girl I loved in Washington, I cabled back that I would be there as soon as I could.

I left Washington for Los Angeles on New Year's Day, wound up my affairs, took out my passport on 2nd January, left on the 3rd, and on the 4th reported at the designated place, a little town in Northern Austria.

On reading the two horrible scripts they gave me, I called up my agency's European representative and announced: "This is ridiculous; I'd better go back. I can't do these two stinkers."

She urged me to calm down and cool off, and eventually they agreed to let me rewrite the scripts in whatever way I chose. When that happened, I stayed on and made both pictures, each running 105 minutes, and bringing the pair of them in at a total cost of $1,050,000, including the producer's phony overhead.

I certainly didn't expect my version of *The Indian Tomb* to be a great artistic achievement, but I wanted to prove to the producers here in Hollywood that a picture which would cost here some eight or nine million dollars could be made cheaply in Europe and still show a large profit. That way I hoped ultimately to persuade them to let me do whatever I wanted.

That turned out to be a fallacious idea. Although the film made a lot of money in Europe, it failed here because the American distributors reduced the two feature-length parts to a composite ninety minutes and added a badly dubbed English-language soundtrack. When I saw it, I was nearly sick.

After that I did another Dr Mabuse picture[1] for the same producer and, although it was a great success, I would rather not have made it. It's impossible to work properly in postwar Germany, just impossible.

Besides, I'm not liked there today. They don't want to hear about the "Golden Twenties". Maybe it's because they can't make any good pictures themselves. There are many reasons for this, into which I don't want to go now— it's none of my business, anyway. I'm told that lately there've been one or two good ones, but one of them was made by a Swiss, and the other by a young man who's spent his whole life in France.

I am, however, greatly liked in Paris. Godard constantly maintains he has learned a lot from my films. When I appeared (as myself) in his movie version of Alberto Moravia's novel, *A Ghost at Noon*,[2] I found that he improvised all the time. I will never forget a four-page letter to the producer which he'd interpolated in the script in place of a scene in which Brigitte Bardot is supposed to take a bath.

"Dear Mr Producer," it said in effect, "I cannot tell you how this scene will play, what the characters will say, or even what chairs they'll be sitting in . . .". I could hardly believe my eyes, accustomed as I was to the American method of strict adherence to a given shooting-script.

Another instance of Godard's penchant for improvisation occurred in a scene in which a very good actor, Michel Piccoli, and I are walking down a mountain path leading

---

[1] *The Thousand Eyes of Dr Mabuse.*
[2] *Le Mépris (Contempt).*

to the ocean. He played Bardot's cuckolded husband in the picture, and we were supposed to be discussing Ulysses and the Odyssey.

Both Godard and myself felt the scene lacked something, but couldn't decide what it was. Then, as the actor and I talked of Ulysses' homecoming and how he kills all the men in his wife's house, I had an idea. "You know," I remarked, "murder is no solution." And Godard loved it. That was the way we worked.

His aesthetic is that of the *nouvelle vague*. They want to shoot everything just as it is. Let us say, for example, they wish to shoot a scene of people sitting at Chez Fouquet, one of Paris's most famous outdoor cafés. They include all the miscellaneous sounds of traffic, of people going by, of random conversations, etc.

Is it art? I spoke earlier about my use of sound. If I sit alone in a café facing the street, I notice the traffic, the girls going by, and the noises they both make. If, however, I'm sitting with a girl I love, I'm no longer conscious of these things; I see and hear only her.

I remember a scene in a *nouvelle vague* picture—I forget which one—showing two people in bed, accompanied by so much noise that I thought they were in the sleeping compartment of a train. Actually, they were in a small room and the noises all came from outside. I personally think this sort of thing is wrong.

So you must admit that I'm correct if, when shooting a similar scene, I leave out extraneous noises or dub them down. My way of shooting is through disciplined selection. I'm therefore absolutely opposed in principle to what the *nouvelle vague* does. I think it is the death of art, which is primarily selection.

But today's youth—and I will always defend youth—have different ideas about art. The older and younger generations have never understood each other. Perhaps the younger people today are creating genuine new forms; I really don't know.

Take Antonioni. I never liked his pictures—until *Blow-up*—because they all seemed negative; they all seemed to be saying, "You can't help it, life is like that." I think such sentiments are very dangerous to put before today's young people who are struggling to find themselves, who are faced with a world which they haven't created but have inherited from older generations and which is not a very pleasant place for them to be in.

I liked *Blowup* very much indeed because I thought I detected in it—for the first time in Antonioni's films—something which is almost positive.

Rouben Mamoulian

In the formal, leafy streets of Beverly Hills, a low-lying white house, gleaming yet discreet; a building of the kind that in the late thirties was felt to be as ultra-modern as Shangri-La. Inside, it seems much larger, with spacious rooms opening on to a garden filled with massed dark green bushes and conifers. The walls are decorated with paintings of flowers, portraits by Mamoulian's wife; and a dining-room has a large, beautifully polished period table that might have been in Blood and Sand *or* The Mark of Zorro. *On either side of the fireplace are china cats, like those which figured in* City Streets *to symbolize the quarrelling of two bitchy women, and we are reminded by them of the fact that cats appear as a trade-mark in all Mamoulian's films.*

A maid in a white uniform shows us in; we are early; and we wait for a long time, listening to various footsteps on the stone flags of the hall. Finally Mamoulian appears, a tall, slender, scholarly figure rather like the Harold Lloyd of the silent comedies, with round black-rimmed spectacles over mysterious stone-grey eyes. He exudes civilized ease and grace, his memory is astonishing, and, over a delicious dinner by candlelight, he reminisces fascinatingly, recalling conversations that took place as long as forty years ago. Later, in the study, this great inventor of the cinema's forms, creator for the stage of the first productions of Porgy and Bess, Oklahoma! *and* Carousel, *relaxes with cigars in a magnificently opulent setting of black and gold and crimson. Only once in a conversation that stretches from nine o'clock until well past midnight does he lose his composure, when—just as he is about to disclose for the first time the secret of the cinematic*

145

transformation of Jekyll into Hyde in his famous version of Stevenson's classic—a black cat, perched high on a bookcase, hurls itself with diabolical fury across the room, onto the tape, and snarls at it with the air of an avenging demon, like Hyde himself reincarnated.

I believe that film is primarily a graphic medium. Sound is secondary. You can have all the philosophy you like; if a film doesn't come across in graphic terms, it falls short. It is closer as a medium to painting than to the stage. And it should, to achieve greatness, be divorced from realism and naturalism. Obviously, poetry cannot be realistic; it's a lot of foolishness really. "The dawn came up like thunder" ... Absurd! But beautiful. Sculpture and painting are at their finest unreal. Film should be poetic, integrating all the components of art. And it should show the inner truth, not merely the "realistic" truth, in a stylized manner. It must also have rhythm. When I was a child, our teacher of elementary physics said: when a regiment of soldiers crosses a stone bridge, it is always ordered to break step, because if it walked in step, the power of its rhythmic vibration would destroy the bridge. It stuck in my mind that rhythm can have great power: if it can destroy, it can also build. And it can build great tension and excitement in a film.

My first professional stage production was in London in 1922, at St James's Theatre. I was twenty-four at the time. I did it in the most realistic style. It was set in Russia, and I had people chopping real wood with real axes and so on; chips flying all over the place. The reviews were good, and I was invited to America as a result, but I wasn't happy, because I realized straight away that realism has too fixed boundaries. I went to New York to work on staging productions for the American Opera Company, and for two and a half years I directed operas of every kind.

Then I directed stage shows at the George Eastman Theatre in Rochester. I integrated dialogue and singing, and it worked; one production I did was *Sister Beatrice* by Maurice Maeterlinck, and this most fully exemplified my musical ideals.

I developed these ideals in my musical *Love Me Tonight*, with Maurice Chevalier and Jeanette MacDonald, made in 1932. The whole structure is musical. I started working on the score with Rodgers and Hart before I came to the book; my idea was to tell everything through singing the words and, where this couldn't be done, through rhyming dialogue also matched to music. Plain dialogue was only used as a last resort.

In the late twenties I did *Porgy*—not the musical, but DuBose Heyward's play—with an all-Negro cast. At the time, Broadway was totally devoted to realism, and David Belasco was the king of naturalists, and Broadway's king. His sets were totally real. With *Porgy* I used a totally stylized technique, and I was on my own.

I had a scene of Catfish Row in the morning: it's waking up, and there is a mounting rhythm of household noises. A man snoring, a hammer, a woman with a broom, sharpening of knives, someone shaking up pillows, and I conducted the whole thing like a symphony: a four-four rhythm, then six-eight, then I syncopated it, and wound up with a Charleston rhythm on the full stage, with every sound fully orchestrated, as it were. The people behind the production at the Theatre Guild thought the heat had affected me, but I went ahead, and I developed the idea in *Love Me Tonight*.

After *Porgy* I did several successful plays, and I began to get offers from studios: Harry Cohn and others. Finally, Jesse L. Lasky and Walter Wanger of Paramount came to me to sign a seven-year contract; during the first three I would learn how to make motion pictures, and act as a dialogue director. This made me laugh, and I said, if I should direct dialogue only, why should I want to leave the stage? I said, "I'll sign for one picture. You'll let me go everywhere in the studio and watch. When I feel I'm ready I'll direct the whole picture." They waited twenty-four hours, and they finally said "Yes".

I started work on *Applause* from the novel by Beth Brown, and Garrett Fort wrote the script: the story of a faded chorus-dancer and her daughter, with a cast entirely new to the cinema. I watched directors shooting, among them Herbert Brenon and Jean Le Mure, I saw the cutting and the rushes, I talked to George J. Folsey, the big cameraman there, and for five weeks I learned. Everything I saw was wrong, and I decided to do the exact opposite.

The camera technique then was to shoot a film as a stage play, with ready-made dialogue. They would put two cameras on the set, and shoot two closeups and a long-shot, then cut them together: all you *could* call these films was talkies! Incredibly, it took two years for some genius to figure out that you could put a camera in a small sound-proof box; in those days they used an enormous camera blimp, a bungalow as big as half this room with a glass front. Inside were the camera operator and the director, and the terrible heat made you feel like an apple pie in an oven. If you wanted to move or pan, it was almost impossible: in effect, you had to move a house! But it didn't discourage me: I said, "We'll just have to move the house, that's all!" And they did!

Finally I began shooting, and ran into nothing but trouble. George Folsey resented me, because I was new from the stage. And the sound and wardrobe department fought me; I wanted wardrobe to make Helen Morgan look blowsy, and in large shapeless pyjamas, and she came on the set trim and natty, and in wonderful shape. I said "Impossible!" And wardrobe said: "She's a star, she has to look beautiful."

As for the soundtrack, when Helen Morgan's daughter arrives in New York, she has just seen her mother cavorting on a burlesque stage, and she's shocked, miserable and unhappy; the mother is unconscious of her daughter's feelings and she puts her to bed and sings her a "lullaby": it's her burlesque song, because she doesn't know any real lullabies. I wanted the girl to take her rosary and say her evening prayers simultaneously. This couldn't be done in those days because there was only one microphone, one channel for recording everything. The mike was somewhere in the middle, and everything had to be correctly distanced or it would sound too loud; you couldn't open a letter anywhere within six feet of a microphone or it would sound like thunder. So how could you possibly hear a loud song and a whispered prayer?

I said, "Why can't we have two microphones, one for the whisper, one for the song, and record it on two channels?" They said, "It can't be done." "Why not?" I asked.

I wanted the whole scene done in one shot, without one cut, with the camera swinging up and down with the rhythm of a lullaby. George Folsey said, "Impossible": there was, he said, no correlation between the focus-man, the marks on the floor, and the guys inside the camera booth. He wouldn't do it, although with a day's rehearsal it could easily have been done.

All this trouble was too much for me. . . . After hours

of arguments I dashed upstairs and I said to a secretary in the Paramount executive offices, "Where is everybody?" She said, "They're having a meeting. You can't come in." I stormed in anyway. Adolph Zukor was there, Jesse L. Lasky, all the big ones, and I told them that unless I was given power to get what I wanted, I'd resign. So George Folsey and the wardrobe and sound men were summoned. Folsey said: "I have the greatest respect for Mr Mamoulian as a stage director. But I've been in motion pictures all my life and what he asks me to do is impossible. I'm trying to save the company time and money."

The others also made excuses. Luckily the bosses told them they'd have to do the picture my way. It was five thirty before we had taken two takes of the scene. I had to tell Folsey where to put the lights; he wouldn't even put them up himself. I went home discouraged, worn out. Next morning when I arrived at the studio, the enormous Irish doorman, in a most resplendent uniform—he always reminded me of Emil Jannings in *The Last Laugh*—took his hat off and performed a deep oriental kind of a bow, saying, "A happy good morning to you, Mr Mamoulian", and he opened the door wide. He'd always looked down at me up to then. I was so young, so new. I said to myself, "What's going on here?"

When I got inside, my stage manager, Earl Reading, whom I'd brought with me from New York, took me aside and said, "I must tell you something. The laboratory was told to print your last night's take immediately, through the night, and to deliver it at eight in the morning. Zukor, Lasky and all the big ones came to see it, and if it had been a mess that was your last day on this picture, or at Paramount. But they are raving about it, and they have given orders to send the sequence to a Paramount sales convention at Kansas City showing next year's product. The order has gone out: "Whatever Mamoulian wants, give it to him!'"

I went on to the set and everybody was smiling. I suppose it was a little bit mean of me, but I thought, "A little dose of revenge is not out of place." It was just a mild case of Monte Cristo, I guess. Folsey, who had said, "It's never been done", now said, "Where do you want the camera today?" And I said, "Well, I think I'd like to shoot the next scene from below, so I'd like to put it three feet under the floor." Folsey said, "The studio has no basement, it stands on a slab of concrete eighteen inches thick, so we can't get below this floor." I told him, "Get electric drills. I saw Third Avenue in New York being torn up. You can tear up this thing just as easily." His men went off and brought the drills, and just before the work was about to begin I said to Folsey, "All right, forget it, that was just my revenge on you." From then on, of course, we all had a wonderful time.

We shot many exciting sequences on location in New York. At the Pennsylvania Railroad Station, for instance: a Gothic cathedral in steel, and it's a crime that it's gone. It was the first time subway scenes had been shot; and scenes on the top of skyscrapers.

Joseph Ruttenberg, who was second cameraman on the picture, would leave fifty feet blank on my orders, and the fifty feet would run on to the next scene, and this would give the illusion of a dissolve effect; we didn't have dissolves then. Every time I see Joe nowadays, he says: "Fifty feet blank!"

In the Pennsylvania Station I had a problem: shooting wasn't allowed there because the traffic would be disrupted. So I said, "I'll take the responsibility; we have to do it, and if anybody is to be arrested, let them arrest me."

We had four hundred extras, and I rehearsed them in the studio to come off a train up a narrow taxi ramp to Seventh Avenue. I said, "If the first take isn't successful I'll wave my white handkerchief. No cameras will be seen; they'll all be hidden behind pillars and posts. When I wave the handkerchief, we'll do the scene again."

Our four hundred extras were in the station among the "real" people and ten special taxi cabs among the others. The first take didn't work correctly, so I waved the handkerchief. And suddenly the whole mass of people turned around and went back into the station. And the real taxi-drivers stood there with their mouths open: four hundred people insane! And then they came back! It worked the second time; but suddenly, towards the end of the shot, a motorcycle with a sidecar roared down the ramp and a man jumped out of the sidecar, stylishly dressed, with a little black moustache. And I said to my assistant, "Who on earth is that? Get him out of there!" And he said, "That's Grover Whalen, the Chief of Police!" We all melted into the woodwork!

Helen Morgan was one of the most wonderful people I

have ever known. Very talented, very sensitive, with an intuitive flair for acting, totally dedicated to her art. The last scene when she commits suicide was very carefully rehearsed: I believe in rehearsal except where you are jumping from the third-storey window on to the pavement; then it's difficult.

There was a gala opening at the Criterion Theatre; I was being treated by Paramount as the white-headed boy by now, and the day before the opening I went to see Lasky and Zukor, Zukor said, "Please sit in my chair." And I said, "Why should I?" But I did. Zukor made a speech about what a great film I had made, saying that I "belonged" to Paramount, and he added, "My boy, I only pray that you don't get a swollen head after this. You are ours. I want you to sign a long-term contract with us, regardless of what happens to the film." Then Jesse Lasky made a speech, and I was deeply moved, and grateful.

Next day the film opened to sensational reviews, which made me highly unpopular in Hollywood. I hadn't done it there, I came from the stage; they didn't like me at all. *Applause* wasn't a box-office magnet, and I didn't hear from Paramount for several weeks. A month, two months ... I went back on the stage and did four or five plays, and then exactly a year later I got a call from Paramount. They offered me a five-year contract, and again I said I wanted a one-picture-at-a-time contract. Finally they agreed and I signed to do *City Streets*, with Gary Cooper. I had been asked to choose a subject, and I couldn't at first find anything suitable; I had met Dashiell Hammett, who was working at Paramount, and I liked him very much; I told him I was looking for ideas, and he put a suggested outline down in four pages.

Dashiell wrote a familiar gangster story, and I accepted it, deciding to treat it in an original manner. There were several murders, and I had them happen off-screen. And I wanted to use symbolism; a term that's anathema in Hollywood. In a conversation between two bitchy women, I simply showed two china cats. I decided to use music for special effect: the *Meistersinger* Overture of Wagner, for instance, at one stage. Most of the music in the studio at the time was in small labelled boxes, as in a pharmacy; fire music, moonlight music, and so on. Different bits from hackneyed themes, mostly.

I cast Guy Kibbee in his first part away from Broadway as the chief villain, and I also made Sylvia Sidney play against cliché by smiling when she was sad and crying when she was happy. The film was a big box-office and critical success.

In adapting my next picture, *Dr Jekyll and Mr Hyde*, I worked with the writers Samuel Hoffenstein and Percy Heath. Hoffenstein was a dear friend of mine; he was a poet, the author of a marvellous book of poems. *In Praise of Practically Nothing.*

Irving Pichel was originally cast as Jekyll and Hyde; I said he wasn't suitable. I wanted someone who could play Jekyll, and Pichel could only play Hyde! I chose Fredric March, and they said, "You're crazy, Fredric March is a comedian! His last picture was called *Laughter!*" I said, "He's a natural Jekyll, he's young, he's handsome, his speech is fine, and I'm sure he can play Hyde." A few days later, B. P. Schulberg, the head of the studio, called me and said grudgingly: "All right, if you're so obstinate, you can have your head, you can have Freddie March." And all that happened was that he won the Academy Award!

I wanted Miriam Hopkins to play the Cockney girl, but she wanted to play Jekyll's higher-class girl friend instead. I said to her, "What's the matter with you? Ivy's going to steal the film." Hopkins said: "She's unsympathetic; I just don't want to act her!" Finally I walked out on her and snapped: "All right, that makes it easy, I'll have no trouble finding someone to play Ivy. Half the actresses in Hollywood would give their eye teeth for the part." She called me back and gave in!

I didn't want Hyde to be a monster. Hyde is not evil, he is the primitive, the animal in us, whereas Jekyll is a cultured man, representing the intellect. Hyde is the Neanderthal man, and March's makeup was designed as such. One problem was to manage the transitions. I puzzled over it for days: could I show the transformation without cuts or mechanical dissolves? Without arrested frames? Suddenly I had an idea.

The secret of the transformation of Dr Jekyll into Mr Hyde in one continuous shot—without cuts and without rewinding the film backwards in the camera to permit the application of additional makeup—lay in the use of colour transparencies which gradually revealed more and more of the actor's makeup. As you know, a red filter will absorb red and reveal all the other colours, and a green filter will do the reverse. Working on that principle, we held graduating colour filters one by one before the camera thus allowing successive portions of March's coloured makeup to register on film. It was all rather primitive—the filters were hand-made—but it worked.

We had a problem with the sequence in which Jekyll takes a drink and is physically transformed: how do you make the audience believe it? I decided to make them feel what Jekyll is feeling. Showing subjectively his demented whirlings round his laboratory. I had the camera revolve around upon its axis, and all four walls of the set were lit completely; this had never been done on the screen. The cameraman had to be tied to the top of the camera: he had to lean down and control the focus from up there. He was as small as a jockey, luckily.

Now that took care of the image, but what about sound? Sound can pull you down terribly. To give an example: I remember a fabulous party Basil and Ouida Rathbone gave in the thirties: Rubinstein was going to play the piano in the garden. A beautiful young blonde in a lovely white dress looking like a heavenly angel was there, and when she heard Rubinstein would play, she was transported. While he was playing someone threw a biscuit to the Rathbones' dog, and the dog dashed up to the biscuit and jumped over the blonde, who yelled "Jesus Christ!" And the whole mood was shattered.

A realistic sound in a magical situation is ruinous, and similarly a realistic sound while Jekyll is being transformed would have pulled you down into the mire of naturalism. So I decided the sound had to be something special. We photographed light frequencies of varying intensity from a candle. I hit a gong and cut the impact off and ran the sound backwards, and, to give the sound a pulsing rhythm, I ran up and down a stairway while they recorded my speeded-up heartbeats. When I say my heart was in Jekyll and Hyde, I mean that literally!

After *Dr Jekyll and Mr Hyde* was completed, Ernst Lubitsch, who was a great friend of mine, and had made a series of highly successful films with Maurice Chevalier and Jeanette MacDonald, announced that he would not direct their next vehicle (I don't know the reason). They called me in and asked me to do it; they said they had no book, no theme, and I'd have to find one in a hurry because they had the two stars on five thousand dollars a week, there was no picture, and the money was mounting up. I refused, because I decided a musical needed a great deal of preparation, and they weren't prepared to give me that.

Adolph Zukor came out from New York and said to me: "We're in dire straits at Paramount. You're one of the family and we need you. Please do it!" And he started crying. Perhaps I was a little naïve then; if I saw tears today, I might be more cautious, but I fell for it. Now I was stuck; what should I do?

Nothing they had on file interested me at all. It so happened that I was on the lot and met a French playwright called Leopold Marchand, who wrote the book for *Three Waltzes*, and had collaborated with Colette: a fat man, a *bon vivant*, a terrific gastronome and gourmet, and the greatest authority on wines I have ever known.

I told Marchand I was stuck; I didn't want to do something just like Lubitsch, with comic royalty and ministers. He said, "I have an idea", and he wrote it down on one long sheet of yellow paper: a tailor in Paris falls in love with a princess who lives in a château in the south of France; he arrives to collect a debt, pretending to be an aristocrat; she falls in love with him, then discovers he's a tailor, and they get together. I liked it, and started planning.

They all thought I was crazy, but they let me do it. Hoffenstein and Heath came to me, after the playwrights Vincent Laurence and Samson Raphaelson had started work on it without success, and we worked out ideas based partly on my memories of childhood fairy tales: the idea of a song travelling from Paris through various people down to the south of France came from a story my grandmother told me, about a prince who finds a piece of embroidery blown by the wind over seven seas and seven lands, and says that whoever made it must be his wife. Finally he discovers her, and she's a princess. Instead of using the embroidery, we used the song.

All the noises of the awakening city of Paris at the beginning, based on my work for *Porgy*, I conducted with the aid of a metronome. I wanted the smoke coming out of the chimneys in "musical" puffs, and they couldn't do it. Joe Youngerman, who is now Executive Director of the Directors' Guild of America, was at that time property man on the picture. He saw me in distress, and solved the problem: I don't know how to this day.

After *Love Me Tonight*, I went on to direct Garbo in *Queen Christina* at Metro. The most famous scene in that film—which was itself the favourite movie, by the way, of both Stalin and Mussolini—was the scene in which Garbo strokes the bedroom where she has been with her lover, so that she will remember every detail. I always divide the world into two: those who like the scene and those who don't.

Garbo works intuitively, and she understood how the scene was to be played. She caught on right away. The scene was choreographed; she played it to a metronome. She had to roll over a bed, and move around the room in what was a kind of sonnet in action.

We did the best we could with John Gilbert. We didn't know who to cast. Originally I wanted John Barrymore, and he was terribly excited; he kept calling the studio from his yacht; but finally I decided he was just a trifle too old. Olivier I tested, and I decided to see if he could sustain his weight in a scene with Garbo. Would she "murder" him? Of course, Garbo hadn't done a test for years, but she had to do this one with Olivier. So I said to her, "Will you do this? I want to see if he can hold his own." We rehearsed it at great length and in full costume, and did an elaborate test, but you couldn't "see" him; he was too callow. Sir Laurence and I laugh about it to this day. He told me in London recently: "I resented it for a long time, but you were right, you were absolutely right."

Garbo would send her director off the sound-stage before she would go on with a love scene, but I told her: "This is impossible. I am on the set the whole time; nothing happens that I don't supervise, direct and witness. It's impossible to do things the way you want." She accepted that.

She couldn't accept any discussion of a scene in logical terms; either she'd got it or she hadn't. I was about to rehearse a scene in which Lewis Stone and Ian Keith were discussing something in Queen Christina's study, and Garbo walks in. It was the first scene we shot, and she told me: "I don't rehearse." I said "What?" She said, "I can't. You just tell me what to do, and shoot it. If you rehearse me I'll be no good, I'll be dull, I'll be stale."

I said, "If you're able to do the scene without preparation I'll be blissfully happy, because this is the director's dream, to get the perfect thing in one take. I'll become famous as 'One-take Mamoulian'. But I have my doubts.

So I'll make a deal with you. You do it right the first time and I'll accept it, but if not you'll rehearse." She agreed.

I rehearsed the others for an hour, she did one run-through, then she was ready for the take. At the end she asked me how I felt about it, and I said, "No good. No good at all. Nothing like what it should be." And she said, "We can't do this film then. I won't rehearse." But I reminded her of the bargain, and I said to her, "I'll print this first take. Then I'll rehearse and print that take when I'm satisfied. You'll see both, and you can go into the projection-room and tell me which you want me to use. Is that fair?" There was no way out for her. I rehearsed her for an hour and at the end, she said, "I'm no good, I'm gone," but she was actually getting better all the time.

We reached Take Eight and printed it. And then she came over to me and whispered in my ear: "Please don't print Take One." After that we rehearsed everything.

There was a scene in which she had to break into uncontrollable laughter. They said to me at the studio, "She cannot laugh." And I said, "Well, that's odd, because in life she has a very childlike infectious laugh, the laugh of a little girl." She herself told me she couldn't do it, too.

The scene is the one in which Queen Christina comes upon the carriage of the Spanish ambassador stuck in the snow. I had to get her to laugh at this. So I went to John Gilbert and Akim Tamiroff and two others and I took them aside, and said, "You know the child's game of 'making faces'?" Finally I got a combination of four faces that, so help me, a stone would have laughed at, it was so funny. I said, "When she comes up, you're under the carriage trying to free it: you look at her and hold that face." I said to Garbo, "No matter what happens go through with the scene. Go into the dialogue, and get it done." And she asked me, "What's going to happen?" I said, "Nothing so far as I know, but go ahead." She rode in and I kept the camera on her; the others were out of the frame, of course. And when she saw the four faces she threw her head back and laughed like a lark.

I didn't want to make *Song of Songs* with Dietrich any more than I had wanted to make a musical when *Love Me Tonight* came along. Dietrich had made a series of films with von Sternberg, and suddenly, for some reason, the studio decided to separate them. She wouldn't consider any director except me, so I had to do it. I said to the bosses, "What's the subject?" "Sudermann's *Song of*

Songs!" they told me. "I don't want to do that," was my reply. "It's old-fashioned, I'm not interested." I was talked into it when von Sternberg and Dietrich walked in and said that the studio wouldn't let me do another picture if I didn't do this one. So I accepted.

It was all right, but there was nothing new in it. I couldn't "open any doors" in it creatively.

As for Dietrich ... she and Garbo are opposite poles. Garbo is intuitive, she's a natural phenomenon, like a geyser, or a stream or a flower; if you touch the right spots—of course, I'm talking intellectually now!—she comes through. Dietrich is not like that, she's a tremendous trouper; no one works harder, no one is more disciplined, and once she's accepted she does exactly what you ask her. With her it's all calculated: with Garbo it's all instinctive. And Dietrich has to be lit very carefully, angled very carefully, you have to be like a painter, using brush-strokes, whereas Garbo's face *can't* be badly photographed; I once asked the cameraman on *Queen Christina*, William Daniels, if he could ruin her face by shooting at an awkward angle; and he tried, but it couldn't be done.

Becky Sharp, originally to have been directed by Lowell Sherman, was my first colour film, based on *Vanity Fair*. Sherman shot for two weeks and then he died. They came to me: I read the script, and saw the two weeks' stuff, and I declined to do the picture; it wasn't my kind of a script, and I couldn't use what had been shot because it wasn't what I would have done. I asked for six or seven weeks to rewrite the script, re-design the sets and start shooting. They agreed, and Robert Edmond Jones—the well-known Broadway designer—did the sets for me. The original contract gave him control over colours. I did not accept that, not because of any vanity—if I didn't play the violin, I certainly would accept Heifetz doing it for me—but I just couldn't let anyone else do it. Luckily, Bobby Jones was a nice man; he said, "I wouldn't let anyone else take over, but seeing it's you, I agree, I give up my control." And he did.

The whole first scene, of a schoolroom, was designed in red. Now that's like starting *Othello* with the murder of Desdemona; how do you build up after it, and what's the point of red, an exciting colour to the eye, in a little schoolroom scene? My idea was to start as close to black and white as I could possibly get, on colour stock, and then start developing more colour gradually as the story's dramatic content increased. I was handicapped by the fact that British officers at the time wore red uniforms, but apart from that I reduced the colours to the absolute minimum.

In one early scene we shot we had red roses and green drapes and a soft beige carpet. When the rushes came back, we saw roses green, drapes red and the carpet was blue! Technicolor is a lithographic process, and at that time terribly wobbly, and we had endless processing problems. But you could correct the colour, which unfortunately you can't today. You can intensify or reduce specific colours, but you can't change them.

The Gay Desperado was a change of pace; a poetical satire, a difficult mode for the screen. I was exhausted after *Becky Sharp*, and I went to Mexico for a two-week vacation. I fell in love with Mexico, its beautifully stylized landscapes, its skies always filled with cumulus clouds. I decided I would never rest until I made a film there.

The first thing that happened when I got back was that Jesse Lasky called me. He was doing independent productions at United Artists; he had the singer Nino Martini under contract and had done one film with him already. He wanted me to do Gounod's *Faust*. It intrigued me; but the script was all wrong. Jesse was desperate: Martini's first film had flopped, and he couldn't think of another vehicle. Then while we were talking, a man called Berinski arrived with the idea for a Mexican film: Mexican bandits see American gangster films and realize how outmoded their methods are and go to the movies as a night school and try to follow the gangster methods of America. A bandit kidnaps a radio singer, who would be played by Martini. The idea caught my imagination: a great premise, and charming as a subject for a satire; but the rest of the story was the dreariest you have ever heard. Jesse wanted to throw the whole thing out but I said, "Let's use the opening scene and the idea."

He said, "If you'll direct it, I'll buy it." I agreed. Wallace Smith wrote it for me, and I loved making the film.

High, Wide and Handsome was a very difficult story to film, about the war between the railroad and the landowners. Tough going, but it was interesting because it had a great deal of Americana in it. It combined song, dance, and drama, and it was based firmly on history.

Golden Boy, Clifford Odets' story of a boxer, played by
Bill Holden, was an idea of mine made at Columbia.
Harry Cohn, Columbia's boss, had been offering me work
for years, but I'd never accepted. After I did *Porgy and
Bess* on Broadway I was fired with the idea of doing a
film version, and Cohn lured me to Columbia on a ruse of
pretending to want to do it. I was furious when I found
he had tricked me, but he lured me back after I'd stalked
out of the office, gave me a cigar and asked me to do one
of three scripts. I rejected them all.

But he charmed me into working for him anyway. I
found the subject of *Golden Boy* in a news-clipping, and I
decided to get William Saroyan to do it. He hated the
studio and gave up. Then someone did another script, but
we couldn't find a star. Finally we got Bill Holden and
Odets, and the whole thing worked out as a good film in a
minor key.

I did *The Mark of Zorro* for Darryl F. Zanuck at Fox.
I had seen the Douglas Fairbanks version, and I was
enchanted by it. I jumped at the chance; it brought back
my youth; because I had fallen in love with California as a
boy through the stories of Bret Harte, and *The Mark of
Zorro* was set there, at a time when it was Spanish, when
it had a great picturesque quality and languor, and wonderful *haciendas* and oak-trees and manor-houses. I was
astonished that Zanuck offered the film to me, because I
had always heard that he had said Mamoulian would
never work on his lot, as I was too independent.

I went to see Zanuck in his classical enormous office,
just slightly smaller than Mussolini's. I said to him, "Why
do you want me, when you've always said I was too
something-or-other?"

He said to me, "We think you're a great director." I
told him I didn't like the script he had sent me—he had
worked with the writers for two years on it and he took
a polo mallet and said, "We won't change it. Out of the
question." I told him what was wrong with it, and give the
devil his due, he told me I had seven weeks to rewrite it.
Then I told him I had heard he always cut his directors'
films, and I told him I wouldn't have that, because I shot
to cut. He told me he couldn't establish a precedent; that
John Ford, for instance, wanted him to do the cuts because Ford wouldn't do it himself, he preferred to go to
Catalina. I started to walk out; he called me back and
asked me how long I needed to cut it. I told him I would

be putting it together as I shot it, but I would like a week. He said he would go to Palm Springs that week, that if he wasn't present on the lot it wouldn't look so bad.

I enjoyed making the film; Zanuck was most pleasant. He was a dream to work with. There was one funny incident: the last scene in the picture shows Zorro holding up the Governor's carriage, taking all the jewels, and then, according to his flamboyant manner, inscribing the letter "Z" on the leather seat with his sword. The governor looks up in panic and says, "Zorro!" I told J. Edward Bromberg, who played the governor, "Instead of Zorro, say Zanuck, with a voice full of terror." He said, "I can't, I'll be fired." But I made him do it.

I did another take with Zorro, but I said, "Don't print the other one, we'll print that later, just print the first one and put it in the rushes for Zanuck to see." Zanuck used to see his rushes with an entourage of about fifteen people, who used to make a nice choral harmony, never a counterpoint. When they heard "Zanuck" spoken, there was a stony silence, and nobody believed their ears. The others were afraid to say boo. So he, Zanuck, buzzed the operator and said, "Run that last scene again." They ran it again and "Boom!" it came back. Luckily, he has a sense of humour and he appreciated the joke. After the film was over he gave me a briefcase, which I still have, bearing the legend, "For M for Z from Z."

I cut the film, and we ran it, and he said it would be great if I followed the cuts he suggested. The cuts were impossible, out of the question: he wanted to eliminate all the love scenes and leave in only the action. I said, "You've got to slow down the story here and there, otherwise it's all sword-fights." I told him that if he made the changes he wanted, my name must be removed from the credits.

He told me he would preview the picture as it stood, and then preview it again with his own cuts. The better preview would win. The film died with the cuts, and succeeded when it was intact. Zanuck told me after the second preview, "You and I, we make a great cutting team. Put everything back and ship it." It was a wonderful gesture on his part. And when I finished *Blood and Sand*, he didn't even hold a preview!

Blood and Sand, about a bullfighter's career, was based on the work of Spanish painters: in the market scenes I used the style of Sorolla; in the luxurious house of the bullfighter's mistress, Dona Sol, Velasquez; in the chapel and the infirmary, El Greco. Anti-realism of course; El Greco couldn't have passed a first-grade examination in anatomy. I had a crucifix which I sprayed blue and grey and green, and I sprayed the sets with spray shadows when you couldn't do it with light. In the chapel scene, when the bullfighter, played by Tyrone Power, came in to pray before the *Corrida*, he and the *quadrilla* came in with normal faces, and they should have had El Greco faces, green and blue. We used gelatines on the lenses and they turned half blue, half green; the assistant director said to me, "This looks terrible." We shot it, and it looked perfect on the screen.

Zanuck said the film had the best colour he had ever seen. I used what came to be known as the Mamoulian palette, with sixteen spray-guns, and I'd come on the set and apply the finishing touches. I had a sequence in Dona Sol's apartment after the bullfight, which was a grand climax of colours, golds and oranges and reds, blood and capes everywhere. How did you cap it? I decided to do the Dona Sol scene entirely in the style of Velasquez, everything black or white, the table, the service, everything. The women in white, the man in black. I came on the set and it was perfect, except that the frames of the chairs were gold and the central bowl of flowers had green leaves. The gold was sprayed black and the greenery black as well.

Koenig, the manager of the studio, walked in and said, "Rouben, are you feeling all right?" He disappeared, and a note came from Zanuck to see him after shooting. And Zanuck said, "What are you doing, spraying flowers black?" I told him: "You liked the rushes, I've been spraying, you liked it, didn't you?" He said, "You know I did," and I said, "All right". So he let me go ahead.

I did *Rings on My Fingers*, a light comedy with Gene Tierney and Henry Fonda, just to fill in time; I saw it the other day on television, and it meant nothing to me. Then I prepared *Laura*, cast it, directed some of it, and Otto Preminger, who was its producer, decided to take over the shooting. I don't want to talk about that episode at all, and it resulted in my leaving Fox.

It was several years before I worked in Hollywood again; I produced *Oklahoma!* and *Carousel* on the stage.

Then I went to MGM for *Summer Holiday,* a musical version of Eugene O'Neill's *Ah, Wilderness!*

I had a conference ahead of shooting with every department, and I wanted to capture the quality of Americana, with the yellows and light greens of Grant Wood and Curry, and similar painters. I didn't want any contrasting colours at all, just tints within a very narrow chromatic range. Cedric Gibbons, the art director, told me he liked the idea but that Louis B. Mayer preferred bright colours; insisted on them, in fact. I told him not to worry.

We had Charles Schoenbaum as cameraman. We had shot half of the picture, and we hit a scene in a bar in which Mickey Rooney as the young boy in the story sees a floozy get bigger and bigger and redder and redder; he's drunk, and she's overpowering to him, she's his first woman. We had to change gelatins, and I said to Schoenbaum, "I don't like that red shadow of the wall." And he said, "I can't see a red shadow at all. It's green." It turned out this top colour cameraman was colour blind! And the sound man at the studio, Douglas Shearer, brother of Norma, was deaf!

Silk Stockings, my last picture, was made at MGM also; a remake of *Ninotchka,* about a Russian girl commissar who discovers love and life in Paris. It was a satire, and the Russians themselves didn't understand it; they just didn't have the right sense of humour. I used dance in the film for dramatic purposes, with Fred Astaire and Cyd Charisse who are both among the great ones. Astaire is a Renaissance man; he works harder than anyone I have ever worked with. I hated making it in CinemaScope—the worst shape ever devised.

Since then, I haven't worked in Hollywood. The trouble is that American films today cannot be works of art, the results of one artist's dreams. Everything is scientific; your whole vision can be changed in the laboratory. Scientists began the cinema, they invented it, and they have the capacity to destroy it as well.

And what is happening in Europe is no solution, either. They have thrown out the old forms—and we needed that, we were becoming too stereotyped—but they have put nothing in their place. The artist today uses the screen the way you'd use a psychiatrist's couch; but he doesn't have any discipline, and he doesn't universalize. Art hasn't got to be just life: it must transform it; it must speak the whole truth. A profile isn't the whole face. I want to *recreate* the face of man, and to show it all.

Lewis Milestone

*Lewis Milestone is one of Hollywood's great motion
picture craftsmen: few can match his awareness of the
power of images in motion, his command of pictorial
rhythm, his ability to integrate sound and movement into a
purposeful kinaesthetic whole. Technically, the key to his
art is editing, the creative juxtaposition of interrelated
shots; thematically, he excels—like John Ford—in the
exploration of relationships within exclusively masculine
groups: the soldiers of his distinguished war films, the
newspapermen of The Front Page, the gangsters of The
Racket, the sailors of Mutiny on the Bounty, the impov-
erished farmhands in Of Mice and Men. The environment
which nurtured his art has also—paradoxically—discouraged it even while making its continued practice
possible. Thus commonplace programme pictures inevitably jostle in his oeuvre with major cinematic tours-de-
force; and now, in his seventies, he seems finally to have
acknowledged the depth of the longstanding rift between
him and commercial film-making. We meet him on a
warm and drowsy afternoon, made even heavier by the
airlessness of the room which, owing to illness, he crosses
with painfully halting steps. There is nothing halting about
his speech, however; his recital discloses a mind as vigor-
ous, outgoing and forceful as the one which brought All
Quiet on the Western Front or A Walk in the Sun to the
screen. The only trouble is that the atmosphere, leaden and
soporific, inhibits a full and immediate appreciation of his
remarks; not until they are played back and transcribed
do they reveal their true character as the testament of one
of the grands seigneurs of American film. This is history,
related by the man who made it.*

I was born in Russia, in the Black Sea port of Odessa. Shortly afterwards my family moved to Kishinev, capital of Bessarabia, a medium-sized city, where I grew up. I arrived in the United States when I was seventeen, and since then I've been here more or less permanently. Whenever I've worked abroad, in England or Australia, it's always been as an American director sent on location.

The First World War got me into films. When I enlisted in 1917, I chose to enter the Signal Corps and, knowing a little about photography, I volunteered for the photographic section of its aviation branch; in those days aviation was just an arm of the Signal Corps. Very soon after that, I voluntarily switched from still photography to motion pictures.

In the army, I started as an editor in a basement laboratory of the Medical Museum in Washington. When the war was over, Hollywood seemed the natural place to go because by then everything had moved out here; so we just followed.

My transition from New York to my first Hollywood job was rather funny. I never thought I'd leave New York. "I'm through with small towns," I told someone who asked me to go to Boston. "I'm in a big city now and I want to stay."

Then, still in the photographic business, I met and became friends in New York with the visiting general manager of the West Coast J. D. Hampden Studios. One day over a drink I asked: "If I come out to the Coast, will you give me a job in your studio?"

This, coming from someone he considered just a good-time Charlie, made him laugh. "What could you do out there?" he said. "In a studio, you know, everything is specialized."

"I know that," I replied. "But there's a particular job I want to do: I want to go into the cutting room and be an editor."

Then he really roared with laughter. "You know what they pay beginners? Twenty dollars a week."

"That's all right," I said. "I'm not looking for money now. I'll take the job and you can pay me twenty dollars a week."

"I'm leaving a week from tonight," he declared. "If you join me on the train at Grand Central Station, I'll know you're serious about this and not just fooling around."

On the appointed day, as luck would have it, my taxi

was delayed on the way to the station and I arrived just in time to see the train pull out. My non-appearance probably confirmed the West Coast fellow's suspicions about me, but I wired him to wait for me in Chicago, grabbed the following train, met up with him and we came out here together.

Despite his promises, I still hung around for a month waiting for the twenty-dollar job in J. D. Hampden Studios' cutting room. Eventually I did get it, but left after a while to work with Sessue Hayakawa. From then on I had a succession of jobs.

One day at Ince Studios I met a director named William A. Seiter, who died not so long ago. Seiter liked the way I was working, and I liked him, so we decided to pool our interests. I resigned from Ince Studios, and whenever Seiter worked I worked too. If he didn't work, I sat around and waited until he got his next job. That suited me very well because it gave me a chance to acquire an eye for detail, to experiment and learn the business.

I cut at night and spent my days with Seiter on the set: that led to my going into direction. Occasionally he would incorporate ideas of mine, and pretty soon he let me pick up certain shots—run-throughs and things like that.

Every time I had the camera to myself, of course, I'd want to photograph an exit or an entrance and I'd bring back half a reel of film with its own self-contained little built-up story. Some of it was used, some wasn't. But that was my beginning as a director.

My first directorial feature film was a thing at Warners called *Seven Sinners*, with Marie Prevost, John Patrick, and Claude Gillingwater. This was a screen original, an idea of mine I wanted to do because at the time there was nothing worthwhile available anywhere, especially for a beginner.

"I know the junk you're going to give me," I told Jack Warner, "but I have a story of my own. If you give me a writer to work with, you can have the story. It's a good one."

"Who do you want?" he asked. I mentioned the name of Julian Josephson. "You must be out of your mind," Warner exclaimed. "He gets $500 per week. I'm not going to give you a $500-per-week writer to start with."

I mentioned another name. "Forget it," Warner said. "He gets $300 per week: still too high."

So I said: "What about that young man who's hanging around the staircase in the vestibule? He's supposed to be some kind of a writer—what about him?"

"If you take him," Jack said, "I'll pay *you*."

"All right," I said, went out and whistled to the guy to come down. "I've just formed a company," I told him. "I'm going to direct. You want to work with me?"

"Anywhere," he replied. "Any time." That man's name was Darryl F. Zanuck.

Zanuck, who wrote my first two pictures, was very ambitious in those days, a man on the go. He knew exactly what he wanted, kept reading the trade papers, the forerunners of the *Hollywood Reporter* and *Variety*. He was very interested in returns, in what each picture did.

"What are you wasting your time with all this stuff for?" I asked. "What do you care what it does?" But he already knew in what direction he wanted to go.

Seven Sinners was a comedy about seven high-strung crooks stranded in an empty quarantined house which they have entered intending to rob because its owners are away on vacation. My next picture, *The Cave Man,* from a story by Gelett Burgess, was about a love affair between a coal-heaver and a jaded lady who, bored with everything, writes her address on one half of a hundred-dollar bill, tears it off and throws it away: whoever finds it can come and claim the other half.

The coal-heaver finds it, and the story develops from there. The role was played by the late Matt Moore, one of the three Moore brothers; the others were Owen Moore, who was married to Mary Pickford at one time, and Tom Moore, who was a big star; Matt was the youngest. The girl was again Marie Prevost.

Through Matt Moore I met the silent star Thomas Meighan at a lunch club. Meighan was at a crucial stage in his career because his contract was about to expire and he had nothing to go on to negotiate a new one. He was looking for a director willing to take a risk with him and an idle crew of forty: all he had was a title, *The New Klondike,* about the 1927 Florida land boom, which I think came from Ring Lardner.

Then I called in a man named Tom Geraghty, an old newspaperman working for Douglas Fairbanks, who by that time was a very good friend of mine. Tom performed a role which at a later date would have been characterized as that of a producer.

"We'll never get anywhere sitting around here," I told him. "We don't know anything about the New Klondike. Why don't we take the company down there and just pick up the story off the streets? There must be stories everywhere."

He thought I was crazy because I had my whole reputation at stake, but two days later Tom Meighan, the crew of forty and I left for Miami to start work.

When we arrived we found they were selling real estate off pushcarts. Men were going through the streets ringing a big bell, and they sold you a lot right off the back of the cart from a map spread out between two sticks. When you went there you sometimes found the land still under water, not yet pumped up.

Tom and I walked around in the daytime picking up local flavour and worked on the story at night. As soon as we had enough material we started shooting. Then he would walk around by himself by day and report what he saw to me at night, when I would go out and look at anything he considered I should see. That was the way we worked.

A story emerged out of all this about a baseball player on the skids who's saved from penury by making a quick fortune in real estate. We housed the crew in the garage of a modest little private bungalow where they'd set up army cots at five dollars a night—this was before motels. Everything was so crowded that local people were making money in all directions, a state of affairs that lasted until the Crash came.

While I developed my love for background on *The New Klondike*, it was with *Two Arabian Knights*, a comedy I made for Howard Hughes in 1928, that I first took up the theme of war in films.

Two Arabian Knights, set in the trenches of the Western Front, was about a feuding sergeant and private who play out their miniature war against a world-war background. During a terrific bombardment they dive into the same shellhole, recognize each other, and knock each other out; coming to, they find themselves prisoners and the whole trench surrounded by Germans.

As prisoners of war they realize that, if they want to help themselves, they must bury the hatchet and present a united front to the enemy. They consequently became friends and together break out of the prison camp; the rest of the film concerned their adventures on the road.

The two men were played by Louis Wolheim—this was his first screen appearance; I brought him out here—and Bill Boyd. I'd seen Wolheim in *What Price Glory?* on the stage, and by the time I got around to using him he was an established Broadway star, having also done *The Hairy Ape* with sensational success.

What Price Glory?, which happened to be one of my favourite plays, had much more of a story that *Two Arabian Knights*. The only resemblance between the two pieces was the animosity of the protagonists: but it was not really animosity, just their idea of humour—to put the other fellow into trouble.

The Racket, which I filmed in 1928 with Louis Wolheim and Tom Meighan, came from a play, one of the first underworld stories to emerge from Chicago. Its author, Bart Cormack, was a kind of society reporter in Chicago, and he beat all the tough guys covering gangland—Charlie MacArthur, Ben Hecht, and Wallace Smith—in their avowed desire, expressed in whatever saloon they were meeting at, to go to New York and write a play.

As a society reporter he'd not only beaten them to the punch but had stolen the thunder of crime reporters, and it caused a big feud between them. But it was a very good play.

At Paramount I then did *The Betrayal* starring Emil Jannings, a triangle story involving a Swiss mayor, a painter, and the mayor's wife: Jannings was the mayor, Gary Cooper the visiting artist.

Jannings was very difficult to work with. You had to know how to handle him. Like most Germans, he could understand a shout, bark or command, but if you tried to be a gentleman with him he would mistake it for weakness.

He always referred to himself in the third person. If he asked you to lunch, and they served soup, he would taste the soup and say: "That's wonderful soup—the best thing for Emil." And he kept telling you that if it was good for him it must be good for everybody.

In those days he had a wonderful woman cook whom he'd stolen from the Rothschilds of France: you couldn't help noticing the respect and solicitude with which he treated her. He'd never think of leaving the house without opening the kitchen door and saying, *"Au revoir, mademoiselle"*, or "I won't be very long; I'll be back soon."

Mrs Jannings didn't rate at all. He treated the cook

beautifully, and I could tell from eating the food that he was looking out for his own best interests.

I refused to put my name on *New York Nights*, a disappointing backstage melodrama, but it got on there anyway. The producer, John Considine, cut the picture all wrong. I looked at it and said: "If this is the way you're going to send it out, take my name off it." They did, but it somehow got back on. By that time it was too late to remove it because everybody knew I'd made the film anyhow.

Universal originally wanted an old-time director, Herbert Brenson, to do *All Quiet on the Western Front*. But he demanded $125,000 for directing the film and they felt it was too expensive. So they started looking around for somebody who would do it for less.

Someone at the studio had seen *Two Arabian Knights* and had been sufficiently impressed—since it was a war picture—to consider me as a directorial possibility for *All Quiet*. My agent in those days was David Selznick's brother Myron, and when I was propositioned to do the film—I'd read the book by then and was crazy to do it—he advised: "We'll ask them for $5,000 per week for ten weeks—that's $50,000, a far cry from $125,000. What we'll end up with is another matter, but the main thing is to make the terms look easy. Whatever happens afterwards remains to be seen."

Well, by the time we'd finished writing the script and preparing and shooting the film exactly nine months had gone by, and they'd paid me $130,000 to the last penny. They wouldn't pay Brenon $125,000 because he asked for it in advance.

All Quiet was, of course, my first sound picture. I'd known about sound coming into general use towards the end of 1928, and, when it did come, there was still a lot of discussion going on dismissing it as just a passing fad. In making silent-film adaptations from plays like *The Racket*, for instance, sound didn't even occur to us. Everybody said, "We've developed quite an art in making silent movies. Nobody's going to go for sound." Well, everybody was wrong.

In a way, sound represented a big advance and in other ways it was a retrogression. People took the easy way out. Before sound, you racked your brain trying to tell the story through pieces of business and pantomime. Then suddenly you didn't need any of that; you could simply say, "Go to the door, somebody's there."

When I was still at Paramount Studios, Jesse Lasky had offered me a picture with a vaudeville team called The Two Black Crows as my first sound movie, at a salary of $125,000. He ran a test he'd made of them and I saw that it was just an old broken-down vaudeville act. "Don't you think they're funny?" Lasky queried.

"Yes," I said, "but they don't need me. They've been doing their act for years in vaudeville, so why don't you simply set up a camera in front of them and shoot? For my first sound picture I want to know something about sound and I know nothing about it now. And I don't want to do it in *your* studio. I want to do it in a studio where I know everybody, and where they know me."

The studio that is now the Sam Goldwyn Studio was such a place. So I turned down Lasky's offer and went there. In most places in those days the sound engineers had decided that they were going to take the business over because nobody knew anything about sound and they did; they made up a kind of cabal. If they were having lunch and you passed by, the conversation dropped to hushed tones so you couldn't hear what they were saying.

At the Goldwyn Studio, however, things were different. There the sound man, whom I'd known in a different capacity, had no qualms about showing me the mechanics of his job. Indicating the monitor up above us he said: "Come on up there. I'll have one man here in front of the microphone and I'll explain the whole thing to you."

Upstairs I saw a dashboard with dials, and, looking through the glass, I saw the man in front of the microphone communicating with the sound engineer by numbers: "Testing . . . one, two, three, four, etc."

I noticed a needle moving on the dashboard. "What does that do?" I asked, and was told it established the volume. "Suppose we did a scene," I continued, "at a volume of seventy; then all I'd have to do in the next scene would be to keep saying 'louder' or 'lower' until I saw a seventy, and that would be it, wouldn't it?" "Yes."

"Thank you," I said. "That's all I have to know", and walked out.

So on *All Quiet* I decreed: "No two cameras, nothing different from before. One camera, and we shoot the way we've always shot." And that—as far as I was concerned—was the big sound revolution; it was that simple. All the long tracking shots, for example, were done with a silent camera unless the scene involved dialogue.

We used dubbing and post-synching not for dialogue but for sound-effects. My top sound man—there was no such animal as a sound cutter then—did a damned good job, although he'd had no previous experience in that kind of thing.

He told me at the time that the hardest sound to reproduce convincingly was a gunshot. "It generally sounds like nothing," he said, "because it's recorded indoors. So we'll shoot off some live ammunition in the hills at night, record it, cut off the first explosion and just use the reverberation; then you'll have some real sound." That way we got enough stuff to put under every battle scene.

We also used a movieola—not, of course, as modern as to-day's. I'd used one way back when I was at the Sennett Studio. I found it in an attic. Nobody wanted it. It was a tiny little thing with a crank on the side through which you pulled the film. The other cutters would observe me with it and tried to shame me by declaring that no self-respecting editor would use a thing like that; they would pull the film through their hands and read it directly with their eyes.

"All right," I said, "when you're blind and I can still see you'll find out that your bravado behaviour will have cost you your eyesight."

I had an instinctive feeling for the material in *All Quiet;* besides, having examined thousands of feet of actual war footage while stationed at the Washington, DC, War College during the war, I knew precisely what it was supposed to look like.

As no Californian terrain exactly matched the European, we went looking instead for some place where we could reproduce the *character* of the terrain, and found it on a mesa in what is now called Newport, this side of Laguna. High on the mesa you don't see the mountains or anything like that to betray the fact that it's in California.

Then, utilizing something I'd learned from watching war footage, I reproduced the smoke of battle by burning a lot of second-hand tyres. They were always on hand, and any time we didn't like the background we obscured it with smoke.

An unfortunate thing happened with ZaSu Pitts, whom we'd cast as Lew Ayres's mother in the film. As luck would have it, the supporting attraction at *All Quiet*'s first and only preview at Santa Ana was a Paramount comedy in which ZaSu Pitts played a madcap maid with her famous comic hand-gestures, etc. No sooner had *All Quiet* come on after the intermission than the audience took one look at Miss Pitts as the mother and howled the roof off.

Despite my pleading that this was a one-in-a-million coincidence the studio insisted on replacing ZaSu Pitts with someone else. So we looked around and eventually found Beryl Mercer; and although her speech wasn't ideal we couldn't do anything about it and were stuck with her.

I think Lew Ayres, formerly a banjo player in an orchestra some place, was really destined to play Paul. He'd been recommended to me initially by Paul Bern— Jean Harlow's husband, who later committed suicide—but at the time his name meant nothing to me.

After a few days, Paul Bern contacted me again and raised hell. "I sent you a young man who I thought would be very good in the film but you didn't even have the courtesy to answer his telephone call. You hung up on him and were very boorish."

"I don't remember anything like that," I said. "Tell him to call me again."

Time passed, and Bern said to me: "Well, you did it again." "Wait a minute," I said. "What time did he call me?" "He always calls you very bright and early in order not to miss you." "Like what?" "Oh, around 7.30 a.m." "Look," I said, "around 7.30 a.m. I don't even speak to myself."

The upshot was that the boy didn't want to come near me. Meanwhile, I'd put George Cukor, who started out as dialogue director on the film, in charge of making the tests for the leading parts because I had so many things to do that I needed outside assistance. We'd meet at the end of each day, and I'd ask him if he'd tested any likely prospects. "Not a soul—nobody," he'd say; he was looking for an unknown to play the lead.

This went on until the day before we were due to start the picture. George and I ran test after test and I had to acknowledge he was right: there was nobody. Suddenly my attention was caught by some medium shots—they were not even closeups—in a scene showing a line of soldiers in front of the field kitchen.

An argument develops: the boys demand double portions because half their company have been wiped out. Food has been cooked for the whole company and the fact that half the company has been lost is, they say, just too bad; they demand double portions. While the argument is proceeding an officer passes by and wants to know what's going on, and a boy steps out of the ranks and tells him.

I looked at that boy, and something about him impressed me, so I ran the scene again. "Don't you notice anything strange or exceptional about this boy?" I asked George, who said he didn't. "Well," I said, "I think he's wonderful. This is the boy we ought to call in and talk to."

"He's all right in the dialogue," George said, "but what about the pantomime, the action that you'll need in the picture?"

"Forget it," I replied. "If he knows what he's saying his face will take care of itself. You don't have to teach him how to make grimaces away from dialogue."

George and I accordingly called the boy in for an interview at nine o'clock the next evening. I tried to upset the guy's dignity in every possible way but couldn't do it. He sat there like a king, with all the confidence in the world.

Conferring with George in the next room, I said I liked Ayres. "Now that I keep looking at him," George replied, "and observing what you were doing to him, I really think this guy has the damnedest presence I ever saw in a very young man."

As a final, acid test I took Ayres in to see George Abbott, the famous stage director, sitting alone in another office. I'd brought Abbott in to see if he could pull the script together, since he was reputedly a great play doctor.

I introduced Ayres and Abbott, and from the young man's point of view it must have been a formidable experience, because here was a man with a background of success and probably three times Lew Ayres's age.

The first question Abbott asked him was: "Do you think you can play this part?"

"I know I can," Ayres answered.

Abbott became a little annoyed at that. "Do you know the shellhole scene?" he asked.

"Of course I do," Ayres replied. "That is one of the best and one of the easiest scenes to play in the whole book."

"Why don't you throw this little bum out?" Abbott asked me, annoyed. "He'll never be an actor, he's just a fresh kid."

"You may be right," I said. "But I noticed that while he upset you, you didn't upset him."

I liked someone who could be that cool, so I took Ayres in to see the big boss of Universal, Carl Laemmle Jr, saying to Laemmle: "For your information, this guy is playing the central character in *All Quiet*."

Laemmle Jr and Lew Ayres were each just about twenty: putting two kids—one an actor, the other a budding executive—in the same room was like a confrontation between two strange fighting roosters.

The studio head got up from behind his desk and said to young Ayres: "Stand up." Lew Ayres got to his feet. "Turn around."

I realized I had to do something about this. "You're not casting a girl in a musical comedy," I said. "You want to see his legs?"

He had to say something, so he looked at Lew Ayres and said: "Your name is Ayres?" "Yes, sir." "I want to change that name." "You're not going to change my name. I was born Lew Ayres and I'll stay Lew Ayres."

Sensing a fight, I said to Laemmle: "Look, Junior, you ought to know better than this. The kid is under age"— they were both under age—"and he has no right to say or agree to anything. His mother has to do it for him. Call Mrs Ayres in tomorrow morning and discuss changing his name with *her*."

The situation thus saved, Ayres and I left. Next morning I tackled Laemmle before he had a chance to see Mrs Ayres.

"What the hell's the matter with you?" I said. "Leave the kid alone. He want's to be Lew Ayres. That's his name. What do you want to change it for?"

Laemmle was considering that there was an actress, Agnes Ayres, with whom he might be confused.

"So what?" I said. "There are Fairbankses all over the place, Pickfords all over the place. Who cares?"

Anyway, we survived that crisis: he went in under his own name, and the rest is history.

We shot six, seven or eight endings for *All Quiet,* and arrived at that final butterfly idea—Paul is shot by an enemy sniper while attempting to seize a butterfly—out of desperation. We did that scene after the whole film was finished and after it had been previewed. We were never satisfied with any of our previous endings, all grandiose ideas derived from the book, such as the armies of the world marching to a common grave, etc.

Reading the book was one thing, trying to dramatize it quite another. Each of our portentous endings seemed worse than its predecessor, and I kept throwing them away.

Finally the scales fell from my eyes. "This is one piece," I declared, "that you cannot finish with a *crescendo*. You have to have a *diminuendo*. You cannot top the whole piece." After that there was nothing to it.

My cameraman, Arthur Edeson, had quit by then, and Karl Freund, a very famous German cameraman who'd done a lot of celebrated films, had just joined Universal. I showed him the film and he raved about it, promising to help me finish it.

"Don't worry about fixing a salary," he said, "because I don't care if you pay me or not. I want to be part of this thing. I feel privileged even to have seen it."

We wanted a simple ending. The book proved rather frustrating because every time you thought you had an original idea and you read it once more you found some suggestion of it—if not the whole idea—in one of its chapters.

Paul was a butterfly collector in the novel. Leaving for the front a second time after a visit home during which he's disappointed and disgusted with everyone's behaviour, he makes his sister a present of his collection. That was the butterfly reference. But it was enough for us: we incorporated it about half-way through the picture to justify his reaching out for a butterfly alighting on an empty bean can in the final scene.

That way, too, he was able to relive his past. It also gave us a chance to dramatize the book's last line: "He died on a day so quiet that the official report read 'All quiet on the Western Front'." We did it by showing that no precautions were being taken, the men were outside the trench, crawling around all over the place on the parapet, and there was no sign of the enemy—until, of course, a lone sniper picked Paul off through his sights.

The harmonica background music we used for this scene just "happened". We were organizing location shooting on what was known as "DeMille's Forty Acres"—the Pathé back-lot in Culver City—when two of our men led in between them, under their arms, a rather stoutish fellow who could hardly walk.

They said they'd found him in a field lying flat on his face and moaning. He started telling me in German that he hadn't eaten in forty-eight hours and that he desperately needed a job. After he'd eaten, I spoke to him again and found that he had a harmonica and knew all the German soldiers' songs. When he began playing them I said: "There is our score. Look no further."

He was a one-man orchestra. I hired him as an extra among the soldiers, and whenever I needed marching songs or nostalgic songs about the Fatherland, he unfailingly obliged. He knew all the repertoire.

The film as previewed was at first rather long. It ran two and a half hours. The studio wanted to cut it and I agreed to let them do it for the film's general release after the New York reviews came out. And that's what they did: it ran the full two and a half hours in New York and then they cut out maybe fifteen or twenty minutes. Nothing significant was lost, and no further cuts were made.

When Howard Hughes offered soon afterwards to let me direct a screen version of the Ben Hecht and Charles MacArthur play *The Front Page*—of which he'd bought the movie rights—I eagerly accepted because I could relate to it, I could understand it, I knew the characters. I made them talk even faster in the film than they had in the play; I don't think anybody has made a picture as fast-talking as that. We added perhaps just three scenes to the stage piece, going outside for the pranks that Hildy Johnson plays on the editor.

The cast was the best we could get. I originally wanted Jimmy Cagney to play Hildy Johnson. Zanuck agreed but Howard Hughes wouldn't accept him—he considered Cagney "a little runt": this was before Cagney had made his mark in *Public Enemy*.

Then I had a chance to get Clark Gable for the part but Howard Hughes rejected him too, saying: "That man's ears make him look like a taxi-cab with both doors open."

It's very easy to make mistakes like that. Once, as Hughes and I were in a taxi going down to the boats on New York's East River, he asked me my opinion of Jean Harlow, whom he'd had under contract since *Hell's Angels* and for whose services MGM were offering him $60,000.

"She hasn't the slightest idea about acting," I told him. "She has a wonderful body, a ridiculous head, and $60,-

000 is much more than you have a right to expect for her contract. Sell it."

He sold it. In Harlow's next picture for MGM she took off like a jet and never stopped, becoming a major star. After that, whenever Hughes reproached me about my judgement, I said: "What about Cagney? What about Clark Gable?" Everybody's liable to make a mistake.

I didn't want to do *Rain* at all. I'd seen Jeanne Eagels do it on the stage and knew that nobody could touch her performance. Also, after she'd played it on Broadway for about three years, you couldn't enter a vaudeville house that didn't feature an act sending up Sadie Thompson.

But Jeanne Eagels was dead, and the front office had arranged for Joan Crawford to play it. As far as they were concerned she—being a big star and a very sultry dame—was the obvious choice. For me, however, the thing had no surprise, no novelty: it was very dated even then.

Finally I compromised and did it. Walter Huston as the preacher was fine, but Crawford wasn't up to it, and the picture couldn't get off the ground—although there were quite a few things in it I liked. I remember audiences greeting with a belly-laugh a scene in which Huston pursued Crawford down a staircase while reciting the Lord's Prayer. They laughed because mass psychology at that particular time didn't favour religion; if we'd waited a few years perhaps the public would have been more sympathetic.

Hallelujah, I'm a Bum, starring Al Jolson, started out originally as an adaptation of a French boulevard play. On my recommendation the producer, Joe Schenck, hired a friend of mine, a Basque named Harry d'Abbadie d'Arrast, whom I bumped into in Paris and who wasn't doing anything, to direct it.

On the first day's rehearsal d'Arrast declared that he couldn't work with Jolson, and wanted Fred Astaire to star in the picture instead.

"You're out of your head," I said. "How am I going to go to Joe Schenck and tell him at this stage of the game that you suddenly want to change the actor? The only reason they're doing it is to be able to write off two million dollars they've paid Jolson. It's impossible."

D'Arrast then walked out and, since I'd recommended him, Schenck put me in his place. The next thing I did was to hire Rodgers and Hart—this was before they hit the big time—and adapt the picture to suit their special musical talents.

The year was 1933, the depth of the Depression, and *Hallelujah, I'm a Bum* was very much a Depression picture: it revolved around some bums in a park, and in the lyrics we referred to policemen as "Hoover's Cossacks". I wasn't influenced by Ernst Lubitsch. He had his own way of doing things—he could only do one type of film—and it would have been silly to try to imitate him. No influence from Mamoulian's *Love Me Tonight* either: I came first, he came second.[1]

John Gilbert was certainly a victim of sound, although there was nothing basically wrong with his voice. The only time his voice went up was when he was over-excited. If he was sure of what he was going to say, and you gave him time to say it, his voice would be absolutely normal. Off-screen he never screeched.

I directed Gilbert in his last film, *The Captain Hates the Sea;* he died shortly after. The big job was to dig him out of his lair and convince him that he ought to return to films, because he was not a poor man. Luckily I knew Jack pretty well, and after much persuasion he agreed to do a test—but only when I promised to shoot it very early in the morning when the studio was practically deserted.

Despite what is in Harry Cohn's biography[2], Cohn, the head of Columbia Pictures, welcomed Gilbert's prospective rehabilitation and promised him star treatment provided he behaved properly. But unfortunately Jack was a little too far gone.

For a week he was perfect; and then he started drinking. That wouldn't have been so bad if it hadn't been for the fact that if he drank one day he couldn't work the next, because by then he had ulcers and he would vomit blood and be very ill. As I said, *The Captain Hates the Sea* was his last film.

Then I did two insignificant musicals at Paramount, *Paris in Spring,* with Ida Lupino and Tullio Carminati, and Cole Porter's *Anything Goes,* starring Ethel Merman. After that I must have gone for about ten or twelve weeks without being given a picture. They were paying me a lot of money under my contract, so I went and complained to

[1] Mr Milestone errs here: *Love Me Tonight* antedated *Hallelujah, I'm a Bum* by a year. (Authors' Note.)
[2] *King Cohn* by Bob Thomas (G. B. Putnam's Sons, N.Y.; Barrie & Rockliff, London, 1967).

Ernst Lubitsch, who was a friend of mine and had recently been appointed head of production at Paramount.

Lubitsch listened sympathetically but said he had nothing suitable for me just then. As he spoke, I noticed a thick manuscript on his desk bearing an intriguing title (which I read upside down): *The General Died at Dawn*. Lubitsch dismissed it as junk, a pulp serial, but eventually allowed me to take it away and read it, in case it might yield a usable idea.

It was easy reading because there were enough adventures in it to supply material for at least fifteen movies. I was about to take the manuscript back to Lubitsch when it occurred to me that the real reason he had been so reluctant to let me read it in the first place was because he feared—correctly—that I would want both to produce *and* direct any film I made from it, because that was in my contract. Then, if anything went wrong production-wise, there would technically be no one for him to blame.

I fixed that problem by going to see an old friend of mine, Bill Le Baron, with whom I'd become acquainted during Tommy Meighans' stint on *The New Klondike*. Bill had been in charge of the studio *before* Lubitsch, and was now one of their top producers. I found him—as I expected—in the Jockey Club at Santa Anita racetrack and announced: "Bill, I'm afraid I've just put you to work."

I explained the situation to him and gave him the manuscript to read that same night. Having read it, Bill conceded it had plenty of action but felt, like Lubitsch, that it was strictly pulp-fiction material. How, he wanted to know, did I propose turning it into a viable movie?

"My idea is simple," I said. "You set up two forces, an American representing democracy and a Chinese general representing authoritarianism. That's the focal point—then we can use whatever incidents out of the manuscript we want, provided we get a writer who understands the political setup."

The writer I recommended was the up-and-coming playwright, Clifford Odets, whom I'd never met; but I'd seen two of his plays and been very impressed. Thus armed, Le Baron and I went in to see Lubitsch who, once he had a producer, relaxed immediately and gave us the go-ahead to make the film. That's how I got to do *The General Died at Dawn*.

The picture's decorative style was dictated by the story: each story is a challenge. I'd done nothing like it before.

Necessity also dictated that scene in which ceremonial swords divided the screen up into several panels of simultaneous action: no one had used that idea until then.[1]

I thought Akim Tamiroff was marvellous as General Wang. To achieve his "Chinese" appearance, I at first instructed the makeup man to superimpose a Chinese-shaped eyelid on him, using the liquid rubber employed by dentists. They tortured the poor guy and blistered his eyelids, all to no avail: he still looked like Tamiroff.

Finally I suggested that they bring in a real Chinese, make a facsimile or cast of his eyelid and then apply it to Tamiroff, using the same principle as in key-cutting. They tried it, and of course it worked; as a result I almost became an honorary member of the makeup men's union.

Bill Le Baron also produced my next picture, *Night of Nights*, which I did to fill in time during the two or three months I was waiting for a studio to give me the go-ahead on *Of Mice and Men*.

Night of Nights starred Pat O'Brien. It was his first picture on loanout away from Warner Brothers. I met him at the racetrack and he suggested I direct it. There was only one problem, Bill Le Baron explained: they'd had to abandon their scheduled film at the last minute because the writer had also sold the same story to another studio, and now they were stuck for a new story while O'Brien, the cast, and crew sat around idle on salary.

To give Le Baron an idea for a story I recounted an incident I had witnessed at the Lunch Club, a famous actors' club in New York, between Louis Calhern and Walter Catlett. It occurred during Prohibition. Calhern entered the club one day, walked up to the bar and ordered a pint of whisky. They'd given him the setup—the glass, and ice and so on—and he was about to take his first drink when in walked Catlett, his closet pal, and stopped his elbow in mid-movement.

"Aren't you opening tomorrow night?" he asked Calhern.

"That's right."

"Well," said Catlett, "what are you doing with this?"

"Mind your own business."

"Look," Catlett continued, "you're a good friend of

[1] Except in Rouben Mamoulian's *Dr Jekyll and Mr Hyde*, 1932. (Authors' Note.)

mine, but if you drink that I'll punch you right in the mouth."

Calhern drank it, Catlett punched him in the mouth, and, in the ensuing fracas, Catlett was knocked out cold; as a result they were both suspended from the club for a month. When Catlett came to, he was very angry and started challenging all and sundry to continue the fight. Just then Calhern made the mistake of returning, whereupon an even worse clash took place; as a result of that second fight they were both permanently suspended from the club.

That incident gave us the opening for *Night of Nights*. I brought in the writer Donald Ogden Stewart, and we spun out the rest of the yarn together, making one of the characters the producer of a play and the other its star actor. I shot the thing as Stewart wrote it.

When *Of Mice and Men* first came out as a story I was crazy about it. Then George S. Kaufman turned it into a hit play, produced by Sam Harris and starring Wallace Ford. I noticed Ford one day in the 21 Club in New York, where I'd gone to have a drink, and his presence reminded me of the play and the film I wanted to make from it.

So I got a friend of mine to call Kaufman, who in turn called Sam Harris, because they were both partners in this venture. Next day I went to see Harris—I knew him quite well—and requested that I be given the right to turn *Of Mice and Men* into a motion picture script. Thus, I argued, the property, which for some reason nobody seemed interested in acquiring, would be reactivated.

I found out the reason for that afterwards. It emerged that Harry Cohn of Columbia had been willing to pay Kaufman $75,000 for the property, although he hadn't read the story, seen the play, or known what it was about. "I don't have to," he told Kaufman. "Steinbeck wrote it, you dramatized it, that's good enough for me."

When Cohn eventually did read it—at Kaufman's insistence—he withdrew his offer; so now Harris and Kaufman were stuck with it.

Harris behaved very generously: he gave me a free option to develop the story into a movie script, on the understanding that, once studio finance had been obtained, we would reopen formal negotiations. And that, for the moment, was where things stood; no contracts were drawn up.

I went ahead and finished the script and took it up to

show Steinbeck, who lived in northern California in those days. Although he said he was delighted with it, I persuaded him to revise it personally; and before my very eyes, by the alteration of a comma or a phrase, it became his.

Meanwhile, after many unsuccessful attempts, I'd obtained studio backing for the picture from Hal Roach. It happened in a rather roundabout way: I'd won a breach of contract lawsuit against Roach, and he persuaded me to accept part finance on a production of *Of Mice and Men* in lieu of damages. My salary, determined in proportion to the rest of the capital invested, emerged as eighteen per cent of the gross.

When I suggested to Roach and his right-hand man, Frank Ross, that we buy the rights to the entire property outright from Steinbeck, Harris, and Kaufman for $50,-000, each of us putting up one-third, they declined. "Too much money," Roach said. "I'm not interested." He'd never believed in *Of Mice and Men*.

We left it at that. The picture was made and released, and for twelve years after that it was never off the screen; it was always being played somewhere.

Several years later I bumped into Steinbeck in New York, and he declared that so far that year he'd only received $17,500 as his share of the picture's profits.

"Are you complaining?" I asked.

"No," he said, "but goddammit, I've gotten used to getting more money every year and this year I only got $17,500!"

I cast *Of Mice and Men* myself. Lon Chaney Jr had played Lennie on the stage here in California; the coloured man who played "Whipper" was repeating his stage role, too. Betty Field and Charles Bickford were both, I think, excellent, but the film's poetic quality derived mostly from Burgess Meredith's performance as George. Meredith had been in several Maxwell Anderson plays, and he modelled his acting style on those. I realized what he was doing but let him go ahead, as I thought it was an admirable idea.

The reason we bleached and redeveloped the first-release prints sepia was mainly because I thought it would make the film look more faithful to the true colour of California in summer: about the end of July everything is burned up.

I ran the completed film for Steinbeck, and he was so delighted with it that, in my copy of the book, he wrote: *"This is a good picture"*, explaining that he wanted to resurrect the word "good" because most motion-picture advertising dealt in hackneyed, meaningless superlatives. We used his encomium in our publicity.

Next I did a couple of light comedies, *Lucky Partners* and *My Life with Caroline*. I started out, you will remember, as a comedy director. After *All Quiet on the Western Front* I had difficulty returning to comedy because, whenever I did one, the reviewers would say, "He's taking a vacation"; they didn't think I worked sufficiently hard on it. Comedies, in fact, aren't easy at all, but to the viewer it seems as if everybody's having a lot of fun.

This particular pair of comedies were of the kind you did if you hoped to stay in motion pictures, in the expectation that the next film might give you a chance to redeem yourself. Everyone in the film industry—writers, directors, actors—has to compromise: you're faced with the alternative of staying out and telling everybody what a big hero you are.

The first time I worked with the late Bob Rossen was on *Edge of Darkness*, a story of the German occupation of Norway, which starred Errol Flynn. Rossen, who later went on to become a notable director, hit on an idiom for the dialogue that had nothing to do with Norway but derived mainly from the language he knew best—the speechways of New York's East Side. Since nobody else knew the difference, the idiom worked admirably.

Edge of Darkness was a very nice job, and had some interesting things in it. An extremely mixed cast gave some damned good performances, Flynn included. Flynn kept underrating himself. If you wanted to embarrass him, all you had to do was to tell him how great he was in a scene he'd just finished playing: he'd blush like a young girl and, muttering "I'm no actor", would go away somewhere and sit down.

Maybe not enough people knew Flynn well. I not only admired him as an actor, I liked him very much as a person. I knew him as a perfect host, a marvellous connoisseur of good food and wine, and as a beautifully behaved guest in my home. His faults harmed no one except himself.

The North Star, written by Lillian Hellman and produced by Samuel Goldwyn, was a much less rewarding assignment than *Edge of Darkness*. It was the only film I've done with Goldwyn—which is no reflection on *him*. I just didn't like working with him, didn't feel in accord with him at all; he was too adamant, too dictatorial, and you had to go his way, because he'd never change his mind about anything. Besides, I was outnumbered: there were too many of "them" and not enough of me.

Poor Erich von Stroheim, who played a German general in the film, lacked a few mechanical, technical things that he should have learned much earlier on the stage, and he now found it difficult to acquire them. For instance, he couldn't pick up a cue quickly enough, couldn't cut in on someone else's dialogue. The previous performer would have to finish his or her speech before Erich could start his. That put great limitations on his performance and on what you tried to achieve in moments of dramatic excitement.

I've done several films with Dana Andrews, who is a friend of mine, and liked him and Farley Granger so much in *The North Star* that I used them again in my next film, *The Purple Heart.* We knew nothing about wartime Tokyo, the setting of *The Purple Heart*, and had to more or less invent it in the studio. As technical adviser I had a minister's daughter who'd lived there a long time, including part of the war, and with her help we tried to prevent our *ersatz* Tokyo from becoming too wild.

I got the idea for the ballad running through *A Walk in the Sun* from my childhood in Russia. War veterans there weren't taken care of the way they are here. There were no convalescent hospitals, no government support or money for them to live on. You were lucky to come out of wars alive. You were crippled—well, you did the best you could: you stood on the corner and sold matches or cigarettes.

Very often, in the town where I lived, you'd see war veterans on street corners who'd become troubadours; they played a bulbous-shaped Russian kind of mandolin and sang ballads about their war adventures—fighting the Turk or something like that.

The problem facing Robert Rossen and me in adapting Harry Joe Brown's book *A Walk in the Sun* for the screen was how to convey its many marvellous descriptive passages without making the film too talky. We racked our brains, and then it occurred to me that in war you apprehend things more vividly through the ear than the eye.

Remembering the military troubadours from my childhood, I proposed that we pluck the interesting bits out of Brown's narrative, have someone turn them into lyrics with music, and make the result run through the film as a kind of continuous ballad.

It took Rossen a little while to buy this idea, but eventually he did buy it, and we gave the job to Earl Robinson and a fellow named Millard Lampell, who together produced nine ballads which we ultimately pared down to four. It worked like a charm.

I showed the completed film to Darryl F. Zanuck, because I wanted a Twentieth Century-Fox release for it. He raved about it, made all the directors on his lot—including Lubitsch, Henry King, Hathaway, everybody—look at it, and enthusiastically recommended it to his principals in New York. We accordingly got the release, and the rest is history.

The ballad in *A Walk in the Sun* created a sensation. Eventually, no self-respecting Western or television series was without one. But my picture introduced the idea. Usually it's very difficult if you're a trailblazer; very few people want to follow. This particular notion, however, caught on in a big way.

Several years later I was about to see *High Noon* in London when I bumped into its writer, Carl Foreman, in the United Artists building on Wardour Street. Foreman apologized because he said I would shortly see something he'd stolen from one of my films, but I replied that, coming from him, that was a compliment, so he didn't have to apologize.

"What the hell did he steal?" I wondered as I went in to see the movie, but as soon as I heard the ballad I knew.

Rossen and I got on together so well that we collaborated again on *The Strange Love of Martha Ivers* for the producer Hal Wallis, who was so impressed with *A Walk in the Sun* that he insisted I do a film for him.

The Strange Love of Martha Ivers was based on the prologue to an original story which Wallis had bought for about $3,500. It was the last of six suggested properties he offered me, and its working title was *Bleeding Heart*. "What a title!" I said. "You're going to produce a thing like that?"

He explained that *Bleeding Heart* was the name of a plant, and persuaded me to take it away and read it. I did so in the company of Bob Rossen, who occupied an office across the street on the Paramount lot. Rossen suggested we use the prologue—slightly altered so as to give us the rest of our story—and throw the rest away. "But don't tell

Hal Wallis that," he added. "Just tell him you'll do it and that you want me to write it."

I did that, and at my suggestion—or rather, demand—Wallis hired Rossen. Our story—the prologue of *Bleeding Heart*—concerned some children who witness one of their number murder an aunt by pushing her down a flight of stairs. The girl responsible and a boy witness swear each other to secrecy and seal the contract in blood.

That was practically a complete story in itself. We had to invent a boy who leaves without seeing the crime and returns to his home town as an adult. We started the adult story with him passing through the town and staying overnight to have a punctured tyre fixed. When the various crooked local political elements learn of this man's return they want to get rid of him because they think he's come back to expose them. By that time, too, the boy who witnessed the murder is a district attorney (Kirk Douglas) and married to the woman (Barbara Stanwyck) who killed the aunt and, as a result of inheriting all her wealth, is now the town's biggest political power. That gave us our whole story.

Barbara Stanwyck is a great trouper and was wonderful to work with; so was Judith Anderson, who played the aunt. This was Kirk Douglas's first picture, and he was obviously new, very anxious to learn and very modest.

The Strange Love of Martha Ivers turned out satisfactorily as far as I was concerned, despite Hal Wallis, who was a nuisance. He was not constantly present on *my* set but he made his proximity felt. After I cut the film, I just left the lot; I didn't think it was worthwhile staying and fighting over it with Wallis inch by inch. The problem was not that he wanted to take things out—he wanted to *add* things. After I left, for example, he had someone shoot big enormous closeups of Lizabeth Scott, which he proceeded to insert in the picture.

My association with Enterprise Studios began when they offered to let me direct *Arch of Triumph* because of my former identification with the work of Erich Maria Remarque. I read the book, found it quite interesting, and accepted their offer.

The basic mistake made in *Arch of Triumph* was that the script was much too long. I wanted to have more time to shorten it, but they refused because they were anxious to duplicate the success of the nearly four-hour-long *Gone with the Wind*, which had just been reissued. Besides, they had paid a lot of money for what they felt was an important story, and they had two important stars, Ingrid Bergman and Charles Boyer; so they wanted a long picture

Well, they got one. It was a long picture, all right, and expensive for those days. One thing wrong with it was that it was supposed to be a realistic piece and it had two major stars in the leads. If you have two stars like that, then half your reality goes out the window; all you have is another film with Ingrid Bergman and Charles Boyer.

That was the first drawback. The second was that, by the time the picture was finished, the bottom had fallen out of the market and they no longer wanted four-hour pictures, so we had to cut the damned thing down to the more conventional two hours, which is easier to do on paper than on celluloid. For all that, I like lots of *Arch of Triumph*. I have a copy of it here.

Next I did a little comedy, called *No Minor Vices*, that we tossed off for Enterprise because they wanted to keep the gates open, and after that I did a much more personal film, *The Red Pony*, in partnership with John Steinbeck, Charlie Feldman—who was an agent then—and Republic Studios. I selected Aaron Copland to do the score because of his previous outstanding work on *Of Mice and Men*.

For the main role we chose Gigi Perreau's kid brother, a little boy who took the first syllable of my own name and called himself Richard Miles. He's now on his way to becoming a very successful young novelist. I saw him here recently and read of the publication of his second novel in, I think, the *Saturday Review*.

Following *The Red Pony* I went back to Twentieth Century-Fox and Darryl F. Zanuck for a number of films, of which *Halls of Montezuma* was the first. That represented a return to the war theme after a more or less enforced break. I liked certain things in it, but it was really just a job, not a true opportunity to state my personal beliefs about war. I wasn't crazy about the overall idea.

Kangaroo was an underrated picture. I suppose the idea of making it in Australia originated in the Fox sales department: they'd accumulated a lot of money in Australia and I suppose the only way they could move the money was to reinvest it there.

I think the reason *Kangaroo* was so unfavourably received by the critics was because of its weak story. I couldn't help that, I was saddled with it by the studio. I spent a pleasant afternoon discussing it with members of the Sydney Journalists' Club, of which I was made an honorary member during my stay in Australia; during the afternoon I bought them all beer.

"I'm sorry the story's so bad," I told them, at the same time asking their help in tracking down interesting locations. They promised to do whatever they could. Next morning a young lady reporter from the *Daily Telegraph* called at the Hotel Australia, where I was staying, to deliver a message from her editor-in-chief, a very famous Australian newspaperman named Brian Penton.

The message said that Mr Penton had heard about my visit to the Journalists' Club and invited me to call on him in St Luke's Hospital, where unfortunately he was very ill with kidney trouble, having just come back from Boston, where he'd gone to see if he could be helped.

So I went and met this extremely intelligent and interesting—but obviously very sick—man, who picked up two books from his night table and, handing them to me, said: "Please take these as a gift. Between their covers you'll find everything I thought worthwhile saying about Australia. You may use any part or both of them in their entirety as you see fit—it's up to you."

I took the books—one was *Landtakers*, the other was *Inheritors*—right over to the hotel and, having read them, realized they would make marvellous pictures of their type. When my writer arrived from America, the first thing I did was to make him read them. Then we tried to persuade the studio by long-distance telephone to scrap the damned scenario they'd sent me out with, which was a joke, and substitute the Penton books.

"It's a lot of gall," I told them, "to ask me to come into a country and do a picture about it without me or anybody in the entire crew knowing anything about it. None of us has ever been here. Now here are a couple of books about the real Australia written by an Australian, and I think they'd make wonderful pictures."

They told me to forget it; trying to convince them from a distance of over ten thousand miles away was hopeless. Then, since Mr Penton had been kind enough to say I could use any part of his two novels, I fell back to my second-line trenches and resolved to narrow down the human story to the minimum and concentrate on the animals' plight during the drought. That way we came out of the venture with *something*, whereas otherwise we'd have had nothing. (Richard Boone did get something valuable out of it, however—the basis for the character of Paladin in the television series *Have Gun, Will Travel.*)

We made our own working conditions for *Kangaroo*, using an Australian crew instructed by my half-dozen key personnel, who ran it like a school. The Aussies blended in fine. I ignored the one studio in Sydney—Pagewood, which had only one sound-stage—and shot right inside houses, saloons, and natural interiors, utilizing as many historic locations as possible; in the country—the "bush", as you call it—we used little pubs and places like that, mainly in and around Port Augusta. We also shot on board a coastal ship.

One of the reasons I wanted to concentrate on Sydney's historic landmarks was to emphasize the fact that we were actually in Australia: out in the wide open spaces you might as well be in Arizona.

By the time I'd finished shooting the picture and had made the first cut, I'd fallen in love with the whole drama of the thing and instructed the music department at Twentieth Century-Fox to accompany my favourite sequence— the cattle-drive—with a soundtrack they had there of Shostakovitch's Sixth Symphony. When they did that, the sequence was really a masterpiece.

Zanuck saw it, jumped out of his seat, brought his wife in and ran it three times. But each time he ran it the original excitement inevitably diminished. Then came the blow: we couldn't use Shostakovitch's Sixth—not because of copyright, because we have no copyright with the Russians, but because, having experienced a lot of trouble when they'd stolen it once before, they didn't want to steal it twice. So they arranged for a new score.

Later, the film was compromised still further. One of the by-products of Darryl's squabbles with the Fox management was his temporary refusal to preview new pictures—he'd just ship them out cold. I urged him to put *Kangaroo* out in front of an audience to give us something we could not get any other way.

"Don't bother about that," he said. "I saw the picture and it's good. Ship it."

We accordingly sent the film out. A couple of months later, Zanuck called me saying that it had been previewed in the East and shipped back here with a demand for a whole new ending.

Then the fat was in the fire. I went in and volunteered my services because I wanted to rescue as much of the film's quality as I could. But we had to do whatever Mr Zanuck wanted. He can be good but, boy oh boy, he can also be very, very bad.

What can I say about my version of *Les Misérables*? It had been done before: I hope it will never be done again. I pleaded with them: "There are fifteen other stories much better than *The Bishop's Candlesticks*. Why do it again? The book has marvellous things. Take, for instance, little Gavroche during the Revolution—this kid's story really has something."

They wouldn't listen. So, having exhausted all your intellectual arguments, you go in saying: "Oh, for Chrissake, it's just a job—I'll do it and get it over with." And that's what I did.

I'd naturally seen the Richard Boleslawski version, made by the same studio in 1934, with Fredric March as Jean Valjean and Charles Laughton as Javert, but you couldn't go by that. Laughton's performance has become history, beyond criticism, but I think it's terrible: he hammed it all over the place.

My "biopic" of Dame Nellie Melba should have been called *Melba* like I should have been christened Napoleon. It had nothing to do with Melba. The script was worthless. It did have one point of interest, however. The tiny stages of Walton-on-Thames Studio in London, the oldest studio in England—where we were supposed to make the picture—were booked solid: the producer told me it was possible to get a stage there for only two weeks.

Having seen the script, I said: "How do you expect me to shoot *Melba* in two weeks in that silly small studio? Forget the studio. Let me find actual locations, natural interiors—they're plenty of them in London—and do it like that."

And that's what we did. The production looks as if we spent millions on it, but I can point out to you one place in Fire Lane, directly across the way from the Dorchester Hotel, from which we managed to extract five sets: a casino upstairs, a restaurant bar as you walk in, and so on. The building, which once belonged to the Rothschilds, is still intact and used as a venue for weddings, lectures, and things like that.

After *Melba* I did another war story, *They Who Dare*, based by the scenarist Bob Westerby on a factual incident told to the producer, Aubrey Baring, by two survivors of a ten-man expedition in the Mediterranean in World War II.

Their mission was to plant high explosives on an aircraft field atop a mesa on an island, from which enemy planes were harassing Allied shipping. They had to load the planes with explosives and blow up the field and every plane on it, landing on the island from rubber dinghies, disgorged by a dilapidated Greek submarine.

Landing stealthily and secretly was no problem; the problem was to rendezvous again with the submarine at an agreed hour, because once the first bomb went off the enemy would immediately realize that someone uninvited was on the island. In the event only two men survived. A lieutenant and a sergeant. I took the story down verbally from the sergeant at the suggestion of Aubrey Baring, who was a friend of his, and had it dramatized. The resulting film was *They Who Dare*.

The Korean war formed the background to my next picture, *Pork Chop Hill*, which was extensively re-edited before release and after I left. I didn't agree with the way Mr Gregory Peck wanted to edit it, so I simply walked out and he edited it the way he saw fit.

The trouble was that the whole Chinese side of it was lost, so that, looking at the film, you say: "Who the hell are they fighting?" I did have the Chinese side adequately shown at the beginning, but not for long. Gregory Peck took it out at the urging of his wife. "You know, darling," she said, "nothing happens until you come on the screen, so why don't you just lop it off?" He thought it was a great idea and lopped it off.

You can take anyone provided they have humour; what is unendurable is people who are like blocks of wood. That's why I so enjoyed working with Frank Sinatra and his gang on *Ocean's Eleven*. They're a very life-loving lot, they like to kid around, and the fun they were having benefited the picture because when I called the shots it rolled right onto the screen—at least it did in my opinion. We shot about half of it—twenty-two days—on location in Las Vegas and the other half in the studio.

Frank is very nice but moody, and if you want to work with him, it's up to you to understand him; he's not going to put himself out to understand *you*. If he likes you well enough, he'll try to see your point of view. I like a lot of things about the man. He's temperamental, however, and if you line up twelve people who know him, you'll get twelve different versions of his character and behaviour. Some people say he's not charitable enough; I think he's charitable to a fault. He does a lot of charitable things that he doesn't advertise.

When I came on to *Mutiny on the Bounty*, after Carol Reed left, I felt it would be quite an easy assignment because they'd been on it for months and there surely couldn't be much more to do. To my dismay, I discovered that all they'd done was a seven-minute scene just before they land in Papeete, in which Trevor Howard issues instructions about obtaining island breadfruit.

Marlon Brando swears he had nothing to do with Carol Reed's departure; that was a matter between Reed and the producer.[1] However, Carol resigned with full pay, which is not a bad way to go.

During my first two weeks on the film Brando behaved himself and I got a lot of stuff done—especially with sequences like the arrival in Tahiti, when I could work with the British actors. I got on beautifully with Trevor Howard, Richard Harris, and the others; they were real human beings, and I had a lot of fun. I've remained very good friends with Richard Harris.

Then the trouble started. I would say that what went basically wrong with *Mutiny on the Bounty* was that the producer made a number of promises to Marlon Brando which he subsequently couldn't keep. It was an impossible situation because, right or wrong, the man simply took charge of everything. You had the option of sitting and watching him or turning your back on him. Neither the producers nor I could do anything about it.

Charlie Lederer wrote the script from day to day. He would bring it on the set in the morning, then they would go into Marlon Brando's dressing-room and lock themselves up there till lunchtime. I don't know what went on, I never went in there.

After lunch, they came out. By then it was about two-thirty and we hadn't shot a scene. You had the option of shooting it, but, since Marlon Brando was going to supervise it anyway, I waited until someone yelled "Camera!", and went off to sit down somewhere and read the paper.

[1] Aaron Rosenberg.

When the picture was finished Brando came to see me, wanting to know why—as he put it—I'd treated him so badly.

"I didn't treat you badly," I said. "You *behaved* very badly. You didn't even want to discuss the scenes, you just took over."

I thought Brando's performance as Fletcher Christian was horrible. I've only seen him act once, and that was on Broadway in *A Streetcar Named Desire:* a marvellous performance. But he was never an actor before and hasn't been one since.

There've been other films which I've only partly directed. Years ago I quarrelled with Gloria Swanson over a picture I did with her called *Fine Manners.* When she started weeping, I told her I'd do anything she asked, whereupon she said it wasn't fair to hold me by turning on the tears; so I left.

Later, in the nineteen-forties, I did about half of *Guest in the House*, starring Anne Baxter, and quit because of a ruptured appendix. I can understand why John Brahm, who finished the film, didn't get on too well with Miss Baxter. The difference between his conception of the story and mine was that I thought we had to scare the characters, not the audience out front. There's a big difference there, and I think she felt the same way about it, because it robbed the actress: he was trying to scare her in order to scare the audience.

Throughout my career I've tried not so much to express a philosophy as to restate in filmic terms my agreement with whatever the author of a story I like is trying to say. I've probably had my greatest successes with war films because I've always tried to expose war for what it is and not glorify it.

I believe strongly in marrying a story to its background because I think that's good dramaturgy; otherwise it just dangles in mid-air. In preparing a film, I work very closely with the art director. As I don't draw, I make sure that we both visualize the scene the same way. Then we try various drawings until it's perfect. Finally he does a polished drawing of it and that's it.

I can see what the scene needs on paper just as well as I would see it on the stage—better, in fact, because I'm relaxed, no one's pushing me, the front office isn't badgering me wanting to know how many scenes I've done so far; I'm working all by myself.

I design the whole picture like that, scene by scene, setup by setup. It stands to reason doing it that way because it saves time during production. If you suddenly have a new idea on the set, it might take two hours to achieve the proper angle, and meanwhile everyone else just sits around waiting for the technicians. It's idiotic not to prepare ahead.

I have three scripts on hand at the moment. One is a comedy based on a piece by Gelett Burgess, and although he's been dead for something like thirty-eight years it seems remarkably modern. It's about a wealthy lady burglar in London who breaks into the home of a famous actor, not to rob it, but to absorb culture from its owner in conversation. Two writers, Arnold Belgard and Sam Perrin, who worked for a long time with Jack Benny, have collaborated with me on this. The other two scripts are respectively a melodrama and a comedy-drama.

Among English directors, I think David Lean is tops. I remember, not so long ago, when it was unheard of to get a leading lady in England: they had a lot of good leading men but no women. Now they have a lot of both: every time I see one of these characters come on, he or she is a star. You can only do that through constantly making pictures.

And the English, who go right on making films, not necessarily looking for the blockbuster that's going to make everybody rich in one go, are really accumulating great capital that way, because they've created stars.

Here, on the other hand, young actors who know next to nothing come in full of Method and what-not, and consider it an insult if you try to show them what to do in logical sequence because, not having been part of the invention, they feel robbed.

So you keep what you want to yourself and you all start searching for it together; only, since you have an ace up your sleeve—having already worked it out—you very subtly push the actors on to the thing that's already been discovered, and they're very happy because they feel they were part of the discovery.

I don't see any room for creativity in contemporary Hollywood. They've dissipated their directorial talents, while their other talents are now quite gone. They're not interested in restoring the commercial medium-budget picture and prefer to recruit their talent from television. That box in the corner is big business.

There are some very competent and clever people here, but conditions are such that you do a multi-million-dollar film—as Bobby Wise did with *The Sound of Music*—or you don't do a film at all; you have to go abroad.

You do television instead. I did six television jobs in order to find out what it was all about: two with Dick Boone, because he's a friend of mine; two with Hitchcock; a *Suspicion* special with Joan Harrison, a marvellous gal and also a friend; and one episode of *Arrest and Trial*.

I did the last one to ascertain how Univeral lives. The experience was horrible, and not only because of the rough schedule.

You say: "These conditions, this slavery that exists—why am I in it? I don't have to do it, I won't be hungry if I don't so it. Why should I do it—so that Wasserman and Stein[1] can cut up another five million?" So I quit.

---

[1] Lew Wasserman and Jules Stein, respectively president and chairman of the board of MCA-Universal.

Vincente Minnelli

Driven to Vincente Minnelli's Beverly Hills house by John Ford's chauffeur, we arrive unwittingly at the servants' entrance of the sprawling, low-slung building, tucked behind the flanking symmetrical palms of North Crescent Drive. A loud barking of terriers—seemingly a whole dog-kennel full—greets our appearance at 4 p.m., and a notably haughty Negro maid shows us through the kitchen to the living-room, where the atmosphere has exactly the expected Minnelli qualities: a suave artificiality, a coolly metallic precision and elegance.

Over the fireplace is the same huge speckled mirror that decorated Jack Buchanan's house in The Band Wagon. *On the marble or glass tables are bowls of metal fruit, copper-coloured, and sometimes flanked with razor-sharp metal leaves that, brushed against, would, one feels, leave a long thread of scarlet on a careless hand. The room is sealed and curtained against the daylight, as beige and still as though it were a set in a slightly faded sepia-tone film of thirty years ago. The grand piano looks like the kind you see in agents' offices in vintage musicals, crammed deep with pictures of family and famous in obligatory silver frames.*

Minnelli enters the room in a kind of sidelong, tentative movement like a particularly stylish crab. His arms, thin and delicate-boned, hang loosely from a cream T-shirt, and his body has a curious tension and frailty, a feeling of being just slightly off-balance, like that of someone caught on an unexpectedly slippery ballroom floor just before he slides into a fall. The eyes are hyperthalmic, black and round and brilliantly intense, just like Judy's. He doesn't enjoy being interviewed, so that the whole experience for

197

him is clearly a struggle between a polite attempt to reminisce and a desire to get the hell out of the ordeal. His head twists from side to side like that of a man bound wrist and ankle in a chair. Yet, as he smokes and sips powerful brews of coffee with incessant unease, he conveys, through a glancing laugh and an occasional thrust of wit, the charm and grace of his brilliant comedies and musicals.

I first began working at the Paramount Theatre in New York. I produced shows for Balaban and Katz when I got out of high school in Chicago, including the preparation of sets and costumes. I became art director at Radio City Music Hall for two years; the policy was to change the film each week, and during the time I was there they only held over one film twice; which meant that every seven days I had to create something fresh.

I began to direct and design Broadway shows. Not only would I handle the performers, but I'd light them and do the costumes as well; I was completely out of my mind! I'd never do that again. The first Broadway production I did was with Beatrice Lillie, a revue called *At Home Abroad*. And then an edition of the Ziegfeld Follies which Billie Burke produced; another thing with Beatrice Lillie called *The Show is On*, and one with Ed Wynn called *Hooray for What?* Harold Arlen wrote the score for that one.

The last show I did was for Jerome Kern and Oscar Hammerstein: *Very Warm for May*. I taught myself as an artist, a designer; I never went to art or technical school. Arthur Freed—the producer at MGM—came to see me in New York, and sold me on the idea of coming out to Hollywood; and for a whole year I had no title or anything. At the studio I just worked in all departments and did some writing and some shooting of numbers. Any producer could call me, and ask me to work on his script; and finally I directed the all-Negro musical, *Cabin in the Sky* for Freed in the early forties.

I directed all Lena Horne's numbers in other directors' films: she came to the studio about then. Pictures of the quality of *Panama Hattie*, unfortunately. But Freed was a marvellous showman, and we worked well together: he had a wonderful flair for getting people out here to the Coast—he was the first to use Alan Jay Lerner, and Betty

Comden, and Adolph Green—people like that—and then he'd let them create.

He wasn't creatively involved himself; we'd talk over everything with him in the broadest terms; only, of course, I had problems with the MGM art department; I had to revolutionize them initially. They were shocked at a lot of things I wanted to do. At the beginning it was rather a strain, but they saw everything my way in the end. Their methods were staid and old-fashioned, and they weren't integrated properly; and I liked to feel that numbers should be given as much importance as dramatic sequences, that they should be woven into the story completely in a way they hadn't been hitherto.

I worked very closely in with the art directors, and I was lucky in having men of the calibre of Preston Ames and Jack Martin Smith to help me with the designs. I always liked to shoot with just one camera, which wasn't all that common. I preplanned the films very carefully; I worked with the writers on the scripts in detail. But there was always an area for improvisation as well. I rehearsed a great deal, and then had the minimum of takes.

And I worked in very closely with the dance directors. Not everything I made I chose myself; I was working for a big commercial studio after all, and I had to accept everything I was given; but there are ways of achieving a certain quality in a film in spite of its lack of promise as a subject; and I hope I managed to raise the level fairly often.

For *Cabin in the Sky* there were a few changes: some new songs by Harold Arlen ("Happiness is a Thing Called Joe" was one of them); and for *I Dood It* as well. Someone else had started shooting that film, and had done some numbers which weren't very good; and I had to go in and save it. I did what I could.

My first colour film was *Meet Me in St Louis*: about the St Louis fair of 1903, a version of the famous *New Yorker* true stories by Sally Benson. The material was brought to Freed, and some people worked on a screenplay, but unfortunately they made a mistake in the writing: they didn't feel Sally Benson had enough "story", so they made up an awful lot of plot and that was a mistake. So Freed called me in, and I went right back to the original material. The people at Metro were very much against the idea I had of following the material to the letter. They insisted: "There's no story, nothing happens."

But Freed and I were determined (and so was Judy Garland, who had hated the way the whole thing had been "written up") to preserve the autobiographical, series-of-sketches flavour.

We all felt that this was a story which should be played and presented very realistically. We recreated St Louis as it was at the time of the Fair; the look of the film was based squarely on period shots of the town. The costumes by Irene Sharaff were marvellously authentic.

The famous Trolley Song scene was originally just a straight-forward number which Judy would sing; but I wanted a lot of suspense in it, such as whether a boy would or would not be able to make the trolley, and so on. It was worked into the plot; it wasn't just a number hanging in the air.

Charles Walters worked on the film with me, and did a wonderful job on the dance direction of the number "Skip to My Lou". What attracted me most to the subject was the Hallow-e'en sequence, when the little girl, played by Margaret O'Brien, is frightened, and there's a wonderful feeling of family. When we first ran the picture, it was too long, and a studio executive suggested we should reduce the length by taking out the Hallow-e'en sequence, which, he said, could easily be eliminated. I nearly went out of my mind, but luckily the Metro people saw the light and changed their views; they looked at the picture without that scene and it was an entirely different and much inferior film, a boy and girl picture, and not a family picture, which was what we wanted. We went back and cut another number with Judy, and a bit more instead, and the length was brought down that way .

We had a problem with Margaret O'Brien, who played the little girl. She was always in war films, and her speciality was crying hysterically. She had been taken in hand by a dramatic coach whom she imitated; so much so that she wasn't like a child—or a human being, even. She was just like Sarah Bernhardt; every gesture was enormous, as in the *Comédie française*. The problem was to have her to act like a child again, and to get her to do so, to be normal, was incredibly difficult; I had to work very hard on her.

The Clock, my next picture, began with another director, and with a beautiful screenplay, which unfortunately wouldn't work when it was filmed. The studio was planning to shelve it. It was the story of a young boy and girl who wander around New York saying banalities to cover up what they really feel; it was very difficult to do that way because the remarks would simply have sounded banal to an audience anyway. So I had to do something with it, and I didn't have much time to save it; I decided at once to make New York another character, and I introduced a number of crazy New York people, subway weirdies, that kind of person, and I used a lot of improvisation, not actually having a new script written but instead developing new ideas, new situations and dialogue as we went along.

For instance, there was a scene of a little boy and a pond; he's sailing his boat, and Bob Walker, who played the boy (Judy Garland played the girl), made friends with him in the original; it was all terribly "darling". But instead I made him kick Walker; and that made him more real, more human.

Yolanda and the Thief was not completely successful; a fantasy that just didn't perfectly come off; but it had a very fine ballet done by a New York choreographer, Eugene Loring. The story was by Ludwig Bemelmans, and the film was made in Bemelmans's paintbox colours, which I think was an effective device. At that time, unfortunately, fantasies of that kind just weren't very popular, and the film wasn't a great success. And Lucille Bremer, who played opposite Fred Astaire in the film, should have been much better: she was a protégée of one of the studio bosses, and was quite unsuitable.

There was a problem in making my revue film, *Ziegfeld Follies*, because you had to use the various stars in it as they became available from other pictures. I should say I directed about two-thirds of it; the best thing in it was the "Limehouse Blues" ballet, danced by Fred Astaire. For that sequence, one of the finest things I have done, I had a pantomime prologue and epilogue painted in two colours only: yellow and brown.

The style of the prologue and epilogue was based on English mezzotints: very dim and foggy. The central Chinese fantasy was done not so much in the Chinese manner as in the style of French *chinoiserie*, furniture designs, panels and so on, of the time of Louis XVI. The French of that period had their own strange conception of China as they had of an America populated by Indians with feathers. Quite absurd, but beautiful in its own way.

I enjoyed making *Undercurrent*, a thriller, with Robert

Taylor and Katharine Hepburn. I was fascinated by the characters' neurotic behaviour, by their psychological inter-relationships. I always am willing to take on a subject that might seem alien to me, to look for things below its surface.

The Pirate, with Gene Kelly and Judy Garland, took me back to the musical; it had been a play starring the Lunts on Broadway, based by S. N. Behrman on an old Spanish work. The style was inherent in the material, the eighteen-thirties in the Caribbean, and the setting was an international port which took its colours from many different countries. Although the film was deliberately stylized, I wanted to create the feeling that the story could easily have happened, in Martinique or an island of that kind. We did actually avoid all locations, so as to ensure a deliberately artificial flavour. Cole Porter wrote the score.

For the "Mack the Black" ballet, in which Gene Kelly as the pirate dances all over a set billowing with flames, we had Robert Alton do the choreography; but Gene Kelly and I provided most of the ideas for it: the fire was our idea.

Madame Bovary was a subject that appealed to me because I had always like Flaubert's novel. The first script was wrong, it was altogether too simple, too pat: you just can't be too logical with a subject like Emma Bovary; so many writers have described her, Maugham, Freud even, and none of them agrees about her. She is a controversial character, open to all kinds of interpretation.

I saw her as enormously complex: she was always living in a dream-world wanting things to be beautiful, and yet she was caught in the mire of ugly areas of living. She refused to accept that fact, and lived beyond herself, beyond her means. Jennifer Jones saw the character as I did, and she was marvellous for it, because she's an Emma Bovary herself, very contradictory, very romantic.

For the ballroom scene, in which Emma is whirled into an atmosphere of dazzling excitement, I asked Miklos Rozsa to compose a very "neurotic" waltz, and it had to be the exact length of the sequence: it was put together with a stop-watch. I shot entirely to the music, so that each cut was timed precisely to the dictates of the score, including the scenes that showed Charles Bovary at the gaming tables in between the dancing. We used various kinds of camera crane, and the idea was for the whirling camera never to let go of the figures.

At the end the windows are smashed to let in air, because Emma is fainting. That conclusion to the scene was, of course, taken from the novel itself. Throughout the picture I kept using mirrors, the mirror in the farm showing her always trying to glamorize herself, dreaming of something she wasn't; in the seminary, where she read the French romantic novels of the time; and then in the ballroom, when she glances into the glass and sees herself surrounded by men in the one perfect image that fulfils her romantic hopes. And then you see her in a dingy hotel room with her lover, and a cracked mirror displays her ruin; it is a recurring image that nobody noticed.

Father of the Bride was based on the book of reminiscences of a banker, and had to be absolutely authentic. I used a simple style to match the simplicity of the subject. Spencer Tracy set the pace of the film; you can't go any higher in comedy than Spencer Tracy, and he was magnificent. It was the first time I had worked with Elizabeth Taylor, and I was surprised to find that she was a marvellous actress with a great deal of depth; it took a lot of sensitivity to play the part of the banker's daughter in the touching way that she did.

In *An American in Paris*, with Gene Kelly and Leslie Caron, the script idea was to precede the multi-coloured ballet at the end with a masked ball. That idea annoyed me terribly: so arbitrary, there seemed to be no point in the ball. Then all of a sudden I thought of using a black-and white ball; I called Freed and he was delighted with the idea, because black and white had the advantage of resting the eyes from colour, so that, when the ballet came on, the colour seemed more fresh and immediate.

The film originated because Freed wanted to do a picture using Gershwin music, and *An American in Paris* was to be the ballet; Alan Jay Lerner was brought in, and we developed the story of a young American artist, Gene Kelly. It was quite daring then to finish the picture with a twelve minute ballet, and have no dialogue at all after it. Everybody at the studio thought we were crazy, but we did it anyway.

We found Leslie Caron like this: there was a girl we had heard of in Paris, and Gene Kelly was in England at the time; we wired him to go over and see this girl, Leslie Caron. Luckily he had seen her, in a Roland Pettit ballet called "The Sphinx", and had already tested her on his own; immediately we saw the test we were very impressed. Her mother was American, so she spoke English well enough.

Apart from a second unit montage of Paris streets early on, the entire picture was made in Hollywood. While we stopped to rehearse the ballet for three or four weeks, I made *Father's Little Dividend* on another set. It was a sequel to *Father of the Bride*, in which a new baby is born to the family: it was all right, up to the baby—but after that it was all clichés. Albert Hackett and Frances Goodrich, who had written *Father of the Bride* based on actual experiences, had to make up the new plot, and it wasn't real.

The Bad and the Beautiful was set in Hollywood: the story of a dynamic producer, played by Kirk Douglas, and the people who love and hate him. The central figure is a composite of many people: Val Lewton was the inspiration for the scene in which Douglas points out that terror is far more frightening if you don't show the source of the menace; and some of David O. Selznick was in the part.

The character of the drunken star (Lana Turner) whose father was a famous actor was based partly on Diana Barrymore; and we had Louis Calhern do a kind of imitation of John Barrymore's voice on a record. I was amazed that Lana Turner was capable of playing the part so well! She responds if you take time and trouble with her; if you don't, she'll just sail along. In the scene when she storms out of Douglas's house after finding him with a floozy and breaks down in the car in the middle of the traffic, we had to have the car revolving round the camera, and we explained the action to her much as you might explain choreographed movements to a dancer. We went over it once mechanically, and then she did the entire thing in one take. She was excellent for the part.

Up to that time, Kirk Douglas hadn't played anything as restrained as the producer and I liked to have him restrained; he's enormously vital, and you have to keep a tight rein on him at all times.

The Story of Three Loves was originally to have had three directors, but I finally directed a larger portion of it, and a prologue and epilogue were added that destroyed the thing completely. For *The Band Wagon*, we had Jack Buchanan as a crazy high-powered producer in a story about backstage.

We weren't sure about him at first: that he could play a

scoundrel, a dominating self-centered person. The man was a cross between Orson Welles, Norman Bel Geddes, and Jose Ferrer, who had at that time done similar pretentious theatrical productions: there was an awful lot of my own remembrance of the theatre in that picture; my days with Balaban and Katz, and at the Paramount. All the out-of-town scenes, the moment when things go wrong at a first night, were terribly authentic, autobiographical. *The Long, Long Trailer* was, like so many of my films, based on real experiences as well: the story of a man who had owned a trailer, and we cast Desi Arnaz and Lucille Ball, who were then in the full, fine flush of "The Lucy Show".

In keeping with my usual style, I made *Brigadoon* entirely on the sound-stage. I studied photographs of Scotland: misty monotones, yellows and greens, and based the film on those subdued colours throughout its length. The central set of the Scottish village was broken up into vistas: everywhere you pointed the camera it showed a different vista.

The Cobweb, like *Undercurrent*, was a psychological story which appealed to me strongly: it was set in a mental institution. John Houseman bought the book, and the original script failed to work, so we called in the author of the original novel, William Gibson, who had based much of it on his own experiences. His wife was a psychiatrist in a hospital: Menninger's, I think. Like *Brigadoon* this film was made in CinemaScope, which presented problems: it was hard to do closeups, they involved distortion of the face, so there weren't as many closeups as I would have liked to have. Luckily, by the time I had made a couple of films in the new medium, they had worked out satisfactory lenses, and these made good closeups possible.

I never did like CinemaScope very much: it's not so much that it's wider as that there's less on the top and bottom. I don't think it's the right composition for pictures.

I wasn't happy with the way *Kismet* emerged. I had succeeded in persuading MGM to let me do *Lust for Life*, but in return I had to do *Kismet* beforehand; I had to finish it in a hurry and get on a plane and go to Europe and start *Lust for Life*: they were keeping a field of wheat alive for me artificially in the south of France until I got there! So I did *Kismet* in a terrible hurry.

We worked in all the places where Van Gogh had

lived: at Arles, the asylum in San Remy, in Paris, at his father's home in Holland, in Amsterdam, the Borinage coalmine in Belgium. The people in his painting "The Potato Eaters" look like no one you have ever seen, and yet they exist, and we found them in Holland.

Kirk Douglas was the only possible choice for the role, first of all because of his physical appearance, which is ideal, and then for his great violence, a marvellous quality for playing for the part, because Van Gogh, like Douglas, was very fierce in his loves and his hates: a wonderful performance. Done to the life.

Gigi was a charming story; I had always wanted to do it. I worked very happily with Cecil Beaton on recreating the world of Colette. The studio wouldn't be persuaded to hire him initially, because he was so expensive, but he was definitely the man for the job. He's a very great artist. *The Reluctant Debutante* was entirely made in Paris: at the time, Rex Harrison and his wife couldn't work in England, as they'd used up the quota of what they were allowed to earn. We did the whole thing in a French studio, and it was developed, rewritten as we went along.

We started *Home from the Hill* at Oxford, Mississippi, where Faulkner lived, then went to Texas and then back to Hollywood. George Peppard got his big start in that picture: he was very much a Method actor, and sometimes that works and sometimes it doesn't: we had to find a common ground for working on and, at first, that was a problem. After all, we started on location, and you can't wait for "something to happen inside of you" when you're losing the sun and have to do a take: it just doesn't work. Finally I had to tell him: "I know you're a seething volcano of emotions, but I have news for you: nothing is happening." When we got back to the studio there was more time to discuss these things, and dig into the character. And he wound up giving a wonderful performance.

I had wanted *The Four Horsemen of the Apocalypse* done in the period of the First World War, not the Second: but the studio wouldn't agree. And then they insisted on dubbing in Angela Lansbury's voice for Ingrid Thulin, because they claimed that Ingrid Thulin's voice could not be properly understood. Ridiculous! And the very bad script had to be fixed as we went along; I didn't like it at all.

In *Two Weeks in Another Town* I returned to the theme of picture people; this time the story was about

Hollywood figures in Italy. It was very badly cut by the studio head, without a moment's warning; John Houseman, who produced it, was in Europe, and I'd been out of town when it happened, and when we learned the news it was too late to do anything about it, because the negative had been tampered with. The man in charge of the studio was fired within two weeks, but it was too late to undo the damage he had done.

The cutting ruined the whole conception: for instance, there's a scene in which the Hollywood star, played by Cyd Charisse, is explaining her philosophy to a newspaperman, and the philosophy is very beastly and brutal. The whole flavour of an orgy scene was lost, and so much else was taken out: the inner motivation of the characters, the pressures that made them act the way they did, the manner in which their lives intertwined and reacted on each other, abrasively or happily. Owing to this picking away at the material, what was profound became shallow . . . it's painful to talk about the ruin of that film even now.

Once again, *Goodbye Charlie*, about a husband and wife who change roles, was damaged by cutting: the studio took out a key scene; one in which Tony Curtis is in the kitchen and delivers a wonderful speech about identity, the monstrous struggle to get along without an identity. He talked about the sordid things we all live by: identity cards, fingerprints . . . records of every little thing we do, of everything until we die . . . and during this, all in one take, as the wife is preparing her own lunch and eating it, very messily, just as a man would do.

I never liked the story of *The Sandpiper*, but I wanted to work with the Burtons, and I did what I could with it, and all you *could* do was make it visually as good as possible.

Sad to say, I never did *Say it With Music*, on which I'd been working for four years. It's three stories in one, covering sixty years of Irving Berlin's music; one story is contemporary, then there's one in the twenties, and another in 1911. You go back and forth in time, as in Thornton Wilder's *The Skin of Our Teeth*. Berlin wrote four or five new songs, and we'd turn all his ragtime songs, twelve to fifteen of them, into a ballet toward the end of the picture. And, as in *An American in Paris*, not just an isolated thing on its own, but a ballet that resolves certain elements in the plot. After all that work and heartbreak MGM shelved the project and I went to Paramount to do

On A Clear Day You Can See For Ever with Barbra Streisand instead.

I find the contemporary film very exciting; there are so many levels, and each time I go to the cinema I find wonderful things. I liked *Blow-Up* enormously, and I wanted it to win at Cannes, which it did. It accomplished what it set out to do, to show England, the world of photographers; it was completely authentic. And I like realism, in all pictures. If a film involves you, and is interesting for what it sets out to do, then I like it.

Making pictures is the same everywhere. It doesn't matter where you make them: once you're on a set, it depends on you: most of my films, although made in a studio, have been in a sense independent films. And freedom is the essential, the one thing none of us can do without.

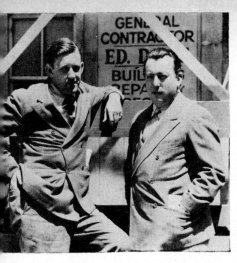

Novelist John O'Hara visits Lewis Milestone (*right*) on the set of *The General Died at Dawn*.

Maureen O'Hara, Finlay Currie, Peter Lawford, Richard Boone and Chips Rafferty in Milestone's *Kangaroo*.

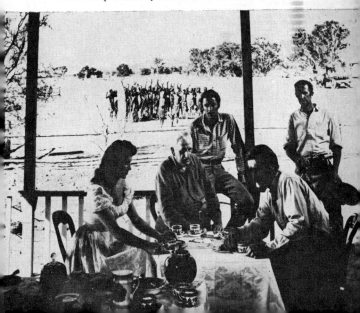

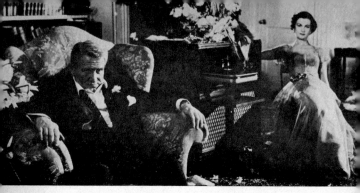

Spencer Tracy and Joan Bennett in Minnelli's *Father of the Bride.*
By courtesy M-G-M.

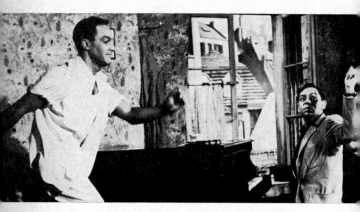

Gene Kelly and Oscar Levant in Minnelli's *An American in Paris.*

Edward G. Robinson and Rosanna Schiaffino in Minnelli's *Two
Weeks in Another Town.*

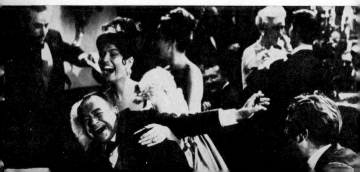

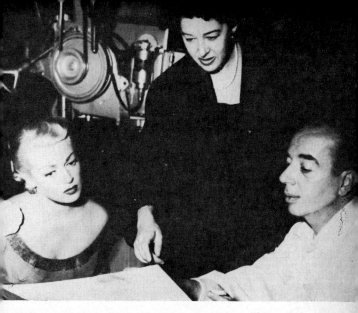

Director Vincente Minnelli and Lana Turner (*left*) during the making of *The Bad and the Beautiful*.

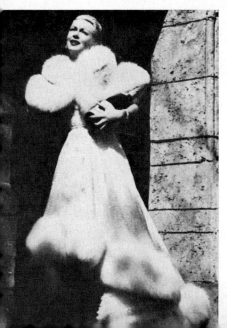

Lana Turner in Minnelli's *The Bad and the Beautiful*.

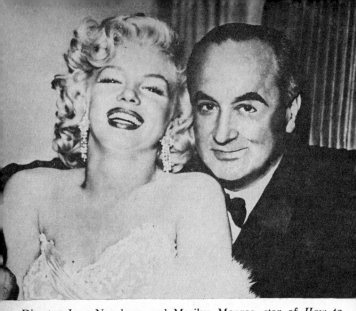

Director Jean Negulesco and Marilyn Monroe, star of *How to Marry a Millionaire*.

Gary Merrill and Evelyn Varden in Negulesco's *Phone Call from a Stranger*.

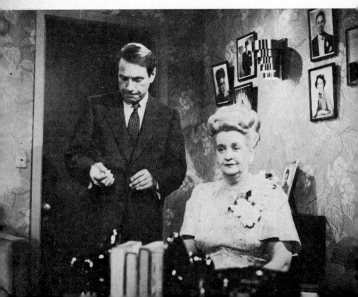

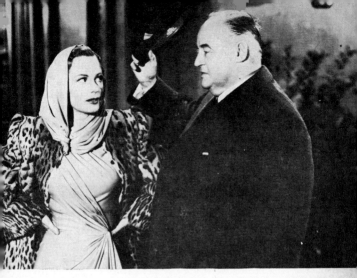

Geraldine Fitzgerald and Sydney Greenstreet in Negulesco's *Three Strangers.*

Jane Wyman (*left*), Agnes Moorehead and Lew Ayres in Negulesco's *Johnny Belinda.*

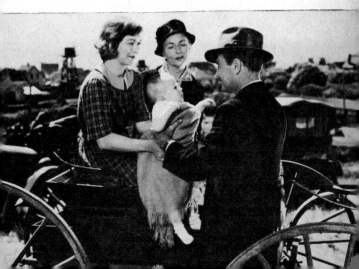

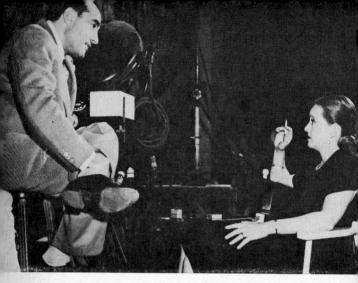

Director Irving Rapper and Bette Davis on the set of *Deception*.

Robert Alda in Rapper's
Rhapsody in Blue.

Paul Henreid in Rapper's
Deception.

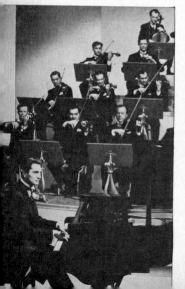

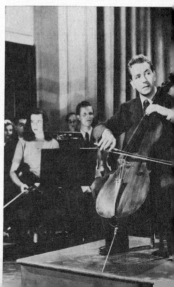

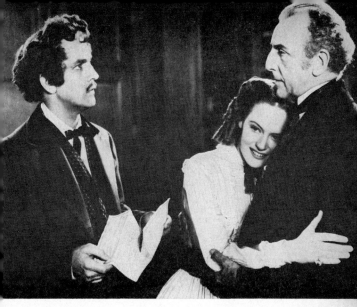

Fredric March, Alexis Smith and Walter Hampden in Rapper's *The Adventures of Mark Twain.*

Claude Rains and Bette Davis in Rapper's *Now Voyager.*

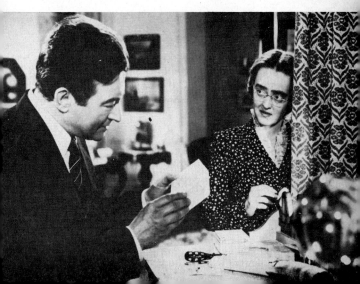

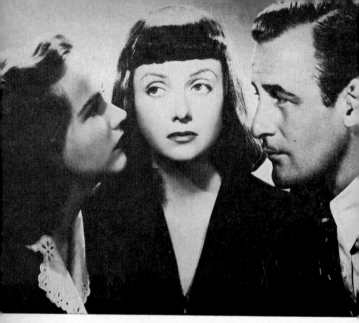

Kim Hunter, Jean Brooks and Tom Conway in Mark Robson's
The Seventh Victim.

Boris Karloff in Robson's *Bedlam*.

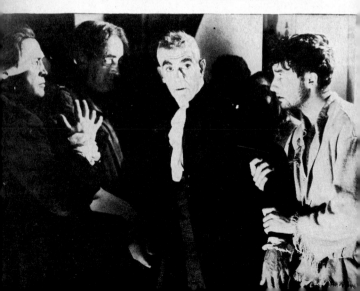

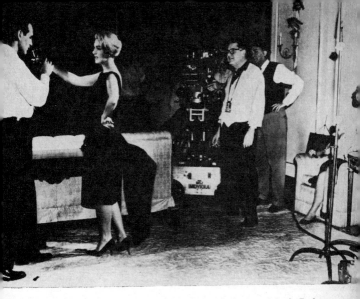

Paul Newman and Joanne Woodward with director Mark Robson on the set of Robson's *From the Terrace*.

Tony Scotti, Sharon Tate and Lee Grant in Robson's *Valley of the Dolls*.

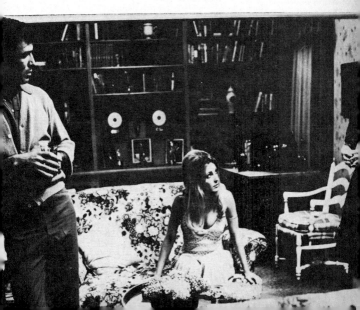

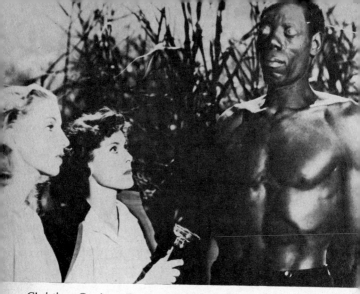

Christine Gordon, Frances Dee and Darby Jones in Jacques Tourneur's *I Walked with a Zombie*.

Jane Greer and Robert Mitchum in Tourneur's *Out of the Past*.

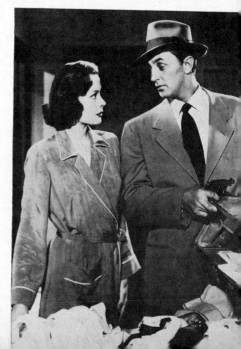

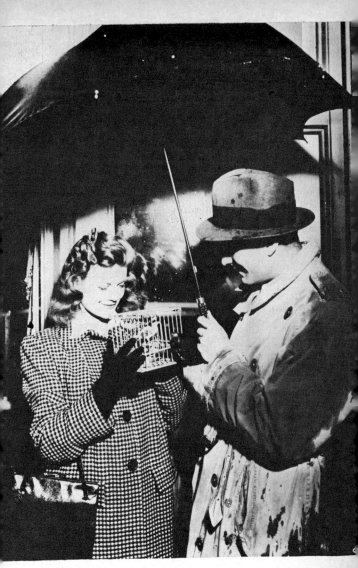

Simone Simon and Kent Smith in Tourneur's *Cat People*.

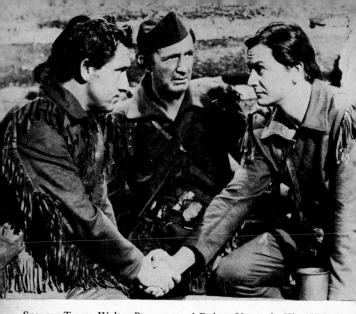

Spencer Tracy, Walter Brennan and Robert Young in King Vidor's *Northwest Passage.*

Joseph Cotten (*center*), Otto Kruger and Harry Carey in Vidor's *Duel in the Sun.*

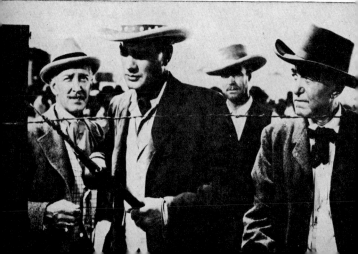

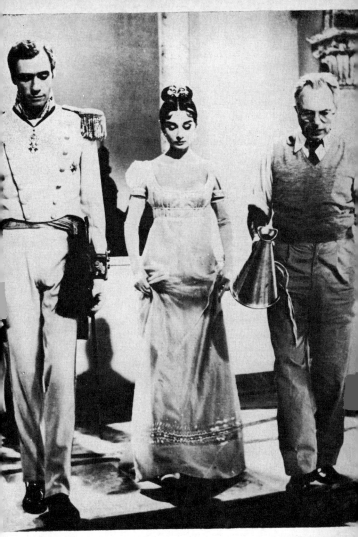

King Vidor (*right*) with Mel Ferrer and Audrey Hepburn making
War and Peace.

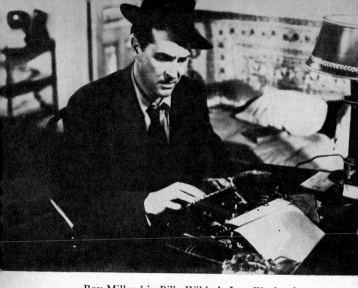

Ray Milland in Billy Wilder's *Lost Weekend*.

Erich von Stroheim and Gloria Swanson in Wilder's *Sunset Boulevard*.

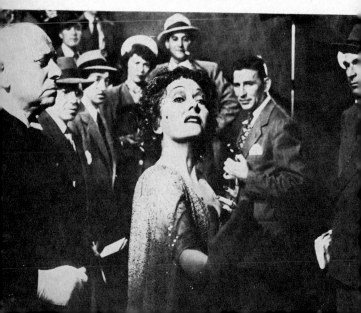

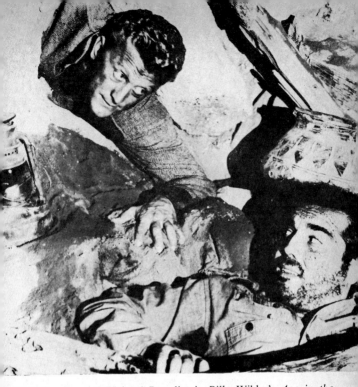

Kirk Douglas and Richard Benedict in Billy Wilder's *Ace in the Hole* (U.S. title *The Big Carnival*).

Tony Curtis and Jack Lemmon in Wilder's *Some Like it Hot*.

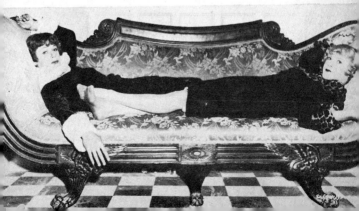

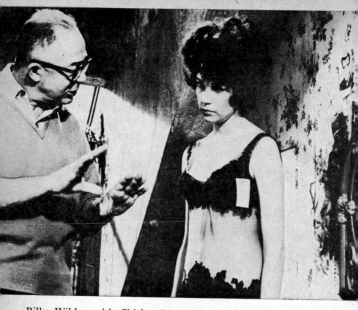

Billy Wilder with Shirley MacLaine, star of Wilder's *Irma La Douce*.

Jack Lemmon in Wilder's *The Apartment*.

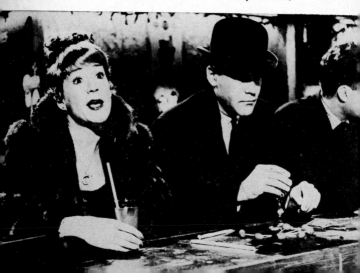

Jean Negulesco

From the Balkans to Beverly Hills via Paris, Jean Negu-
lesco's progress has taken him to the point where he now
owns not one but three splendid houses in the most lush
residential district of Los Angeles, together with other
properties and apartments in sundry world capitals. Arriv-
ing at one of his homes late in the afternoon, we discover
his wife, the former model and Columbia contract player
Dusty Anderson—whose appearances graced such forties
extravaganzas as A Thousand and One Nights, *and whom*
he married in 1946—conducting a lively real estate argu-
ment on the telephone. Real estate, not surprisingly, is her
hobby. Her husband's, to judge from the surroundings, is
pictorial art: besides Toulouse-Lautrec posters, the rooms
and corridors carry his own elegant line drawings and oil
paintings, reminders of his Parisian artist youth, spent
largely in the company of Modigliani. On the mantel
broods the same idol, Kwan-Yin, Chinese goddess of mer-
cy, that figured memorably in Negulesco's moody black
comedy of 1946, Three Strangers. *The director proves a*
delightful host, animated and charming, looking, with his
dark hair and lively brown eyes, some twenty years young-
er than his age (he is in his late sixties). A true cosmo-
politan, he has lately been endeavouring to set up an
Iranian film industry, journeying frequently to Teheran for
consultations with the government and putting at its dis-
posal the fruits of more than thirty years' movie experi-
ence. In this, as in all he does, Jean Negulesco displays a
civilized urbanity that is immediately appealing. Holly-
wood success, he demonstrates, need not result in kidney-
shaped pools, fur-lined toilet seats and pink Cadillac con-
vertibles; it may also mean a heightened pursuit of culti-

vated pleasures, a life-style of opulent yet unaffected good taste.

I was born in Romania, and before coming to America as a successful painter in 1929, I lived and worked as an artist for fifteen years in Paris. Brancusi was my teacher, and about 1918 I got to know Modigliani, spending a lot of time in his studio; he only started to paint, incidentally, because he found it too expensive to sculpt.

I began my motion picture career at Paramount in the early nineteen-thirties as technical adviser on a rape scene. The film was *The Story of Temple Drake,* an adaptation of William Faulkner's *Sanctuary,* starring Miriam Hopkins.

I did some drawings showing how the scene could be managed so as to pass the censors—it was suggested with hands, fingers and so on—and the picture's producer, Benjamin Glazer, liked some of my sketches so much that he made me his assistant.

Being an assistant producer was a little more complicated than being an assistant director. I acted as sort of a go-between between the producer and the director because they were usually feuding. However, I gained an extraordinary amount of experience through that, because I sat in on every story conference, fought over the cutting of pictures with the editor in the cutting-room, and examined all the rushes in detail.

I worked on all Benjamin Glazer's films: the Maurice Chevalier pictures, the *Big Broadcast* pictures, musicals. My first assignment was to do the opening of a musical called *This is the Night.* That was also Cary Grant's first film. Frank Tuttle directed, and Lily Damita was the star. After about two or three weeks they contemplated dropping Cary Grant from the film because of his pronounced Cockney accent. Fortunately they didn't, and he went on to become the great success he is.

Then I started doing second-unit things, working mainly on camera angles because of my painter's pictorial sense. I arranged camera angles for all the musicals, integrating the songs rhythmically with the movement of the images.

My biggest such job was the second-unit direction on Frank Borzage's 1932 version of Hemingway's *A Farewell to Arms,* with Gary Cooper and Helen Hayes. I did the battle scenes in that and had quite a torrid time, because I was trying to act as a director without having had a director's experience. I dressed the way I thought a director should, imitating Josef von Sternberg with his cravats and night-time working habits.

Borzage was a strange man. He'd have a scene with, say, three hundred extras, and all he'd be interested in was the way water would drip from a leaf and the way you'd see Gary Cooper passing by through this dripping water in the big retreat from Caporetto.

There was an amusing episode here. We had a wonderful unit manager who always considered every director to be a trifle crazy, requiring constant humouring. If the director was a foreigner all you had to do was say, "Yes, sir", and not to try to question anything.

We were working at night. I called him and said: "Charlie, I've been reading in the book about this exciting retreat from Caporetto, and among the refugees on the seven trucks bearing away the children, the old people and peasants and nuns, were the occupants of the evacuated Caporetto whorehouses. What a wonderful touch! Those painted whores holding children in their arms ... Charlie, tonight on each of those seven trucks I want to have between five and seven whores."

There was a big silence. "Did you hear me?" I asked.

"Yes, Jean," he replied. "You'll have them."

I arrived on the set that night looking every inch a director with a big coat, a hat, a little cane, and a spotted cravat. "Well," I inquired, "where are the whores?"

"We're trying our best," Charlie said, "but I don't think we can fit seven on one truck."

I looked around and they were pulling horses onto the trucks.

"I didn't say horses," I exclaimed. "I said whores!" They laughed their heads off after that.

My second-unit work at Paramount and Universal so impressed a Warner Brothers producer of short subjects named Gordon Hollingshead that he hired me in a similar capacity on a picture dealing with the nineteenth-century Red Cross.

That was followed by a lot of dramatic and musical shorts at Warners, including some orchestral shorts and the first ballet films ever made, featuring the Ballet Russe de Monte Carlo, with Leonide Massine, Tamara Toumanova, and Danilova. They included *Capriccio Espagnole* and *Gaîté Parisienne*.

Then I had a chance to do a feature. Jack Warner, who was brilliant at knowing how to find things, said:

"Why don't we get some new directors with fresh ideas to make pictures for $300,000 or $400,000? With those small budgets, we can't lose."

So when they asked me what I would like to do—Hollingshead was supposed to be the producer—I said, *"The Maltese Falcon."* It had been nominally made twice—the previous versions had starred respectively Ricardo Cortez and Bebe Daniels, and Warren William and Bette Davis—but neither version paid much respect to the book. Neither was really *The Maltese Falcon*.

When you have a good property, a successful property, why spoil it? It's like when I saw Artur Brauner recently. He wants to do *Passion Flower Hotel*. I read the script, which was competent enough. But I said, "It's not going to be as good as the book. Good or bad, the book is a success. The public likes it, it has a certain quality: use it, don't lose it. Why do you want to apologize for it, to dilute it?"

And this is one of the greatest sins of the moving picture scene everywhere. Producers, or people getting great salaries, want to "lick" a story, and in the process of licking it they change it.

But to return to *The Maltese Falcon*: I started work, and after about two months they called me saying: "It's too bad, but somebody else wants to do *The Maltese Falcon* and you'll have to go back to doing shorts."

Naturally I was miserable. Then I found that John Huston was doing the picture as his first directorial feature. I liked John, had a great admiration for him. "Good luck to him," I said. He did a beautiful job, too, following the book closely; my handling of the film would not have differed significantly from his.

One night soon afterwards I was playing gin rummy or something with a group of people that included Anatole Litvak. Over a drink Litvak said to me: "I heard that you were trying to do *The Maltese Falcon* and they took it away from you."

"Please," I said. "I knew nothing about John Huston's plans to do the film. I've now seen what he did and it's magnificent."

"Well," Litvak said, "I have a present for you. There is an Eric Ambler story that everyone has been trying to lick. It's called *The Mask of Dimitrios*, and when you've read it you'll be just as eager to do it as you were to do

The Maltese Falcon." (It was then called *A Coffin for Dimitrios.*)

I gave the story to Henry Blanke, the same producer who'd done *The Maltese Falcon*, and we sat at home three nights in a row, pasting up pages of the book, and that's how the script of the picture was made.

Then the time came to test actors for the film. My idea at that time was to let actors do whatever they liked in tests to find out how wrong they were. You either said, "It's wonderful"—because every actor is intelligent and has a few tricks—or stopped them.

So I made a test of Peter Lorre and Sydney Greenstreet. Peter was a joker—he and Humphrey Bogart were a great pair of clowns—forever perpetrating gags. When Lorre and Greenstreet monkeyed around during most of the test, I didn't say anything; I just let them go.

The next morning the producer, Blanke, came to me after looking at the rushes and said: "I saw the rushes. They are terrible. I want to tell you something, Jean. This is your first chance to make a picture. But if the first day's rushes are as bad as the test I've just seen, you won't be doing the film."

"Henry," I said, "I let them ruin the test just so I could see what they should *not* do. Let them monkey around for the time being; I don't care."

"Jean," he said, "I am worried."

Fortunately, next day I had quite a good scene. They liked the rushes of that and the picture proceeded smoothly. It came out very well, I thought.

But that was a tight spot because, when you wait fifteen years for a chance to do a picture and the producer tells you that the tests are so bad that you might be taken off next day, you are naturally upset—especially since I'd already been taken off two films that I'd begun (one was called *Singapore Woman*) and been demoted back to shorts.

In *The Mask of Dimitrios* I established a sombre, low-key mood that I followed in a number of subsequent films. I learned that the public loves to share the actor's situation, to be a vicarious part of the action. It's curious that when you see actors moving and talking in semidarkness it's always more exciting than seeing them plainly, because you identify with them more.

In 1946 I made *Three Strangers*, from John Huston's original story; Wolfgang Reinhardt produced it. Huston, however, was not responsible for two of the film's best scenes: the one around the idol Kwan-Yin, and the one in which Geraldine Fitzgerald stubs out her cigarette on the hand of her husband who has unexpectedly returned. The cameraman was Arthur Edeson, who'd photographed *The Maltese Falcon*; he was my cameraman on five or six consecutive films, including almost all those I made with John Garfield.

Three Strangers had some very weird scenes—such as that of Rosalind Ivan communing with the spirit of her dead husband through his portrait—that I thought impressively eerie, but the picture was not the success we expected.

When I told Jack Warner that I wanted Peter Lorre to play a romantic lead in it he laughed and said I must be crazy. But as the film cost almost nothing and I had no other assignment, I went ahead anyway.

Lorre was the most talented man I have ever seen in my life. If you watch *The Mask of Dimitrios*, you'll find that the whole picture, its entire mood, is held together by him. Without him, you're a little bored by it.

I think his chief asset lay in the element of surprise. When you expected him to be quiet he was loud. When a scene in *The Mask of Dimitrios* threatened to run down, for example, this little man would shout for no reason at all; and as you were slowly recovering from the shock he'd ask mock-innocently: "Did I scare you?"

He was wonderful. When they were measuring his distance from the camera with a tape-measure—and everybody was just sitting there bored stiff—he would scare the bejeezus out of the man measuring with a sudden yelp and the poor guy nearly dropped the tape; that's the kind of thing he did with his scene in *The Mask of Dimitrios*.

I allowed Lorre complete freedom to improvise. Sometimes he went too far, and then I think it's the role of a director to step in and say: "I think it's wonderful, it's very funny, but it's not in keeping with the mood and style of the rest of the film." Something similar happened in *The Mudlark* with Alec Guinness, who was so good, so different, that the rest of it was thrown a little out of balance.

But it's generally a good idea for an actor to improvise, because it keeps him thinking about the role; he stays at home with it, he wants to improve it. And, because a modern actor who has achieved a certain standing in the industry is a human being who reads and collects and listens to music, he has certain valid notions about his part or about the significance of the picture.

Sometimes it can be terrible. Lately we saw three great personalities come together disastrously in *A Countess from Hong Kong*. Two of them were impressed with the third, a genius, and, having great respect and admiration for this man, tried to imitate him; and of course the thing came out very weak.

Joan Crawford didn't improvise in *Humoresque*. She is a very effective actress, and so much a star that her acting spills over into her private life. If she is a mother, she *acts* like a mother, the best mother in the world. If she is a mistress—which I don't know about—she probably acts like the greatest mistress in the world. Everything for her is acting; this is her life, her food, her drink. She gives herself completely to any part she has to play, whether it's sad, or gay, or whatever.

After we'd been making the picture for about a week, Jerry Wald, the producer, came to me saying that Joan had entered his office weeping and complaining that I didn't want to talk to her.

I asked him what he meant. "Well," he said, "you don't explain any of the scenes she's doing to her."

"What is there to explain?" I asked. "We've had no scenes yet to discuss. Everything she's done so far she's done admirably. After all, you can only walk into a room three ways, fast, slow, or medium. You open the door or you don't open the door; you break it down or you push it open."

"Anyway, *talk* to her, whatever you do," he said. "Do something to improve her morale."

I went home really quite worried. How could I talk to her? How could I get through to her? I couldn't serenade her with a violin or anything.

Then my wife Dusty said, "Why don't you do a portrait of her?" And I did a wonderful portrait embodying what I thought the *Humoresque* character being played by Joan should be, highlighting the lips, darkening some portions of the face.

When I gave it to her she cried with happiness, saying: "*Now* I know what you mean. You don't have to spell it out in words."

"Joan," I said, "I'm sorry, but I'm not an eloquent man.

This is what I think the character should be." And we were very good friends after that.

Humoresque was a very successful picture—it played one Mexican theatre continuously for three years—but I have occasionally been criticized for some of the fancy dissolves I used in it: the blind-roll dissolving into a piano keyboard, the soda-water dripping from the siphon and dissolving into a wave, etc. This was a period in which I was trying to be "clever" and when such arty effects were all the rage. Later they became so over-indulged that people looking at them today exclaim, "My God, that's so banal!"

That's often the fate of films that once seemed original. Not long ago I saw Ernst Lubitsch's *The Smiling Lieutenant*. It looked terribly old-fashioned because many of his wonderful touches have become so familiar through over-use that by now they are clichés.

Some of the technical effects in *Humoresque* were very elaborate without being showy, such as the scene of the ice-skaters being reflected upside down at Rockefeller Centre. That was all a beautiful piece of mechanical trickery. We were never in New York, just as there were no actual sea scenes in *Titanic*. Everything was done on the stages.

There *is* an inverted mirror at Rockefeller Centre. We made a complete process plate of the whole background scene and had our characters in the foreground. We started our shot at the process screen and then moved back to the characters; the illusion of actually being in New York was almost perfect.

The shot through the brandy glass at the beginning of the party sequence wasn't technically difficult to manage, although the cameraman at first said he couldn't do it.

"Try it," I said. "What can you lose? If necessary we can cut it out later." And it worked.

I chose to do that because I like to tell a story through the eye, and shooting a party through a glass seems to me to lend it more of a "party" feeling than just doing it conventionally with long-shots; I think it sets the mood quite effectively. You move when things get static; that's the secret of picture-making.

However, the most elaborate technical trick of all in *Humoresque* was the matching of John Garfield's fingering on the violin to the music pre-recorded by Isaac Stern—and, believe it or not, this is a *genuine* Hollywood story! It was very complicated and we made two or three unsuccessful attempts before getting it right.

First we tried it with a mask. This was during the war when there was a great shortage of rubber. I suggested putting a John Garfield mask on a real violinist and photographing him playing in long-shot. When I broached this idea to the makeup man, Perc Westmore, he said: "We'll try it, but I have a better idea. We'll get an actor who resembles Garfield, build up his face a bit, keep him in semi-darkness and let him play the violin like that."

On the first test we made the man look like Fred Clark. The next one was no better, so finally on my pleading they made the mask and clapped it on the chosen musician. Unfortunately you couldn't shoot with it for more than five minutes at a time because it somehow inhibited the wearer's breathing.

We gave the man a violin, started playing the pre-recorded music, and signalled him to start his imitation fiddling: whereupon some incoherent mumbling was heard coming from under the rubber mask. "What is it?" we asked. "Mumble, mumble ... " he went. So we took the thing off and he exclaimed, "I'm not a violinist, I'm a piccolo player!"

Then the prop man suggested: "Why don't you take *two* real violinists?"

So we made a big hole in the elbow of John Garfield's coat, and a real violinist's hand came through it and fingered the violin. Another violinist was behind him—there were three guys—doing the bowing, and John Garfield was in the middle.

It was perfect!

The really extraordinary part of this magnificent fake concert was that John Garfield couldn't even hold a fiddle! It was all done by two people stationed behind him, and the effect was fantastic. He told me later that everywhere he went people would ask him to give concerts. They'd bring him a violin and he'd protest, saying: "No, no, I don't feel well ... "

I did the same thing with Maurice Chevalier's guitar playing in *Jessica*; I had two men behind him. Since it's pre-recorded, it doesn't matter if the playing and the music don't match perfectly, as long as it looks more or less right.

The use of Wagner's *Liebestod* in the final sequence of *Humoresque* was not my idea but Oscar Levant's. Franz

Waxman, the picture's musical director, fought bitterly over it. "Let's listen to it," I said. We did listen to it and it was so beautiful that I suggested doing it as a violin concerto. The melody was just right for it, and the record afterwards sold immensely.

For *Deep Valley*, made the following year, I used Big Sur and Big Bear locations. It was all done on location, as a matter of fact, which was unusual at that time; everybody wanted to remain studio-bound.

There was a strike in progress in Hollywood then, so they sent us away with instructions not to come back for the time being. Someone had to be shooting something, and so we started to improvise and to build sets. Despite falling snow, we had to make the locations look spring-like with artificial flowers, especially at such moments when Dane Clark and Ida Lupino were looking at some fish in a stream.

The picture wasn't very successful at the box-office but it was very successful for me personally because Darryl F. Zanuck hired me on the strength of having seen it to do a film called *Road House*, also with Ida Lupino. He'd made every producer and director on his lot look at it to see how a movie should be shot on location. This was one of those occasions when, under pressure and force of circumstances, things of great quality sometimes emerge.

I love *Johnny Belinda* more than anything I have done, not only because it was my most successful picture, but also because I had a completely free hand in making it.

I'm very grateful to one man for landing the assignment, and that man, strangely enough, is Errol Flynn. I'd been assigned to do Flynn's *The Adventures of Don Juan*, the most expensive and sought-after project on the Warner lot. I had unorthodox ideas about Don Juan: I thought he should have been a victim of women rather than their victimizer. Flynn didn't agree with me at all because he still wanted to be the wonderful guy who jumps out of the window pursued by the irate husband saying "You made love to my wife" and all that.

After about three months, Flynn approached Warner saying: "I'd love to do the *Don Juan* picture but not with Negulesco." Whereupon Warner called me and said: "Johnny, I cannot make *Don Juan* without Errol Flynn but I *can* make it without you."

"You're absolutely right," I said.

"Why don't you go to Jerry Wald?" Warner suggested. "He has so many scripts."

Jerry gave me three scripts to read, and the first one was *Johnny Belinda*. Vincent Sherman went on to make *The Adventures of Don Juan* and subsequently lost his job at Warners, which was ironic in view of the fact that I lost my job there too after *Johnny Belinda*.

Making it, however, was the happiest experience of my life. We all loved what we did in it. This was the only time in my career when everybody connected with the film—including actors, cameramen, still-photographers, etc.—felt themselves an integral part of the project.

We stayed back at night, met every evening to discuss it. Actors would say: "You don't need me in this scene; the scene should go to so and so." That was the first time I'd seen actors altruistically trying to improve a picture at the expense of their own parts. The still-men would be up at 4 a.m. to get shots of the fields, long-shots with offbeat compositions. Then they'd develop them and bring them to me asking: "Is this what you meant?" And, by God, they were right! We were all together, all a part of this project.

We went on location north of San Francisco, seeking a landscape similar to Nova Scotia, the setting of *Johnny Belinda*. We found it at Fort Bragg—nothing was shot in Nova Scotia itself—the same place where they made *The Russians are Coming*: the same street, the same church, everything.

Jane Wyman lived and studied for two weeks with deaf-and-dumb people in preparation for her role. We had a technical adviser and also an actual deaf-and-dumb girl, who was like the girl in *Johnny Belinda*. Jane watched her all the time.

The trouble was that during tests and closeups you could see by the expression in Jane Wyman's eyes that she could hear what Lew Ayres and others were saying. So we consulted a doctor who had developed a combination of waxes which, when inserted in Jane's ears, rendered her quite deaf. You could have shot a gun off behind her and even in closeup it wouldn't have registered on her face. This is one of the reasons why the thing was so real and natural.

At Warner Brothers they didn't like *Johnny Belinda*. I don't know why. Maybe they felt it was too preachy. Maybe—and although this now sounds a little wild, it did occur to me at the time—Warners, having introduced talking pictures, didn't like the idea of a film about the deaf and dumb.

In fact, they took the camera away from me before I'd finished shooting it. The last shot of the film, according to the shooting script, is supposed to be of three people coming home, but instead of that they used an old shot of the doctor (played by Lew Ayres) alone. But that is one of the hazards of picture-making.

Jack Warner was opposed to offbeat pictures at that time. For example, he disliked *The Treasure of the Sierra Madre*. That appeared the same year as *Johnny Belinda*, and both were enormous successes. Yet he fired me.

If you'd been in his place, you'd realize that it wasn't difficult for a man like Warner—as indeed he admitted to me afterwards—to make that kind of mistake. It's not their fault. They're involved with so many things, have so many decisions to make. They might be in a bad mood one day and, looking at a picture like *Johnny Belinda*, will say: "Who is going to like this?"

They approve of a project. They approve of a cast. They look at the rushes. They let you go ahead. And sometimes they're maybe too hasty in finding faults.

After *Johnny Belinda* had received twelve Academy Award nominations, Warner called me long-distance and said: "Well, kid, we did it again!" By that time I'd not only been fired from Warners but I was working on *Road House* at Fox. Yet he said "we", and added: "Next time we do a picture we're going to get fourteen nominations!"

Zanuck would often make similar errors of judgement. When I used to play croquet with him at Palm Springs, we'd stop every Friday at San Bernadino on the way there and preview a film. I saw pictures on those occasions that were so funny, so successful with audiences, that people were in the aisles.

"This is going to be the greatest success of all time!" Zanuck would exclaim, and he'd wire Spyros P. Skouras, head of Twentieth Century-Fox, lengthily in those terms; and the picture would go out and be a big flop. That happened with a Jimmy Stewart picture called *Jackpot* and also with others. They all enjoyed extraordinary previews but failed on general release.

Working at Warners had been wonderful because it was a very tough training-ground. They had strict schedules which you couldn't exceed by so much as a day. I had to make shorts there at the rate of one reel daily; often I had to make do with existing sets and invent stories of my own. Budgets were very tight. Jack Warner kept a short economical rein on everything. *The Mask of Dimitrios,* for example, cost under $400,000.

Fox was very different to work for from Warners. It was not as tight or as strict; it was much more liberal. If they liked what you were doing, there was no limit to your budget, no restriction on your way of shooting, on your casting or anything.

Whereas Jack Warner was a difficult man to enthuse—he told you what to do and how to do it—Darryl Zanuck was a man who, if you could spark a little enthusiasm in him, would get twice as enthusiastic as you were. Not only that: if you made a mistake, he wouldn't hold you responsible. He'd say: "Don't try to be a hero."

We made a picture in England which was quite bad, called *Britannia Mews*. The critics crucified us, so I wrote him a letter saying: "I'm sorry, Darryl. I liked the cast, I liked the story, I thought I did my best. I promise I'll make it up to you somehow."

To which he replied by letter: "Who the hell do you think you are, playing the hero like that? I okayed the picture, I bought the book, I okayed the cast, I saw the rushes and approved them. Sure, you made a mistake, but so did we. Don't try to be a hero, just don't do it again, that's all."

I came to work for Zanuck from India, where I'd gone with my wife Dusty, feeling very low after having been fired from Warners over *Johnny Belinda*. Charlie Feldman, my agent, called me back saying he thought he could get me into Twentieth Century-Fox because they had a commitment with Ida Lupino who'd starred in *Deep Valley*, the film which had so impressed Zanuck.

From the beginning of our association, Zanuck was very fair with me. Handing me the script of *Road House*, my first Fox film, he stated with unusual honesty: "This is a bad script. Three directors have refused it. They don't know what they're doing, because basically it's quite good. Remember those pictures we used to make at Warner Brothers, with Pat O'Brien and Jimmy Cagney, in which every time the action flagged we staged a fight and every time a man passed a girl she'd adjust her stocking or something, trying to be sexy? That's the kind of picture we have to have with *Road House*. Now take it and do it like that."

I did, and it was very funny, some of the funniest lines going to Richard Widmark and Celeste Holm.

After that I did quite a number of films at Fox. One of the best was *Titanic*, which involved some tremendous technical problems. Firstly, I wanted to make it in colour, but these were the days just before the introduction of CinemaScope, and, owing to economic restrictions, I had to make it in black-and-white. Also, since the audience would be anticipating a catastrophic climax right from the beginning of the picture, I wanted to make the build-up, the preliminaries, as gay and light as possible, without hints of darkness; I wanted to play against the climax.

But it was difficult for the special-effects men, because sometimes they had to telescope seven or eight scenes together for technical reasons. So often I had to adjust my shooting schedule to fit in with their schemes. I'd shoot, say, part of a scene and stop, then pick it up somewhere else maybe the next day, and do it in pieces like that.

My favourite film I made at Fox is *Three Came Home*, starring Claudette Colbert and adapted from the book by Agnes Newton Keith. I like what I did with camera style in that. It was my first film with the writer and producer, Nunnally Johnson, with whom I made altogether four pictures. Florence Desmond, who was so good in it, was a friend of Nunnally's and the wife of an executive of Lloyd's of London. Sessue Hayakawa gave a beautiful, dignified performance as the prison-camp commandant, although he often forgot his lines. David Lean used him in *Bridge on the River Kwai* on the strength of his appearance in *Three Came Home*.

Under My Skin was the last film I made with John Garfield. He led a rough life and burned himself out. Playing single tennis one day, he collapsed on the court, foreshadowing his approaching death.

A film that cost little money was *Phone Call from a Stranger*, although it received a Lion of Venice award for its script, the work of Nunnally Johnson. I'll never forget Bette Davis in it: a complete professional, she'd come on the set and transform herself as if by magic into the bedridden invalid she played; she really "became" that woman.

I was nearly thrown out of the movie industry over a dispute on *The Last Leaf*, a segment I directed for the episode film *O. Henry's Full House*. Union rules declared that three painters were required to paint a leaf on a wall! Jean Peters, now the wife of Howard Hughes, gave a touching performance. She never wanted to be an actress. She would much rather have been a teacher; in fact, I think she had a slight inferiority complex about it. I used her also in my remake of Jean Renoir's *Swamp Water*, called *Lure of the Wilderness*.

My initial tests for *How to Marry a Millionaire* were done in 3-D. Then, when Fox officially adopted Cinema-Scope for all its films, I switched to making it in that. It brought numerous problems. How, for example, were you going to do intimate scenes on that great wide oblong? And this was supposed to be a comedy!

On the first day of shooting there was no viewfinder and the cameraman, the late Joe MacDonald, had to guess the composition of the images. Also, the film stock was heavy and had little scratches running through it. Because of our unfamiliarity with the new process, we did the opening scene between the three girls—Betty Grable, Lauren Bacall, and Marilyn Monroe—nine times.

Soon, however, we acclimatized ourselves to Cinema-Scope and I quickly went on to do *A Woman's World*, which I shot at short notice and at tremendous speed in twenty-two days, because Zanuck wanted the picture to open at a certain time. Then came *Daddy Long Legs*, a musical with Fred Astaire and Leslie Caron and marvellous costumes designed by Tom Keogh. Shooting of that film was saddened by the death in the midst of it of Fred Astaire's wife.

I also did a remake of Clarence Brown's *The Rains Came* called *The Rains of Ranchipur*, with Eugénie Léontovitch in the part originally played by Maria Ouspenskaya. I'm afraid Louis Bromfield, the author of the novel on which it was based, wasn't very happy with it.

From my film version of Françoise Sagan's *A Certain Smile* people seemed to expect a "dirty" picture, but the writers made it instead into quite a gentle, rather advanced love story.

The Best of Everything was my final film with Jerry Wald. Jerry's energy was fantastic, and his creative contribution to the films he made considerable, though often indirect. His death came as quite a shock to me. I remember receiving the news with two other friends of his, Clifford Odets and Oscar Levant.

One of my main problems on *The Best of Everything* was to persuade Joan Crawford to accept a non-starring role. I did it by having a scene written for her that was not to be included in the film. But a script-girl told her and spoilt my plans. Nevertheless Joan did appear in it.

Lately I've made most of my films abroad, starting with *Three Coins in the Fountain* and *Boy on a Dolphin* in the mid-fifties. When I make a picture abroad, I always go to the best book store in town and look through every photographic book about that particular country. Usually foreign photographers do better work about a town or country than native photographers. For example, in Sicily the most exciting things are done by the Germans: they came and "found" things. It's just like a French painter who's never been on the Eiffel Tower; he has all his life to do that, whereas a foreigner does it immediately.

For some of these books, photographers have sometimes spent as much as two or three years trying to capture the atmosphere, and we just try to reproduce it. When you show it to a motion-picture cameraman it's easier for him to understand what you are talking about. Occasionally they don't understand, not only because they're unable to do what I ask, but also because my accent is so thick that when I get excited or nervous nobody can understand me.

My most recent project has been *The Heroes*, a jewel robbery story shot on location in Iran and starring Stuart Whitman and Elke Sommer. It's been very exciting. Luckily I still have a great enthusiasm for movie-making. I hope I never lose it.

Irving Rapper

Irving Rapper's apartment is set high in a glistening white building in the very heart of Hollywood. Only a stone's throw from Hollywood Boulevard, with its seedy spangle of light-signs, its driven restless sixties people, and its ever-skulking hustlers, Rapper inhabits a seemingly sealed-off forties world. As so often in Hollywood, fantasy and reality seem one, so that as you enter the hall, where a super-efficient blonde announces your arrival directly from the reception desk to the host's telephone, you could easily be in a scene from a vintage Betty Davis picture, and you half expect to see her charge stormily at any moment through the glass swinging doors, ready for an argument with David Brian or Bruce Bennett—those lost figures of Hollywood's past.

*Chez Rapper, the atmosphere of that past persists. Comfortably plump and relaxed, with an elegant and cultivated personality, he is utterly unlike the brisk new generation of grey-suited, fiercely efficient Hollywood men. His best known films were made with Bette Davis—*Deception *and* Now, Voyager *among them—but his unacknowledged technical skill, his tremendous flair for the cinema, were perhaps more formidably displayed in his biographies:* The Adventures of Mark Twain—*a tour de force of historical reconstruction—and* Rhapsody in Blue, *a ritzy, glittering account of the career of Gershwin. Like so many Hollywood talents, he has been put firmly—and one hopes only temporarily—on the shelf by the newest generation, but looking round the apartment— a cross between Gershwin's in* Rhapsody in Blue *and Bette Davis's in* Deception—*you see the compensations: Chinese lampstands "fit for a museum" (the phrase was Paul*

225

Henreid's in Deception), *magnificent paintings crowded tightly up the height of a wall, a louvred cocktail recess, an atmosphere of spacious, glossy luxury. And beyond the great windows and the penthouse balcony, the whispering traffic, the horn-bleeps and the diamond shine of an ocean of lights: Los Angeles.*

I went to Warner Brothers for a job in the mid-thirties as an assistant director, and they told me at first that my stage experience—I had worked extensively in the theatre —was unsuitable. They said that since they didn't do Molnar plays, they had no idea where they would fit me in!

I went home feeling very distressed, and then, by chance, I found a clipping which reviewed a play I had directed in stock called *Crime*. I took it back, and when the Warners people read the rave account of my work on the play, they engaged me immediately.

I began working on a horror film called *The Walking Dead*, with Boris Karloff and just about the entire stock company of Warner Brothers. It was a bad story, but it was directed by the great Michael Curtiz, who was my mentor and guide for many years, and to whom I owe my knowledge of the cinema.

I was on two or three pictures a year from then on. *Kid Galahad* began my association with Bette Davis, who had just come back from England after losing a court case against Warner Brothers, and we became great friends. We are still friends, although strangely enough, I haven't seen her in more than fifteen years; we write each other letters, and speak on the telephone, but we haven't gotten together in all that time.

I was on *The Life of Emile Zola*, with Paul Muni, and *The Story of Louis Pasteur:* all the great biographies Warners did at the time. Then *All This and Heaven Too* and *The Sisters*. Many of these pictures were made for the producer Henry Blanke, the most sympathetic, versatile and intelligent producer at Warners.

These films were made very slowly, very painstakingly, because the great stars needed the most careful photographic attention, and their cameramen had to treat their faces cosmetically with light and shadow: it would take hours to set up the shots. And the stars would often be deeply involved in the direction in a creative sense: Bette Davis, in particular, had a marvellously probing intelligence, which gave great strength to the director working with her.

Sometimes, of course, you'd have to correct her. I remember when I was making *The Corn is Green* with her: at the end of the second act, which we retained in the film, there is a moment when the school-teacher in the Welsh mining village conveys to the audience that she has dreamed, that she somehow clairvoyantly knew, that her star pupil's main historical question at the big examination would be all about Henry VIII.

Bette tossed the moment away, and there was a bit of an argument; I simmered down for five days and finally I said to her, "Bette I saw the cut stuff, and I'm very sorry to tell you that wasn't the way it should have been done." And she said, "Do you really think so?" and I said, "Yes." And she agreed to do it again. You could get through to her, although she had enormous power at the studio; she was its queen.

In this early period I started to preplan my pictures— my first was a small film, with James Stephenson and Geraldine Fitzgerald, called *Shining Victory*, in which Bette Davis as a joke appeared in a bit part as a nurse— but I didn't preplan quite in the sense that Hitchcock does. I'd plot out the opening and closing of a sequence, and its highest dramatic point only. I'd sometimes begin with fully detailed plans and sketches, but then Bette or someone would yell out, "Why did you do that?" And I'd throw them all away.

I would improvise a good deal, but I always followed the scripts I was given to the letter. At Warners they would give you a finished script, and if you refused to do it, you were out on suspension. Your contract specified that you must do anything you were assigned to. If a camera movement took an unusually long time, I would improvise a phrase or a line, but broadly speaking there would be no major reconstruction.

I was known as the rebellious director at Warners: Bogart used to say: "Skippy, you have one more suspension and you'll be on the San Francisco Bay Bridge." I had ten suspensions in seven years! I would refuse, say, a crime picture I wouldn't even know how to begin, or some Nazi picture when I thought people were tired of them, or non-literate scripts.

Luckily, Bette and others were in my corner, which helped. Of course, sometimes I had to do a film I really didn't want to do: and one of those was *The Adventures of Mark Twain*, with Fredric March. It was the only time in my life I dined with Hal Wallis, who was a sort of benevolent dictator at the studio, and he told me: "Irving, I admit it's not a perfect script. But it will have prestige. It may not be the box-office thing you want, but it won't hurt you." I made it finally because I had to be busy or be drafted! So I did it! And I'm not sorry I did, because friends of mine call up and say to me, "I cried last night during the last scenes. It was on television. . . . "

I always felt that this and my other major screen biography, *Rhapsody in Blue*, lacked the integration, the close feeling of progressive excitement that a script should have: they are too sprawling, too episodic. There were things I liked in *Mark Twain*: his feeling for youth, and the magical scenes of his death, with all the cats around his body, and the body coming out of the bed and listening to little Huckleberry Finn calling him in the clouds, and the little boys going fishing with him.

Rhapsody in Blue—the story of Gershwin—was another rambling story, a little too sentimental at times, although written by some wonderful people, mainly Clifford Odets, with far, far too much music. The person who should have played it was Tyrone Power. Jack Warner originally suggested John Garfield or Cary Grant, and I said, "I can hardly see Cary Grant down in a fish market for the early scenes, or having a Jewish family, or Julie Garfield as a high-hat socialite going up Carnegie Hall. So I'd much rather have an unknown." It's a tragedy that Ty was in the Marines; he had those marvellous eyes, which could have been a poet's or a pianist's, and he had the most intriguing manner of a gentleman, which Gershwin was.

When they asked me at the Gershwin home, "Would you like to see some pictures?" I said, "No, play a record of his voice. I'll get the whole thing out of that."

In other respects—that is to say, apart from the casting of Robert Alda as Gershwin—I was happy with the film. I was greatly aided in making it by a great cameraman unfortunately no longer with us: Sol Polito. He helped enormously with the visual pattern of the film, its whole construction. I've always had a rule: keep the camera moving, make the movements as fluid as can be. Coming from the theatre, which is composed after all in a permanent still picture, or series of still pictures, I've wanted to avoid stillness in films, and I gave my cameramen an order: keep the flow.

And I have a rule that I must have the greatest cameramen in the world to work with: I had Jack Cardiff on *The Brave One*, of course. I would rather argue with Bette Davis, the greatest star in the world, than with my "eyes".

On *Rhapsody in Blue* I was lucky in having the great choreographer Le Roy Prinz to help me with the whole production. He did wonderful things for me, like the shadow of the band on the wall in the orchestral Première of *Rhapsody in Blue* itself, a sequence that he choreographed, and the whole of the *Blue Monday* sequence, an episode with an all-Negro cast that came from a musical of Gershwin's which flopped, but which later became the foundation for *Porgy and Bess*.

But much as I liked *Rhapsody in Blue* (for its incidentals rather than its script and story and general development) I much preferred *Now, Voyager*, which was my first really big picture at Warners. I was given a finished script by Casey Robinson: it's possible that Bette Davis may have done some work on it as well, but I knew nothing of that, it must have all happened long before I was called in.

My mother, I remember, died the year that I made it; I had intended going to Europe for a few months to get over that, but Hal Wallis said I must do the picture or be suspended. I made *The Gay Sisters*, with Barbara Stanwyck, and then rushed straight into *Voyager* with less than two weeks to prepare it. And one whole week of that was swallowed up with test scenes of Paul Henreid, who had just arrived from Europe and couldn't get used to English, and Bette Davis had to get used to him. Of course, I had the problem of getting him used to Bette as well!

My great teacher, Michael Curtiz, was originally supposed to have directed this picture, but he didn't like it as a subject and preferred to do an action picture. I insisted on casting *Voyager* myself; I was starting to sail high, and they gave me my head. So I hired Claude Rains to play the psychiatrist, and Gladys Cooper, whom Hal Wallis had never heard of, to play the mother, and Ilka Chase and Bonita Granville, who was the vicious prying niece in *These Three* to needle Bette Davis, who played a sad spinster released from her inhibited and repressed life in a Boston family.

Hal asked why I cast Ilka Chase and Bonita Granville, and I told him, "These are the only people I can find who will needle Bette Davis." Bette Davis on the receiving end for a change, and it had to be very poignant and dramatic! And she said when she heard that, "Oh, Irving, you son-of-a-bitch!"

The story wasn't that good, more or less *Cosmopolitan* magazine level, but what made the picture great was brilliant acting.

With *Now, Voyager* I began my trademark of having rain; right at the beginning in that instance, and on the windows of the pianist's apartment in *Deception*; rain in every film I've made, like Hitchcock's comic appearances, and Fritz Lang's hands, and Vincente Minnelli's party scenes. Rain adds so much to a mood of tension: whenever I was doing an examination as a kid, it was always raining. . . .

One scene was cut from *Voyager*: when the girl, played by Davis, is on a boat on an African cruise with her mother when she's young, and she sees herself dressed like a princess, and a beautiful young ship's officer comes to invite her to a dance, and she becomes aware for the first time she's wanted; it was all done with pillars mounting into the night sky. It was shot silent, and it was probably too long; so it was cut.

For *Deception*, we had a trash-can outside the elevator on the way up to the apartment of the central character, played by Bette Davis. And Bette said, "Why the trash-can?" And I said, "Well, Lennie Bernstein's first penthouse was like this." The apartment was exactly like Bernstein's, the big studio windows and so on: everyone remembers that set.

Deception was the story of the love affair of a pianist played by Bette, and a cellist, played by Paul Henreid, and the tension that results from the jealousy of her teacher, the great composer Hollenius, played by Claude Rains. Henreid couldn't play the 'cello really, so we tied his hands behind his back, and the two hands of a real instrumentalist came out from behind him and played. In *Rhapsody in Blue* we did the same thing with Robert Alda at the piano, and there I think it was too obvious; I always squirm every time I see it for that reason. But the average person couldn't see it. As long as shots like this are done on movement, no one ever notices.

Deception ends with Bette shooting Claude dead and

going to prison, but it should have been concluded as a comedy, and the writer, John Collier, intended it that way. It was supposed to have a gay, light, natural, "So what?" ending. The three people walk off as friends. But Bette wanted a dramatic conclusion; she insisted on it; and I didn't care very much either way, so I gave in. The dramatic scene gave her a greater chance, and I will say she seized on it!

For *Deception*, I used Ernest Haller as my cameraman instead of Sol Polito, my usual one. The late Sol Polito was a no-nonsense technician, whereas Ernest Haller is almost a cosmetician's cameraman, very concerned with making the stars look beautiful. And that brings me to a story which has been told very, very often; it is supposed to have concerned Dietrich or Garbo, and it didn't. Bette insisted on Haller, and I insisted on Polito for *Deception*, but I let her have her way because I didn't want her to be worrying about the camera work: it might affect her playing of the part.

Five days after we started, she said: "Have you seen the rushes?" And I said, "Of course, I see them every day." And she said, "What do you think?" And I said, "Bette, you're giving me a marvellous performance." And she replied, "I'm not talking about my acting. How do I look?" "Bette," I told her, "you sound like Paulette Goddard." "Don't be funny!" she told me. She stormed into the projection room, and I came in and there was a big argument going on between her and Haller. And she said to him, "Ernie, you photographed me in *Jezebel*, didn't you?" And he said, "Yes, what about it?" "Can't you photograph me like that?" And he replied, "Bette, I was seven years younger then."

But seriously, Ernie did a very good job; he used those wonderful deep-focus shots that gave the story so much weight. The whole thing rested on two people, Bette and Paul, who were on screen in every scene, so the depth of the shots was essential.

I always try to get the best composers as well as the best cameramen: I had a terrible row with Ray Heindorf, the musical director at Warners, about the title music for *Marjorie Morningstar*, with Natalie Wood. I told Milton Sperling, the producer, that it didn't create the right mood; we started with a camp and water at night, and it didn't put me in the right nostalgic mood. When I used to go to camp as a child and heard the bugle over the water, it did something to me; but there was nothing in this at all. He said, "Oh, you want all that old-fashioned stuff." And I said, "It's appropriate." So Sperling brought in the people who wrote "Love is a Many-Splendoured Thing". And at the third line I said, "It's wonderful", and it was: it was one of the five that was nominated for an Oscar that year.

On *The Miracle* ... the main trouble there was casting. The girl who played the nun was thrust on me without a test. I was furious, I was floored. The whole thing was unspeakably bad because of her. I didn't even talk to her.

Another film that worked out badly was *Anna Lucasta*, from the play by Philip Yordan, with a white cast. Susan Hayward was supposed to have done it, but Paulette Goddard produced a letter promising her the part and it was too late for anyone to get out from under; we'd all signed to do it.

Compromises all the time; but one picture of mine in recent years wasn't compromised: *The Brave One*.

My friends, and my agent even, advised me against making it—the story of a boy fighting bulls in Mexico, which won for Dalton Trumbo, who was then blacklisted, an Oscar under another name.

They all said, "What do you see in it?" And I said, "It's so simple, it reads like a fairy tale." And it cost $430,000 to make, and grossed eight and a half million. After that, I'll follow my own judgment, all the time.

Mark Robson

Smooth and diplomatic behind executive hornrims, Mark Robson occupies a comfortable ground-floor office on the Twentieth Century-Fox lot, its relatively unpretentious furnishings somehow inconsistent with his blockbuster image: for this specialist in glossy wide-screen escapism has repeatedly made cash-registers jingle around the world with adaptations of racy national best-sellers like Peyton Place, From the Terrace *and* Valley of the Dolls. *His speech is measured, low-pitched, almost pedantic; and as he talks, politely parrying or evading awkward questions, he stares distrustfully at the microphone, fully aware that his utterances are being irrevocably preserved. From somewhere a record player bawls the theme tune of his latest smash-hit movie, and we reflect that he has come a long way since the days when he helped edit Orson Welles's early masterpieces* Citizen Kane *and* The Magnificent Ambersons, *and directed some of the most widely admired horror fantasies of the late producer Val Lewton. Like Robert Wise, another Lewton alumnus, Mark Robson has graduated from inexpensive B pictures to those with seven-figure budgets and correspondingly colossal grosses. Does he ever, we wonder, yearn for a return to less grandiose but perhaps more artistically satisfying subjects? His list of planned projects, all costly and star-studded, provides the answer: there can be no question for him at least of "selling out", for this man has clearly arrived at his intended goal, and he is perfectly satisfied, artistically and otherwise, right now.*

When Orson Welles came out to California in 1939 after having done his sensational *War of the Worlds* broadcast in New York he became interested in doing various projects, one of which was Joseph Conrad's *Heart of Darkness*.

Robert Wise and I, who formed a sort of team in those days—he was a film editor and I was his assistant—went to work at RKO on *Heart of Darkness*. Time went on, shots came in, and then one day we found ourselves looking at some film that took place inside a projection room. "What the hell does this have to do with *Heart of Darkness?*" we wondered.

We found out within a few days that this was a totally different film, that he had started production on *Citizen Kane* without anybody knowing it. The studio executives all thought he was doing the Conrad story.

That was the beginning of my association with Orson Welles, editing *Citizen Kane* with Bob Wise. After that I worked with Bob on *The Magnificent Ambersons*, and I was also the editor of *Journey into Fear*.

While we were editing *The Magnificent Ambersons*, Orson was down in South America making *The Raft*, a segment of a three- or four-part film to be called *It's All True*, and he had Norman Foster in Mexico doing another segment, *My Friend Bonito*. Jack Moss, Orson's executive producer, was left in California, and under him we continued editing *The Magnificent Ambersons*.

Finally Bob and I took it out to preview, and I guess in one fell swoop about a quarter of the theatre audience got up and left. Then about five minutes later another quarter left, and then finally the last half of the audience left, until there were about two or three people remaining in the theatre and many angry patrons waiting for us outside.

So we figured we had quite a lot to do. We took the picture back and continued re-editing it throughout maybe ten or fifteen previews. Towards the end, Jack Moss, Bob Wise and I were no longer looking at the film but at the audience, watching to see if any of them left. We'd say: "Maybe this fellow's just going to the men's room." And a little later: "Oh, here he is, he's back."

Finally the picture was played so that nobody left the theatre. That is basically the film that is now called *The Magnificent Ambersons*.

I must say that the original version was simply marvellous: it was truly *The* Magnificent *Ambersons*. Theatrically wonderful; photographed by Stanley Cortez superbly. But it was so advanced, so ahead of its time, that people just didn't understand it. At least an hour was taken out of it for release, although I don't recall specific sequences. It was a kind of chopped-down version of Orson's original conception.

He never participated in the editing—although he honestly had the right of final cut on the picture—because he'd left the country in a hurry. It was the beginning of the war, and he'd been assigned to this South American film that was somehow connected with inter-American relations. It was no one's fault but his own. Don't blame any of the executives or the people who invested in *Ambersons*. It was clearly Orson's fault because he was not present. He was escaping in one way or another.

Something similar happened on *Journey into Fear*. Orson produced it and acted in it; Norman Foster was the director. They made an incomplete film; that is to say, the film was finished but it had no finish. It had wonderful things in it, but it also had much that was very silly.

Orson left the country without fulfilling his obligations as producer and actor. On returning to America, he didn't even want to see the film. When he did see it, he wanted everything put back that the studio had taken out. This was wartime and would have involved a million or so feet of film in release prints.

I was on very good terms with him and asked him if I could try to put *Journey into Fear* back into some continuity that would please him. He agreed and I did. He was quite pleased with the results and only then consented to come in and make a finish to the picture.

I don't know if Orson in effect directed it, as has often been said. Norman Foster was the official director, and a very talented one, but plagued by bad luck. In *My Friend Bonito* he did, incidentally, magnificent work, foreshadowing Irving Rapper's *The Brave One* in its story about a boy who sees a fighting bull born and grow up and enter the ring in Mexico City.

When Orson was, so to speak, "evicted" from RKO—he was given a few hours to move out—most of the people who had been associated with him were punished: because of our love for him, because of our hopes for him. I was sent down into the B picture department. In that department was a man called Lew Ostrow, who had been a great film editor, a "film doctor", at one time at MGM, and later an executive producer at the same studio.

Now he was an executive producer in charge of the B films at RKO and, having taken a liking to me and my work, he asked me to sort of look around at the films that were being made in his department and see if I could help them in any way.

Val Lewton at this time was a story editor for David Selznick, and Lew Ostrow, knowing of his marvellous talent, made possible Val's move to RKO as a producer. Val didn't know much about film, physically speaking. He knew stories very well; he had a great fondness for directors and writers. But he was fundamentally a writer, a poet, a novelist-poet, an historian.

I was assigned to Val's unit as an editor: to show him something about film and to help guide that department involved with his films. He thought of his unit—and he had his own little horror unit—in terms of the producer, the writer, the director, and the editor; a kind of team in which we all worked extremely closely together.

Jacques Tourneur, the very wonderful director son of Maurice Tourneur, was Val's first director. They'd worked together at MGM on the second unit of Selznick's *A Tale of Two Cities*, and he directed Val's first three films. Now in the development of those films the editor was with them at all times, even at story conferences. My job wasn't in the cutting-room until the film was in production. My job was in the office with them discussing story, special effects, casting, all kinds of things like that.

When Jacques was finally promoted into more important films—or, rather, higher-budget films; I don't think they were more important, just more expensive—they needed another director, and Val wanted me to become the director for his unit.

The "brass" at RKO, the president and the executives, knew me because I had acted as a kind of "diplomatic courier" between them and Orson Welles—they weren't speaking at the time—during the final stages of *Journey into Fear*. So when Val asked Lew Ostrow, the department head, whether I could become his unit director, Ostrow thought it was a great idea, and when he put it up to the company front office, they readily agreed.

I was signed as a director at RKO at two hundred dollars per week and my first picture was *The Seventh Victim*. That picture achieved some kind of notoriety in England after the war, as I discovered when John and Roy Boulting came out here about that time, wanting to meet the fellow who had directed it. They used to bicycle a print of *The Seventh Victim* around London, among them Carol Reed and Cavalcanti and people like that, thinking it an advanced, weird form of film-making.

I was very flattered to hear it. I was still occupying the little office I shared with Bob Wise. It must have measured about eight feet by eight, and we had an arrangement whereby the first man entering in the morning got the desk and the chair; the other fellow had to pace up and down for the rest of the day.

The Seventh Victim was a very low-budget film for those days; I think it cost about $100,000. I don't remember much about it now. I do remember however that it had a rather sinister quality, of something intangible but horribly real; it had an atmosphere. I think the actors and the director had to believe very strongly in the possibilities of disaster: that something *was* there. We believed it ourselves. We talked ourselves into believing it. We had a kind of fidelity to that feeling. We had the characters speak throughout in a deliberately quiet, polite and subdued manner, engendering a very calculated undercurrent of *possible* disaster. That technique, which I guess today appears rather funny, was very daring in its time.

In each of these films we had what we called the "bus", an editing device I had invented by accident, or possibly by design, on *Cat People*, that was calculated to terrify people and make them jump out of their seats.

It derived from a sequence in *Cat People* in which a girl was walking through the transverse in New York's Central Park, imagining that she was being followed by somebody or something one supposed could be a cat of some sort, a leopard possibly, though one couldn't tell. Looking over her right shoulder in terror, this girl backed away from the mysterious sound, ready to accept anything that might jump on her. From the other side of the park a bus came by, and I put a big, solid sound of air brakes on it, cutting it in at the decisive moment so that it knocked viewers out of their seats. This became the "bus", and we used the same principle in every film.

We used it in *The Ghost Ship*, with Richard Dix, which incidentally was *not* based on Jack London's *The Sea Wolf*, nor was it similar; and we used it in *Isle of the Dead*, which was an interesting project because here we took a painting, Boecklin's "Die Insel der Toten", and imagined a story around it.

All these films, in fact, were screen originals. I remember one evening we were up in the office until two or three in the morning devising a non-stop horror sequence for *Isle of the Dead*. We were hysterical with laughter because one of our central characters was trapped and had to go through a tunnel. Every time he went into it he became terrified and had to run out of it, then into it again, thus giving us our "unending" horror sequence, our "perpetual" horror scene! It was a riot.

That brings to mind a little anecdote. By the time we made *Isle of the Dead*, Mr Ostrow, whom we adored, was no longer our executive producer; he had fought with the company and left. Our new executive had as his assistant a very important man from the theatre division who said, after listening to our story deriving from the Boecklin painting: "I could spit on a marquee and make more money than you fellows could!" And shaking his finger in my face as I left, he added: "And remember—no messages!"

Back in my office I called this man on the phone and said, "You know, I'm terribly sorry but there *is* a message to this film." "What is it?" he asked. *"Death is good,"* I replied. He took it quite straight. However, the department head was a much more gentle sort of man and also had a sense of humour. I recall his asking Val to tell him what the story was all about in just a few words. "It's very simple," Val said. "It's the story of a woman driven insane through the natural process of premature burial."

"Ah, yes," the man said. "That's quite simple."

We tried something quite unique on *Isle of the Dead*. Nowadays when we have so much money we're apt not to use our imaginations. I recall on that film having to take Boris Karloff through a battlefield. And I had an idea: I noticed a great backing, a rather large cyclorama left over from *The Enchanted Cottage* or something like that, with dirt on the ground and everything rather folksy. I knew that if one could light the backing dimly then the line between the backing and the ground became the horizon line.

The only way to judge distance was by relative position with the foreground. So, if you put a wheel in the foreground, you could move an actor past or behind that wheel and use the same background, and put some other object in the foreground, and you had a different place.

With that in mind, I took about six or eight of Goya's drawings of the Iberian campaign from his *Disasters of War*, got a number of extras, posed them in the grotesque

positions in which Goya had drawn his figures, and made
a dolly shot with these people in the foreground and Boris
Karloff walking behind them against this grey background.

Now, that technique is certainly valid, and we should do
more of it. One sees it somewhat in contemporary films
where the budget is restricted, but too seldom in major
productions.

In *Valley of the Dolls* recently I needed a street in San
Francisco. We calculated the cost of going up to San
Francisco with a full crew at around $78,000. One could
almost make a film for the cost of moving the company.
Then I said, "Let us build the street here at the studio."
So they submitted drawings and the whole thing came out
to around $23,000.

That would have been a big saving. But it just hurt me
to think of spending $23,000 for a set that was going to be
on the screen only a few moments. So I said to the art
director: "We're going to do this whole thing for $4,000.
That's all we have. Now let's just use our imaginations."
As a result of that, we found a spot on the lot here and
did a whole street for $4,000. It looks very realistic and, I
think, rather beautiful.

This stemmed out of that early experience on *Isle of the
Dead*, a typical Val Lewton project. Equally typical was
Bedlam, which originated rather strangely. A Hearst paper, the *American Weekly*, used to run a Sunday supple-
ment featuring offbeat articles like for example, "Secrets
of the French Police". One day I noticed in this supple-
ment the name Tom O'Bedlam.

I'd never heard this name. Out of curiosity I looked it
up in some research books and found that there was a
word, "bedlam", and that the word had something to do
with the St Mary of Bethlehem Hospital for the Insane,
and that it was the first truly organized insane asylum.

From there it was only a short step to reproducing
much of Hogarth's *The Rake's Progress* in our film; in
fact, we virtually used Hogarth as our art director. The
dialogue was an amalgam of all kinds of eighteenth-
century characters, including Lord Sandwich and various
others.

All this time I'd been making films with ghouls, so to
speak. I'd never done a film with real people. These were
all very low-budget movies, experimental in their time. I
even made an experimental western, *Roughshod,* which
had practically no gunplay or shooting.

An exception was *Youth Runs Wild,* picked by James Agee, whom we all respected very much and who seemed to like our films, as the best film of its year, the same year that *Going My Way* won everything at the Academy Awards. It was a story of the dislocation of people during the "swing-shift" period of the war: the effect on youth when families are broken up and there is insufficient parental care.

At that time I had a new executive producer at RKO who didn't quite understand what we were doing, and after the film was completed, he chopped it up. As a result of that, we had a terrible fight and I was fired, only to be re-hired shortly after.

Dore Schary was then the head of RKO. He had lots of friends, but he didn't seem to have the will to force me upon any of his important actors. So when the time came for them to pick up my option, I was dropped.

Then I did other things: started coaching actors, making tests, working on stories. Finally I made a couple of films, and within about a year and a half I was back at RKO at some outlandish fee, about ten or twenty times my former salary, on a film I never even made, one of Jerry Wald's. The irony was that if I hadn't been fired, they could have continued paying me my old salary for maybe ten years.

Stanley Kramer had seen a lot of the films I had done for Val Lewton and wanted me to do a film called *So This is New York.* I read the material and didn't care for it. Dick Fleischer did it. Then when the time came for *Champion,* Kramer called me in and we did that.

The boxing *milieu* of *Champion* appealed to me because, when I was a young man, my father, who had a gymnasium with a rowing machine in our home and who used to have a physical education trainer come in and give him exercises, taught me and my brothers a little boxing. By the time I went to prep school I was a pretty good boxer, though never very serious about it.

While *Champion* was still in production, Kramer and I got together and decided to make *Home of the Brave.* That was a rather daring film, the first of the Negro cycle. Stanley was very clever about getting the finance for it: he had John Stillman or some lettuce people on the hook for a lot of money and just went ahead with the project in secrecy. It turned out an enormous hit, a bigger hit financially than *Champion.*

The Kramer outfit at that time was a quite independent, very small motion-picture centre, with no conventional "front office". Carl Foreman was a tremendous contributor to that group, as was George Glass, who was in his time one of the great press agents. Carl, Stanley and George: they were the company.

They were very interested in screen credit because they were trying to build themselves up. At that period I had three films playing on Broadway simultaneously: *Roughshod, Champion* and *Home of the Brave.* The credits on the last two films read: "A Stanley Kramer Production. Produced by Stanley Kramer". There was no director credit on either of them. Carl Foreman was named as writer but there was no mention of Mark Robson.

Finally, George Glass was called in, because contractually you can't do that, and eventually they got a plate with my name on it and kind of smudged it, so that you couldn't read it. That really happened. They were young people trying to get ahead, and I guess nobody was going to stand in their way.

Stanley is, I think, a fine producer, an imaginative person, adventuresome. He has faults, lots of faults, as a person, but everybody does. He is still potentially one of the great producers. In spite of the strange things he did, I would have stayed with him, but I got an offer from Samuel Goldwyn and went to work over there.

That was one of the worst periods of my career. I didn't care at all for the films I made with Goldwyn. They were awful: *Edge of Doom, My Foolish Heart, I Want You,* etc.

Goldwyn was quite different from anyone I'd been accustomed to. He would say, "All I know is: get the best talent", and he would go out and get "the greatest writer" and "the greatest designer" and the "greatest" this and the "greatest" that, and I would say to him: "But what do you want *me* for? Let everybody else do the work."

Away from Goldwyn, I made what I think is a very good film, *Bright Victory*. It was interesting because it provided another confrontation with the Negro problem. It was the story of a boy from the South, with the normal intolerance of people from that part of the United States, who acquired human perception after he was blinded. While I believe it was a disaster financially, it won the New York Critics' Award for Arthur Kennedy in the main role, and a lot of awards all around the world.

In the picture, Kennedy wore corneal lenses through which he couldn't see; and we also used a number of real blinded veteran soldiers from Valley Forge General Hospital, among whom we interspersed a few actors.

I made two films with Jerry Wald, *The Harder They Fall* and *Peyton Place*. He was a remarkable man, and he had many faults. He was kind of a "buckshot" producer, blasting out in all directions at once. But he was also one of the most stimulating of all movie people; I liked him very much. You'd be working on a Wald project and suddenly you'd get a memo about Shakespeare, for example, sparked off by something he'd read somewhere. In fact he was an avid notewriter, producing hundreds and hundreds of memos.

John Michael Hayes did the *Peyton Place* screenplay; it went through at least eleven drafts. The first one I read was about two hundred and sixty pages. While it was imperfect, and structurally wrong, still one could see that it was possible—with hard work—to pull it together. Jerry was tireless, and John Michael Hayes worked extremely hard; on a weekend he would rewrite a whole script. The final screenplay was written on the stage as the film was actually being made.

We found it difficult to start *Peyton Place* properly. Then a couple of location trips I took to New England yielded a whole new view, another look at the story in terms of *telling* it. I was able to bring photographs back and say: "This is how you could start it." And gradually it shaped itself up very well.

Jerry was most ambitious in his desire to make good films. For example, he sent me a memo saying, "We must do something about the churches in New England"—that's all. He kept writing me notes about churches: "There are lovely churches in New England", etc. In effect, he harassed me with churches.

As a result, I found myself looking around at churches, and one day I saw a Martin Buber quotation displayed outside a Methodist church. "Maybe I should photograph some of these churches," I thought. And that's how the montage of people going to church on Sunday was conceived, aided by the late Franz Waxman's lovely score and locations, taking in the whole area around the town of Camden, Maine; we went as far as Belfast, I believe, for some of it.

Searching for the ideal Peyton Place, I went first to

Woodstock, Vermont, and made a survey. A public relations man there seemed very delighted with the idea of using the town in the film, but before I could go much further we were thrown out because some of the town's church groups didn't want to have anything to do with *Peyton Place*.

On my return to Los Angeles, I received a cable from the Governor of Maine, saying: "Please come to Maine where we are broadminded." So the next day the art director, Jack Smith, and I went east to Maine.

Ironically, looking around New England on *Valley of the Dolls*, I recalled what a magnificent town Woodstock was and went back there trying to remember the exact place where I'd met the public relations man. The town is now very much the same as it was. I walked by accident into the same shop I'd been in some ten or more years before, and a man turned round and looked at me. "Not you again!" he exclaimed. "What do you want now?"—as though I'd only been there the week before.

"You know, it's a strange thing," I said, "but I have another problem book. It's called *Valley of the Dolls*." This man had been in the thick of all the previous trouble with the church groups, involving the mayor and the whole community. Now he wanted to wash his hands of the whole thing. "Here's a brochure," he said, handing me one, *"but don't talk to me!"*

I made quite different use of New England in *Valley of the Dolls* from the use I made of it in *Peyton Place*. Here again we didn't quite know how to start the film. Finally we opened it much in the style of the novel, which tells of a girl's feelings on coming to New York, and examines the steps leading up to it.

Accordingly I photographed the true incidents of the interior action recalled by the girl, framed within the present action of her going to New York. Her recollections were done in a very strange cinematic style of stills and slow motion and stop-motion and colour, going back and forth in time. We saw her during the credits and the opening narrative coming down to New York from her beautiful New England home town, remembering its railroad station and skating-pond and the interior of her house.

In the rest of the film, I employed a cross-cutting style in keeping with its three or four parallel basic stories. I tried to do fresh things: the episode of Neely's sojourn in the insane asylum, for example, was photographed in such a way as to give an effect of having been vignetted in oil. I also used some interesting light changes, stop-changes, from exterior to interior, and some unorthodox cutting devices, like employing a dissolve where normally you'd have a straight cut and vice versa.

I've often worked with William Daniels, the veteran cameraman of *Valley of the Dolls*. He uses a lot of quartz-iodine lights, his own inventions. One of his lights— I don't know what he calls it—is in a frame, and it puts out at about 25–50 feet about 700-foot candles, enabling one to achieve tremendous illumination with great mobility.

Often we used a panafocal lens, a development of the Panavision company, involving an extension of a crane-shot fitted with a zoom, so that frequently our lens was being changed rather unconventionally in the middle of a move, from a 95 maybe to a 50, or from a 50 to a 75. We also used some interesting zoom shots with moves from a 500 to a 50.

Following *Valley of the Dolls*, I did *Daddy's Gone A-Hunting*, starring Carol White, and now I'm working on Irving Wallace's *The Plot* and, after that, Jon Cleary's *The Long Pursuit*.

Jacques Tourneur

Arguably the only person in the world to smoke a pipe and a cigar with alternate puffs, Jacques Tourneur is an extremely amiable, comfortable-looking, plump man whose appearance never suggests the sinister imagination of his best films: Cat People, The Leopard Man, *and* Night of the Demon. *He speaks slowly, diffidently, modestly and carefully, anxious at all times to make every point absolutely clear. His "apartment" is a self-contained duplex house, tucked away between tall buildings in the very heart of Hollywood, furnished with quiet but exquisite taste that by its feminine touch suggests his wife's rather than his own hand: a delicate impression of framed portraits, a French clock of unusual form, beautifully designed armchairs. The staircase comes right down into this tall, cool living-room, which the visitor walks straight into without any intervening hall. A place far removed from the overpowering opulence of Mamoulian's or the modern ritziness of Frankenheimer's, but in its charming reserve and good taste no less impressive a reflection of its owner's personality. Curious to think that this very pretty domicile once belonged to Scott Fitzgerald, who died there.*

My career in Hollywood really began when I was working on *A Tale of Two Cities* at Metro for David O. Selznick. I was on contract to Metro on a week-by-week basis and doing very small B and C class pictures. Selznick put me in charge of the second unit on *A Tale*, which involved handling all the Revolution scenes. He introduced me to the writer Val Lewton, who was to be a major presence in my career: the producer of my horror films at RKO. Lewton and I had a separate unit at Metro, and together we wrote a separate script of about fourteen pages for the Revolutionary sequences entirely independent from the rest of the film. We worked on developing the material—Mr. Selznick chose me because of my name: he thought I must be right for a French subject—and Val Lewton and I struck an immediate *rapport*; and finally Selznick put my name on the credits because, since it sounded so French, it would give a look of greater authenticity to the picture! Later, when Lewton went to RKO, we continued working together.

Val Lewton's mother was for many years the story editor for Metro-Goldwyn-Mayer in New York. She was a very literate and highly cultured woman. Val was a wonderful person. He had a Russian background, and he was a dreamer and an idealist. I am a realist: I always brought him back to earth. You need that in a partnership. He'd go off into flights of fancy and I'd say, "Well, look, this can't be done." I'd pull him down and he'd bring me up. That was good. Without me he would have been out of the business: he was so impractical. He was a sort of Danny Kaye fey character out of Papasvili, and lived in another world. Every afternoon we'd have tea and stop everything! For an hour we'd talk about everything except the film: Pushkin and the old steppes and the snow.

We were making so much money on our films together that the studio said, "We'll make twice as much money if we separate them." So they pulled us apart. It was a mistake: we belonged together. He was a perfect gentleman: if I suggested doing something stupid, he would accept it nicely and then arrange not to do it. We *never* had any arguments.

He would originate the ideas for our films, and then call in the writers, myself, and the editor, Mark Robson, and we were encouraged, over cups of tea, to say anything "wild". And gradually ideas developed: it's fun to work that way. Val was so conscientious! I'd go to a film or a theatre downtown, and my wife and I would be driving back to the San Fernando Valley at half past one or two in the morning. And always, as we passed the studio, we'd see a light in that corner office of his, and he'd be alone working, correcting what the writer had written; he could only work at that time of night. Next day he'd hand the work to us. That conscientiousness killed him; he was overly wrought up; he was one of those people with a very calm exterior, rather stout, but seething inside. And that killed him, I think.

He left RKO because the studio chief, an intelligent, sensitive man called Charles Koerner, died, and the new people who came in were tough businessmen. He switched to Universal, but he didn't live long.

Val Lewton called me up at RKO one day and said, "Jacques, I'm going to produce a new picture here, and I'd like you to direct it." He said, "The head of the studio, Charles Koerner, was at a party last night and somebody suggested to him, 'Why don't you make a picture called *Cat People?*'" And Charlie Koerner said to Lewton, "I thought about it all night and it kind of bothered me." So he called in Lewton and asked him to make the picture.

We started talking, and a young man called DeWitt Bodeen—he's a writer, a very talented playwright today—suggested ideas, and we suggested others. The whole film, including the scoring, the cutting and everything, cost $130,000. And I got three thousand dollars flat fee for it. We made it very quickly.

We worked out the story of a girl who is obsessed with the idea of cats, who herself turns into a cat. In it is a scene everyone talks about: there's a girl, the heroine, in a deserted indoor swimming-pool at night, and her enemy, the girl who becomes a cat, a leopard, prowls along the side of the pool howling, and the shadows are on the walls, and there's a feeling of terror. To get the right feeling of claustrophobia, we purposely selected a pool in an existing apartment building here that was like the inside of a shoebox: white walls and low ceiling, with powerful light reflections from the water.

Now, I had a friend in the San Fernando Valley who had a swimming-pool and kept two pet cheetahs. On hot days when he was working, I'd go there in the afternoon all alone. I'd dive in and swim around. And one day I'll be damned if one of the cheetahs wasn't out of his cage and starting to prowl around and growl in a low way, and I thought, "Oh my God, here I am feeling naked, I can't scream," and I was going round in circles in the nude, just as the girl did. Luckily, the cheetah was afraid of the water. And eventually, from way back on the property somewhere, the gardner came with a rake and shooed the cheetah back. But for a while there I had a frightening feeling.

We believed in suggesting horror rather than showing it. The shadow you saw of the big cat on the wall of the swimming-pool was actually my fist. We had one big arc light with a diffuser on it in the pool and we had to shoot the sequence in one morning. We tried the effect every possible way to get the right diffused shadow, and then finally I made the shadow myself. That's the way to make films: improvise. If you're too well organized, it's no good.

My only complaint about the scene was that the girl threatened in the pool wasn't feminine or diminutive enough. She was built like a wrestler! Too bad!

Later on in the picture there's another famous scene in which a woman appears in a restaurant before the heroine, and reminds her that she belongs to the cat people. We wanted a woman who looked like a cat, and we searched and searched until we finally found this very thin model, and all she had to say was one word, meaning "Sister". I wasn't too happy with Simone Simon's performance as the cat girl. They had a contract with her at RKO and we evolved the story about a foreign girl because she had an accent.

The picture was made during the war, and during war, for some mysterious reason, people love to be frightened. Subconsciously we all enjoy being afraid, and in war that feeling is intensified. Wars release our needs: young men can rape with sanction, plunder without retribution. We all love wars and love to be frightened, and in wartime people had money from the plants, money to burn, and they loved that kind of film.

My next film, *I Walked with a Zombie*, had a horrible title for a very good film—the best film I've ever done in my life. It was poetic, and took place in Haiti, which meant we could take advantage of the theme of voodoo. We were lucky in finding a man called Sir Lancelot, an improviser of Caribbean songs, and we used him as a Greek chorus, wandering in seven or eight times and explaining the plot. And we had a very fine cameraman, Nicholas Musuraca, who managed a beautiful visual quality.

This was a *Jane Eyre* set in the tropics: about a girl in a house where there's an insane wife.

We had a dance group from Haiti, and they gave a stylized version of the voodoo ceremony. The story was childish and primitive—a man whose wife is a zombie, those things don't exist—it doesn't make any sense, the walking dead, the dead wife. But the whole thing had the consistency of a legend, something you're telling to children.

In this film, as in others, I made the people talk very low, as I think this indicates sincerity, and I always sit in on the dubbing and hold it very quiet. A lot of people don't like that, but it makes for the effect I want. I'll have an actor replay a whole scene as though he's just talking to me in a normal voice, and it's effective.

I didn't like my next picture, *The Leopard Man*. It was too exotic, it was neither fish nor fowl: a series of vignettes, and it didn't hold together. There were some startling things in that story about a series of murders in a Mexican town by a man dressed as a leopard: the blending of the shriek of the leopard and the shriek of a train, and the blood of the girl attacked by the cat going under the trestle of a door, and her mother on the other side unable to let her in. But there were too many bad scenes, and even though we used an effective Mexican birthday song, the overall effect was spotty, uneven.

Another film I made in that period, and one I liked better, was *Experiment Perilous*, a period melodrama about a frightened wife, set in the early years of the century. Warren Duff, the producer-writer, picked up a lot of fascinating details. There was a very fine sequence—a wonderful sequence—that was cut out: it took place in a department store, with the old baskets with the wires for delivering money. It showed Hedy Lamarr followed by a detective: she couldn't be sure if she saw him or not.

In the music we used all the old themes: "Glow-Worm", French songs, and so on. We had beautiful snow scenes in the streets. Of course, the look of all these films at RKO was due to the wonderful work of the art department. This was one of the last family studios; normally in the studios there's a man and a half for every job, and if there's a cutting down of personnel, everyone hides, but at RKO everybody was exactly fitted to his job, and no one was after anyone else's. Each man was a specialist: there was a wonderful plaster shop, for instance; the best decorators; a wonderful property room: this was a family studio, like Disney's. Everyone had perfect taste: the art directors, Albert d'Agostino and Van Nest Polglase; the design man, Darryl Silvera.

I went on to make a Western, *Canyon Passage*; the

bigger your canvas the easier the scenes are, and I found this easier to direct than my "indoor" pictures. When you have three or four people in a small room, that's the test of a director. *Out of the Past* was a film I enjoyed making: it opened in Paris last year for the first time: the names in it, which were unknown at the time, have become important: Kirk Douglas, Bob Mitchum. The script was very hard to follow, and very involved; often in this type of film the audience is deliberately confused, because if your story becomes too pat then it's often dull. *Berlin Express* I liked too: for its time, 1947, it had a message: we based the central character of a European intellectual (played by Paul Lukas) upon Thomas Mann. We even used things that Mann had said. It was a story set in postwar Berlin and I think it had some cogent points to make about the changes that were taking place at the time.

Easy Living, a story about professional football players, was a hard one for me: I'd never been to a football game, I've never played football; I'm not interested in any sports. I didn't like *Days of Glory* either, a war propaganda film set in Russia; what those poor guerrillas went through! It was unreal, stylized, and I don't like unreality, stylization.

In all these pictures, I've never had the right of final cut: the right to supervise the final editing of a film. I see a rough cut, make notes to a stenographer, and then go away: after that the studio can do what it likes, restore scenes I've cut, re-edit others, anything. I can't do anything about it, so there's no point in worrying, is there? I used to be an editor in Europe before I became a director. So it annoys me.

I believe in improvisation. I believe in instinct. I believe that when I write something, or paint—I draw and paint— it's subconsciously inspired: we're not doing it *consciously*. There's a book I've been studying, *Graphotherapeutics*, about therapy with graphology, and I've two hours a day now with the man who wrote it; he's correcting my handwriting, and it's altering my whole personality, because he says—and rightly—that your subconscious is writing, not your conscious. And faults in your personality are disclosed in the application of details.

I don't believe in doing everything in advance, as Hitchcock does. I began working in France, and there everything is without a schedule. I'd go on the set and say to the cameraman, "Look, come on over here, and let's look at it from this point of view." That's how we worked! I believe great things come from that great reservoir we have within us of past experience, which is all available. But I do work very hard on the dialogue before we shoot, because I consider the poor actors: once you change the lines, you throw them. I sometimes get new writers brought in, to ensure that the writing is quite perfect.

The director in America is slowly becoming a clerk. He does what he's told as fast as he's told—three days to do a half-hour show—and that's not the way a director should work: he should stamp a film with his own personality. Then you have an entertaining film. But outside of ten or twelve—Hitchcock, the big directors—that big army of the others is an army of clerks.

Night of the Demon, from a story by M. R. James, was a film I liked doing: about a diabolist in modern England, and the attempt of an investigator (Dana Andrews) to track him down. I never read the original story, and the script was rewritten many times. The one thing I didn't like was the introduction of a monster, the demon itself, which appears in the woods at night and terrifies members of the cast. I had an agreement with the studio that they wouldn't do that to me, but they put the monster in after I left. They wanted to cater for the children, you see.

Making a film in London, as this one was, is a director's dream: the man who played the evil central figure[1] was wonderful, and the bit players were all so perfect, so professional. I like a lot of things in the picture: the wind-storm, the comic séance and so on: and that idea of the casting of the runes, with the sliver of paper fluttering when it is placed in the hands of the man who is to become the devil's victim: very good fun. Of course, the scene in which there's a man who's a victim of a catatonic trance state and is examined by doctors must have made physicians wince: it was so childish, my God! The man comes up to the stage to examine the tranced figure and it's all wrong medically, but it was enjoyable.

The storm which the diabolist summons up to impress his adversary with his magic, and a scene in a farmhouse when the investigator is threatened by some grim rural people, were favourites of mine.

I had a fight over the staging of the storm scene. We

[1] Niall MacGinnis.

had to rent twelve aerial engines from World War I. We were on an exterior location, and there were great big trees, and if we'd had half a storm it would have been inadequate. We had truckloads and truckloads of dead leaves, and we set the radial engines whirling—cost a fortune, no one would talk to me. They said, "We'll do it with generators, electric machines," and I said, "No, it's got to be a hell of a storm; it's got to blow over the prams and the nurses in the garden, and all the chairs." So we had all these huge engines going; there was so much damned noise you couldn't hear anything.

I wasn't too happy with *A Comedy of Terrors,* and don't want to talk about it, not on record, anyway. For *City Beneath the Sea* I wouldn't go under water! For *The Giant of Marathon* again I wouldn't go under water! The last was one of those pictures where the actors speak three different languages on the set; it makes the film unbearably static; the young girl speaks in French, Steve Reeves answers her in English, and so on.

Recently, I've been doing television; an episode with Gladys Cooper of *Twilight Zone* I did enjoy doing, but largely I hate doing television; it's horrible. It's against everything I believe in; if you don't bring some of your individuality and some of your experience and sensitivity to bear on a subject, you don't get more than a mechanical result. You do what you can. You can't rehearse, you can't prepare. On one series I worked three days on one episode, and on the evening of the third day the producer gave me the script which I would read in the night and then I'd go into the next episode on the fourth day, and I'd find cast all ready chosen and wardrobed, people I'd never met before. I'd ask each one what he or she was going to play! I did twelve like that, back to back, without a respite. I made a lot of money, but what the heck! That's no way to create, to bring personality to the art. . . . And I believe in individuality, always.

King Vidor

A poet of Americana, his films celebrating the fields and lakes, woods and plains of an irrevocably vanished rural past, King Vidor lives today in a large and far from rustic Beverly Hills home, its study—where he receives us— housed in a smaller, separate building close to the high- way. Glimpsed briefly in David Butler's 1949 Hollywood- based farce It's a Great Feeling, *the director displayed much of the pep and drive and energy one might expect from the maker of* Duel in the Sun *and* The Fountain- head. *Some of that ebullience is missing from the white- haired, rather patrician figure advancing down the path from the main house to keep our appointment—and no wonder, since he is now in his eighth decade. But during a long and fairly exhausting taping session he seldom falters, and we afterwards share a joke at the expense of the author of a recent movie book who solemnly excluded King Vidor from the land of the living. We also admire his paintings hanging on the study walls, mostly sriking panoramic landscapes which include most notably a distant overhead view of the immense city of Los Angeles, as formally stylized and geometrically complex as an image from* The Crowd *or* War and Peace. *Films and paintings are recognizably products of a single vision, pure and deep and intensely lyrical, and often achieving true grandeur. These are all unfashionable qualities right now, but an artist of King Vidor's stature can afford to scorn fashion, for his place in motion picture history will remain perma- nently secure.*

My first films were made in my home town of Houston, Texas, when I was seventeen or eighteen: two or three half-hour, two-reel, broad slapstick comedies. This was an era of very short films. The comedies starred Edward Sedgwick, a comedian who later worked for MGM in Hollywood. They cost no more than the stock and lab costs, about ten cents a foot: approximately two or three hundred dollars each. We didn't spend a dollar outside.

I recently had a similar experience when my class of nine graduate students at USC made two half-hour films for four hundred dollars, only this time there were no laboratory or developing and printing costs because all that was done at the college. The main expense was purchasing the film; the rest cost us only twenty-five dollars.

Following the comedies—two of which were nationally distributed from New York—I made two or three documentaries: one was about title guarantee and business, another was about the sugar industry. By that time we had a camera of our own mounted on a surveyor's tripod and costing no more than a hundred and twenty-five dollars, and finally we put together a laboratory. Our open stage consisted of some telephone poles with cloth stretched over the top.

At that time, I didn't know if I was going to be an actor, a cameraman, a writer, or what. There was no planning; it was a hand-to-mouth existence, whatever you could scrounge.

Then I landed an assignment as newsreel cameraman for our local district, and tried to get the Ford Motor Company—which operated a newsreel for which they paid sixty cents a foot—to finance our proposed trip to Hollywood by selling them my material.

Well, we didn't get much—I don't think the trip cost us more than sixty dollars—but it was enough to make our first down-payment on a Ford, which at that time sold for about five hundred dollars, and we got out here that way, arriving in California with about twenty cents. There were three of us: myself, my wife Florence Vidor, who later became a star, and a boy from Texas who didn't stay on.

At first, in Hollywood, I did a little bit of everything. I would do anything just to get inside a studio and watch directors working. One way I did that was by appearing as an "extra", for which you got a dollar and a half lunch allowance. I wasn't choosy. In one picture, for instance, I had a "bit" as a chauffeur.

Then I obtained a job as a script-clerk, which was a little different from today's script-girl: you almost had to keep accounts. I remember having to look after the magnificent cash sum of twenty-five dollars!

There were no guilds or unions in those days, so we'd just go to each studio department looking for a job. Finally I got one as a writer in the story department at Universal. There I met a man named George Brown who was making a series of half-hour films. Although I hadn't directed, I told him I had, so he sent me out as a cameraman for two or three days on one of his projects. I did know how to operate a camera, however, and had in fact sold one of my short two-reel comedies ot the Vitagraph Company for thirty dollars.

Soon after that, George Brown left Universal, founded his own company and hired me as a director. I must have made about fifteen or twenty half-hour films for him, mainly stories concerning juvenile delinquency.

Then I tried to get a job as a director of so-called "features" by putting three of these short films together to make them look as if they were one picture. That didn't work, so I wrote an original scenario which I refused to sell unless I could direct it.

The people who had backed George Brown's short films—they were doctors and dentists, not really motion-picture men—became interested in my scenario, and nine of them put up one thousand dollars each to form the Brentwood Company and make the film. That's how I came to do my first feature, *The Turn of the Road*.

The Turn of the Road was a metaphysical, more or less religious type of film, inspired by the teachings of Christian Science. It was about a man (played by Lloyd Hughes) whose wife dies in childbirth. This tragedy makes him run away from his home, his friends, and his family, and wander the world in search of truth.

We didn't have enough money to shoot abroad—in India, for example—but we did show his return home. Thrown off a freight train, he sleeps in a barn and there meets his young son, who teaches him that truth is within us—symbolized by the fact that he found it at his own fireside.

The boy was played by Ben Alexander, who later became Jack Webb's policeman buddy in the television series *Dragnet*. Webb has now replaced him; but at that time he was a lovely little blond-haired athletic type of six-year-old boy.

The Turn of the Road was an immediate success. It ran

in Los Angeles for eleven consecutive weeks, which was unusual for that time, and then the print—we only had one print—went to New York. All the big stars and companies made me offers, but out of loyalty I stuck with the Brentwood Company for a year. We had no budget to buy stories so I wrote my own, drawing on things that had happened to me and things I'd seen.

The doctors who ran the Brentwood Company had at first objected to *The Turn of the Road*'s Christian Science theme, but when the film became a big success they wanted my next one to have a similar theme. I declined because I didn't want to make just that type of film. So I had to promise that my third film for them would return to a Christian Science subject, which allowed me to make my second film as a straight comedy.

One of the offers I received after the initial success of my first movie came from First National Exhibitors, a large exhibiting chain which was eventually taken over by Warner Brothers. They offered to finance three films to be made by me. I went to New York, signed the contract, and came back an independent producer. At that time I don't think I even owned a house.

My first film made under this arrangement was called *Jack-knife Man*. Then, when my studio began losing money, I had to close it up, and it was a relief to be able to go over to Thomas Ince Studios to do *Love Never Dies,* a melodramatic love story climaxed by a train wreck.

That was followed by a group of romantic melodramas starring my late wife, Florence Vidor. They included *Conquering the Woman*, an *Admirable Crichton*-type of yarn about a woman sent off to an island with a man; *Woman, Wake Up*; *The Real Adventure*, about a woman in business; and *Dusk to Dawn*, which was a dual-personality fantasy about the soul of a girl in India transmigrating into an American girl: when the latter went to sleep, the other girl woke up in India. Florence Vidor played both parts.

I next undertook a film version of the very successful sentimental Irish play *Peg O' My Heart*, which Laurette Taylor had made famous on the stage and which had been bought by Metro. We used Miss Taylor in it, and although she was then forty-five years old, we had her playing an eighteen- or nineteen-year-old girl: miraculously, we made her look quite convincing.

I'd been hired for Metro by a man named Major

Bowes, then a studio executive and later host of radio's Comedy Hour, an amateur talent programme. I was trying to get an option on a story called *Three Wise Fools* when he offered to buy it for the studio and let me direct it for them. I accepted, and subsequently spent twenty years at MGM. I never signed long-term contracts, only for terms of two or three years; that's why I missed out on MGM's pension plan.

I was very enthusiastic about *Three Wise Fools*, a story of three older men and a young girl, released in 1923. It gave me a chance to explore these people's deeply human feelings, a theme which I've been told runs through all my pictures, although I haven't been too aware of it myself. I've only been conscious of what stories interested me, of the kind of stories I like.

We next went all the way to Florida to capture the intense atmosphere of Joseph Hergesheimer's book *Wild Oranges*: one of the first films I know of for which a company travelled that far. Strange as it may seem today, when we shoot movies all around the world, nobody thought in those terms then. If you talked atmosphere, if you talked of the importance of a film's ambience, they'd say: "Why do you want to go all the way across the country? What's wrong with Griffith Park?" That's what the title of my book[1] is about: "A tree is a tree, a rock is a rock: shoot it in Griffith Park."

Hergesheimer's book described such things as Florida's oppressive heat, the moss on the trees, the tropical foliage, things like that. We went all over Florida trying to capture this atmosphere, and that's what made the picture so successful. Reviewers hailed the break-away from the studio which *Wild Oranges* represented as a milestone in the art of motion pictures.

Unfortunately, this film and others made then were done on rapidly disintegrating old film stock, so I'm not sure whether copies still survive. MGM doesn't seem very interested in preserving them: perhaps the Museum of Modern Art has copies.

Following *Happiness*, an unimportant film with Laurette Taylor, and *Wine of Youth*, a Jazz Era/Flaming Youth exploitation piece with Eleanor Boardman, I directed *His Hour*, a sex story written by Elinor Glyn, author of *Three Weeks* and inventor of the term "it", meaning sex-appeal.

[1] *A Tree is a Tree*, by King Vidor. Harcourt Brace, N.Y. 1953.

Miss Glyn, who was present throughout the making of *His Hour*, was quite weird, probably the weirdest person I've ever come across. Her dress, her talk and her appearance were altogether strange. She had false gums that startled you by turning purple under the copper-hued vapour lights whenever she smiled, and she was overly interested in tiny details that made no difference to the film.

She worried, for example, whether the seating arrangements for the story's aristocrat characters were correct according to protocol, because it was set in Czarist Russia which she had known and still remembered. They were just extras as far as we were concerned, but to her they were real princes and princesses, counts and grand dukes, and she would fuss over details of dress or furnishings that were not being photographed. We humoured her, however, because it did no harm and maintained her interest in the picture.

In those days we'd put a lot of effort into films that would come to town and play for only a few days and then be forgotten. There weren't any neighbourhood theatres all over the city as there are now, and films would just play briefly in one Los Angeles theatre and then vanish for ever.

I wanted to make films like D. W. Griffith's *Birth of a Nation* that ran longer. So I suggested three themes to the young MGM studio head, Irving Thalberg: war, wheat, and steel. We decided I should do a war picture first, so I began reading war synopses. Meanwhile, Thalberg had seen Laurence Stallings's play *What Price Glory?* in New York, and wired me that he'd spoken to the author who was available to write a picture for me if I wanted him.

I accepted immediately, and Stallings, who'd lost a leg in France in World War I, arrived here shortly afterwards with a five-page story. I spent about a week discussing it with him, then accompanied him back to New York to work out the plot. Eventually, he returned here to live, and until his recent death he was a neighbour whom I still saw frequently.

I wanted to make an honest war picture. Until then they'd all been very phony, glorifying officers and warfare. There hadn't been a single picture showing the war from the viewpoint of ordinary soldiers and privates, not one with some feeling of anti-war, of realistic war. Thalberg was attracted to the author of *What Price Glory?* because he detected some of these qualities in his play.

The Big Parade, as we called our story, was not originally planned as a big film, but that was what I really had in mind. I brought it in at $205,000 and then, when I was on another picture, they increased it by getting a director named George Hill to shoot some additional night battle-scenes which didn't involve any cast members.

I shot the main battle sequences in a park near here called the Legion Park, right next to Griffith Park, and one of them at a Santa Monica airfield called Clover Field. Some of the scenes involving four or five thousand people and two hundred trucks were done near San Antonio, Texas.

The famous scene in which the girl, played by Renée Adorée, clings to the back of the truck was done not with one but with three trucks, which we kept circling around the camera; we shot it in Griffith Park near Glendale. Renée Adorée was wonderful. I was mad about her. She was actually French—not at that time a star, perhaps a minor young MGM contract player—and because of her background there was never any argument against using her.

John Gilbert, on the other hand, *was* a star, and, in order to get him to appear in *The Big Parade*, they had sold it to exhibitors among a series of his "star films". I won't say I didn't object to him, but using him was part of the deal. When the picture was finished and became a smash hit, they had to go around and cancel and buy out those contracts in which it had been included as just another John Gilbert starring vehicle. It became a big "special" film, sort of put MGM on the map.

It put me on the map, too. As a result of *The Big Parade* I signed up with MGM for quite a while. There were no Academy Awards at that time, but, had we had them, I probably would have swept the whole field. It was a tremendous triumph.

Before the film was released, we anticipated that its attack on war might arouse opposition. Strangely enough, one of the Duponts—I'll never forget it—who was visiting the set one day, undertook to supply a big tent in which to show *The Big Parade* if exhibitors refused to handle it; and Duponts are supposed to be big war material manufacturers! But as soon as we held our first sneak preview in San Diego, the film's huge commercial success was instantly acknowledged.

For my silent version of *La Bohème,* starring Lillian Gish, we drew more on Mürger's original book *La Vie de Bohème* than on Puccini's opera. The situation was— and I think still is—that while the music, which could have been played in the orchestra, was protected by copyright the book was in the public domain. MGM have a print, in good condition.

I didn't much like *Bardelys the Magnificent,* a Rafael Sabatini story that attempted to establish John Gilbert as a Douglas Fairbanks-type swashbuckler. I was a little ashamed of it, and it wasn't very successful.

It was followed by one of my favourites among my own films, *The Crowd.* In fact, I have a copy of it here, and recently saw it again. *The Crowd* was an original idea of mine. It derived from my subjective approach to *The Big Parade,* which I conceived as the vision of one man observing all its happenings. When Thalberg wanted to know how I proposed to top *The Big Parade*'s success, I suggested the theme of a man observing everyday life, and then went home and wrote *The Crowd.*

I shot probably half the film on location in New York: we went all around the city with hidden cameras, which was way ahead of its time. Mostly we shot out of the back of a truck through a hole cut in the flap, and occasionally out of a camera hidden in a packing box. Nobody knew, and we didn't have to pay press agents or get publicity releases or anything like that.

Those larger-than-life-sized sets in *The Crowd* were the work of the recently retired Arnold Gillespie, who was then in charge of MGM's trick department. He did them in association with the art director, Cedric Gibbons. I was probably influenced by the Germans on that, by such silent films as E. A. Dupont's *Variety* and Fritz Lang's *Metropolis.*

For the scene in which the camera seemed to ascend along the outside of a building and then enter it through a window, Arnold Gillespie and his staff had to construct a whole horizontal thirty-foot-long miniature building and then have a bridge with the camera on it roll up outside it. Today, of course, you'd have a zoom lens and it would be nothing.

But in those days we had no zoom lenses or booms and had to let the camera down on a movable platform with cables. As it went forward on a track it had to be lowered, and we went right up into a closeup with this thing. Later, on location for *The Texas Rangers* in the nineteen-thirties, I remember we constructed a boom out of a telephone pole.

While working on *The Crowd*'s original story I envisaged its hero as a sort of nondescript—but not negative—individual, the sort of fellow you could like and with whom you'd be sympathetic, but not too aggressive, not too active.

One day, I was standing on the MGM lot talking to someone as a bunch of extras went by. One of them said, "Excuse me", and walked between us. I caught a glimpse of his face and realized at once that I had found the fellow I was looking for. I chased after him, and caught up just as he was getting on a bus. I asked him his name—he told me, but I forgot it immediately—and requested him to come and see me next day for an interview.

He didn't show up, so we had to go through that day's list of extras until we came across the name I realized he'd told me, James Murray. Even when we called him he didn't appear; he didn't think it was worth his while. Eventually we made a test of him by paying him as an extra, and that's how he came to play the lead in *The Crowd*.

Murray had been a doorman in New York and had come to Hollywood hoping to work in movies, even if only as an extra. He did make a few films after *The Crowd*—one of them with Mae West called, I think, *The Men in Her Life*—but then he became an alcoholic bum.

At the time I made *Our Daily Bread*, I saw him again and told him I might be able to offer him another large part provided he sobered up and lost some of his beer fat. "Oh, screw you," he replied, "the hell with you." And that was the last I saw of him. I got a letter a while back informing me that he'd either been pushed or fallen into the East River in New York and drowned; it had happened while he was drunkenly clowning around.

The Crowd, which cost around $325,000, didn't actually lose money, but its success was mainly *critical*. The studio had been unwilling to let me have very big stars for what Thalberg regarded as an "experimental" film. Also, they didn't have the advertising facilities they have today, such as television, which might have enabled them quickly to fill a big theatre on the strength of the stars' names.

As a result the theatres, which were all very large, would be maybe *half* filled with a lot of very enthusiastic people. *The Crowd* would have been an ideal art-house film, attracting the nineteen-twenties equivalent of the audiences that now patronize Fellini films, but we didn't have art-house chains then; they were slow developing.

Next I collaborated once more with Laurence Stallings, with whom I'd become good friends, on turning a play about newspapers into a strictly Hollywood romp called *Show People,* starring Marion Davies. I'd already done a Marion Davies comedy called *The Patsy*, and the Hearst press was sufficiently powerful to compel MGM and me to make another.[1]

Show People utilized the old Mack Sennett Studios and a lot of Sennett's old-time comedians. I saw it again quite recently, and it still has a lot of humour.

All the incidents for my all-Negro film *Hallelujah!* derived from my youth and childhood in Texas. My father owned sawmills and lumber-mills, and we frequently used to witness religious meetings and mass baptisms among Negroes. The mass baptism sequence in the river in *Hallelujah!* was suggested by a smaller one I'd seen as a child in Arkansas.

We staged that in Memphis, Tennessee, in the environs of which I shot most of the picture. The man's death in the swamp was shot in an actual Arkansas swamp. Although *Hallelujah!* was my first sound film, much of it, including all the travelling shots, was shot silent and the sound dubbed in later. That gave us all the freedom of a silent picture.

At that time sound equipment was immobile; it still is, practically. I was so anxious to do this film that I just went ahead and shot it silent as I'd done all my previous pictures. If we'd been using synchronized sound, all those elaborate travelling shots would have been impossible.

Post-synching *Hallelujah!* was a madhouse. They had no equipment for doing it—movieolas or things of that kind. We had to run the thing in a projection-room equipped with a buzzer which, when pressed, flashed a light which acted as a signal to the operator to put a grease-pencil mark on the film.

[1] Marion Davies was William Randolph Hearst's mistress for many years. (Authors' Note.)

Of course, by the time you'd pressed the button and the light had flashed on he'd put the pencil mark four or five feet away from where you'd intended. It was maddening. We did a lot of closeups back at the studio because of that. I think the six months we spent post-synching the picture hastened the sound-cutter's death.

I found Nina Mae McKinney, who played the female lead in *Hallelujah!*, in the chorus-line of the New York musical revue *Blackbirds of 1928*. I'd just come from Chicago where I'd tested many people for the film, and was scouring New York's churches, theatres, and dance-halls looking for additional Negro performers, some of whom possess a naturally bubbling personality. Nina Mae certainly did: I was immediately struck by her looks, very pretty and attractive and rather sexy, with a not too black, sort of *café au lait* skin.

The man who played the male lead was Paul Robeson's understudy in the stage production of *Show Boat*. I really wanted Robeson for the part and had written it with him in mind, but he'd left the show by then and gone, I think, to Russia.

Hallelujah! opened simultaneously in two New York theatres, one in Harlem and one downtown. The exhibitors' problem in selling it was to try to avoid attracting a large percentage of Negro patrons into the theatre, and I had to go around personally and endeavour to upset that.

The big Chicago theatre-owners refused to show the film, so a fellow in a small side-street theatre booked it, gave a dinner-and-black-tie opening, and after that the theatre was constantly sold out. Only then did Balaban and Katz, operators of the large movie-houses, agree to show *Hallelujah!* We always had to break the barrier like that.

The same thing happened in the South. I'd make a bet with an exhibitor that the film would do as well as his current attraction, and it did; but the trouble again was that they were afraid that the theatre would be filled with Negroes, and they didn't want that. It didn't necessarily mean that it *would* attract only Negroes, but that was their problem.

It was an artificial problem, too, because people in the South were genuinely interested in the Negroes and in their life; certainly there were no racialist objections to the film at all. The Negroes themselves loved it. Whether they would today is, of course, another matter.

My 1930 wide-screen version of *Billy the Kid* was the first 70 mm. film. It was shot in both 70 mm. and 35 mm. because we only had a few theatres equipped for the large gauge. I've always had the photographic eye, and had always been interested in exterior scenery and in photography, and so was determined to take full advantage of the unusual pictorial opportunities the wide screen offered.

William Fox made a wide-screen revue-type film about the same time, but since the industry was still paying for sound equipment he and the MGM executives got together and withdrew the wide-screen system because of its extra expense.

Years later, when I was making *Duel in the Sun*, the inventor of the 70 mm. camera suggested I do a wide-screen colour Western using his cameras, which were then idle. But just about the time I began looking for suitable stories, out came Cinerama, and shortly afterwards the whole industry took up the wide screen in a big way.

For *Billy the Kid* I sought out isolated locations all over the West and spent a day at the Grand Canyon and Zion Park, trying—with the aid of contemporary photographs— to duplicate the look of the New Mexico landscape which formed the backdrop to the true story of Billy the Kid. In fact, we deliberately copied old photographs of Lincoln County, New Mexico, even searching out matching geography, and completely avoided the hackneyed device of using existing Western studio streets.

I based my conception of the central character as much as possible on history, although of course the only surviving photographs of William Bonney are rather funny-looking old tintypes. I more or less stylized the leading actor's clothes; put him all in black.

The role should have been played by a tough young kid, a Jimmy Dean or a young Cagney. But the studio had this football-player[1] under contract, and, after three years of trying to find him a suitable starring part, they let me do the film only if I consented to use him in the lead.

Finally I gave in, but it wasn't good casting on my part. He wasn't sufficiently sharp or incisive. I didn't particularly want Wallace Beery as the sheriff either, but he had enough individuality and personality to dominate the character and that turned out well.

---

[1] Johnny (Charles) Mack Brown.

The concessions in the casting were in fact so bad that I have no desire to run the movie even today. I haven't seen it since it was made.

The crime of the early days of sound was that they thought you had to do stage plays and photograph them "straight". This practically set movies back twenty years, I suppose. So, when faced with the challenge of bringing Elmer Rice's one-set play *Street Scene* to the screen, I realized that you could make a terribly dull thing out of it by using uninteresting camera angles.

I didn't want to spoil the stage play by going into interiors or moving away from the front of the house, nor did I want to photograph it deadpan: that was the challenge. I wanted to preserve the play's purity and still have what used to be called "action".

My solution was to do it by change of camera setups, by change of composition: the composition became the action. We had a street built on the Goldwyn lot and didn't leave it at all except for one scene inside a taxi, from which the characters walk out into the front of the house; but that wasn't really an interior scene in the strict sense.

This was a pure experiment—I didn't know if it could be done successfully—but it worked, as I confirmed just recently on seeing *Street Scene* again.

Next I did *The Champ*, a child story starring Jackie Coogan. I used to feel I could alternate between an experimental film and a conventional film. *Street Scene* followed by *The Champ* was one of those alternations. It turned out well.

Bird of Paradise, however, was just a potboiler, but *Cynara*, which starred Ronald Colman and derived from a stage play, was a little more interesting. Samuel Goldwyn, its producer, had big ideas; he was always aiming very high, but films like *Cynara* are not the sort I feel best represent me.

I have an intense feeling for the earth, for rural life; the earth is a recurring theme in my films. It interests me photographically, too. I have some of Grant Wood's paintings and also own a ranch—although I'm afraid I don't get up there too often.

Originally I was interested in the Middle West: Indiana, Illinois, and all those states, the centre of America and American life. I used to have a map of the United States marked with pins to indicate the settings of my movies. I regard America as a kind of microcosm of the world: you have African, Russian, and practically all other kinds of people here, and in my films I tried to represent communities from New England to the South, and from the South to the West.

The Stranger's Return, for instance, was set in Iowa, although it was shot out in the country beyond Pomona here in California, because Iowa was too far to go at the time. We built an Iowa-type barn on farming land out there and it looked quite convincing.

Americana was the chief interest, too, in *The Wedding Night,* made for Sam Goldwyn and starring Gary Cooper. It was set among Connecticut tobacco-farmers, despite the fact that tobacco-fields are usually thought to be all in the South. I'd never done a film about Connecticut before, and this was a chance to capture some of its atmosphere.

In the middle of the Depression I read a little article on co-operation and co-op living which spurred me on to make the second segment of my War-Wheat-Steel trilogy, of which *The Big Parade* had been the first.

This was *Our Daily Bread,* a study of the fruits of the earth, for which I have a special affection. I borrowed money on just about everything I had in order to do it. Irving Thalberg said he would have liked to do it but couldn't convince the studio[1], so I ended up financing it myself and just about broke even.

It was shot out Sacramento Valley way, and to introduce a bit of "lift" and sex—because there just wasn't the audience for too much down-to-earth stuff—we brought in the extraneous character of the blonde floozy.

The insincerity of it is quite obvious now, but it represented a hangover from the just bygone heyday of the Mae West/Jean Harlow type of platinum blonde. We did it purely for box-office.

For *So Red the Rose,* a Civil War story, I returned to the moss-covered atmosphere of the Deep South, for which—having come from the South myself—I had a strong feeling. This was exactly the same story as *Gone with the Wind,* although made before it. It starred Margaret Sullavan, about whose acting I was very enthusiastic.

The Texas Rangers was set even closer to home, but it was mostly shot around Gallup, New Mexico, because it

[1] MGM.

was more convenient than actually going all the way to Texas.

After *Stella Dallas*, a successful soap opera, and *The Citadel*, which I shot in England, I undertook a film version of Kenneth Roberts's historical novel *Northwest Passage*, about Rogers's Rangers in eighteenth-century America, but we only filmed the book's first part, which was really a prologue to the main action in Part II. The second part was never made because of the producers' lack of courage. In the first part Rogers (played by Spencer Tracy) was a tremendous hero, but the second part showed his going to pieces, his disintegration, and I guess they feared that audiences of that time wouldn't accept it.

Anyhow, we kept enlarging the first half so much that it became a full-length picture, and it was always anticipated that I would continue on to do the second part: we even kept the actors on salary for a couple of weeks.

But that was not to be, and someone else—Jack Conway, I think—shot the picture's ending. That was in New York. The producer[1] called me up and asked if it was all right. I was so disheartened about not being able to film the whole story that I reluctantly gave my consent.

We shot *Northwest Passage* on location at Lake Payette, near Boise, Idaho. It was terribly difficult. Spencer Tracy had a doctor and a masseur—we were taking good care of *him*, wouldn't let *him* stand in the water too long—but the extras and most of the crew would stand in the water all day. I sent them into the river only up to about their waists; any farther would have been dangerous, and you couldn't take a chance on losing someone.

We shot the scenes showing them in the centre of the river on the MGM studio lake, which was equipped with a safety device. The only other "faking" was to have lighter boats for dragging over the hills and through the forests and heavier ones for actually using in the water, but there were no backdrops or process-shots or anything like that.

Coming after *Northwest Passage, Comrade X*, an insignificant light comedy, represented a change of pace, but I was very interested indeed in the picture I did after that: *H. M. Pulham, Esq*, based on John P. Marquand's novel. Marquand delineates his New England characters with

[1] Hunt Stromberg.

such depth and penetration that I tried using some new, experimental techniques in filming the novel.

I used direct cutting, for example, and instead of the conventional insert of a letter, I used the letter-writer's voice. I noticed in a recent film, *Two for the Road*, that the automobile bearing the two main characters would vanish offscreen, and then the characters would come walking in from the other side of the screen. Now, I'd used that technique in *Street Scene*: as people would go out the other characters would come in—sort of a human and temporal cycle. The putting together of sequences in *H. M. Pulham, Esq* has a lot of this sort of thing, of going to one point that carries you, by a kind of overlapping process, to the next moment, the next part of the film.

I thought Robert Young was fine in the lead, but Hedy Lamarr was miscast. The book called for an attractive American secretary, and Hedy Lamarr's accent gave the part a wholly different image. But as a type she was all right.

The final segment of my War-Wheat-Steel trilogy, *An American Romance*, was a big love of mine for many years. One of my ideas was to illustrate the story by the use and development of colour. That's when I started painting in earnest, although I'd actually begun painting on *Pulham*, which was of course a black-and-white picture.

That was one idea. Another was to bring in the concept of "lift", of rising from the earth up into the air: first you have the earth, the heavy earth and iron ore, becoming progressively more refined until finally it flies up, up into the sky as an airplane, taking in all of America. We started in New York and took in most of the states right across the country to California.

I wrote *An American Romance* for a star cast consisting of Spencer Tracy, Ingrid Bergman, and Joseph Cotton, and at one time the studio promised to let me have these people. When I finally came to do the film, I had none of them: I wasn't enough of a lunchroom politician to prevent someone else taking them over, and so I received secondary casting.

I compromised by taking Brian Donlevy and a girl[1] they wanted to develop, justifying it to myself on the grounds that I'd become a kind of "company man" at

[1] Ann Richards.

MGM and had been on salary for a year without making a picture.

But neither Brian Donlevy nor the girl was very exciting, and that, combined with wartime conditions and studio cutting, spoiled the film. I cut a lot out of it to begin with, and then the studio cut more. I'd discovered, when taking it out on the road in the Middle West, that it was too heavily loaded on the documentary side at the expense of the human side, and wanted to cut it accordingly. Well, the studio did the reverse: they cut out the human story and kept all the documentary stuff. Then, to avoid having to redub the music, they made further cuts according to where the music ended, which was of course nonsensical and ruinous to the film. That's when I became very annoyed and left MGM for good.

I shot much of *An American Romance* at the mills of United States Steel in Gary, Indiana, because I'd seen them from a train window and realized it was the biggest, most spectacular, most photogenic plant of its kind in the country, bigger even than those in Pittsburgh, which I also looked at.

Shooting close to naked flames was extraordinarily difficult, because we quickly became enveloped by sulphur fumes and steam and couldn't see anything for a while. Sometimes we had to stand quite still while a running river of molten steel ran right alongside us. The only consolation was that it warmed us in the prevailing cold weather.

My original conception of *Duel in the Sun* was of an intense, *High Noon* type of thing: all that bigness and blow-up was added later by the producer, David O. Selznick. He got me to run *Gone with the Wind* some time during the shooting and stated that he contemplated blowing *Duel in the Sun* up like that.

And blow it up he did: he added the prologue, narrated by Orson Welles, he added a big spectacular opening, he called in other directors to shoot additional sequences, he had at least three cameramen at different times throughout the making of the picture, and he kept constantly augmenting the cast.

Selznick thought in grandiose terms: the more people he could hire—the more cameramen, the more second units—the better he liked it. Maybe he was trying to buy up competition. He certainly had no sense of economy at all.

Even during shooting he had other directors working on the picture besides himself: Otto Brower, Sidney Franklin, William Cameron Menzies; the last two did a couple of days each, working mostly on scenes not involving the principals.

Selznick was a great one for second units spread all over the place because they could take more time and wouldn't hold up the actors. But all the second unit directors consulted with me about the way I visualized the shots. This is quite normal, provided consultation takes place with the director who has planned the scenes and who can assign the subordinate directors to appropriate sequences. Sidney Franklin, for example, was good with animals, another fellow was good with action; so you let them do it, provided they got together with you beforehand to draw up little diagrams of how you wanted the sequences to go.

Two days before the end of shooting I had an argument with Selznick and quit. That's when he called in William Dieterle, for whom he wrote additional scenes, such as the big opening in the Presidio Saloon with Tilly Losch's dance and the spectacular trainwreck later in the picture. My opening scene showed Herbert Marshall in gaol.

In addition, Selznick had Dieterle reshoot some of my scenes the same way I'd shot them and using identical dialogue, so that afterwards, when the Directors' Guild appointed a committee to adjudicate on credit for the finished picture, it was sometimes impossible to tell the difference between Dieterle's scenes and mine. They ran the film while the cutter and I sat in, and finally decided that I was entitled to credit on all but five, eight, or perhaps even ten per cent of the total.

My quarrel with Selznick was over my allegedly being behind schedule—although it was his fault. At first we were good friends but that didn't last long. He would rewrite and retake for no apparent reason; he wrote most of the picture, in fact. He'd come and ask me to re-shoot a scene I'd already done that day with a slight difference, just to please him, and then complain that I was behind schedule.

But *he* was the writer and producer, not me; and whenever he sent someone to complain about my being off schedule I'd say, "Well, keep David off the set and we'll be right on schedule."

One day his production man had given the camera and

crew to one of the second units so I couldn't shoot
the thing I'd rehearsed. David came out and made a big
scene: "Why aren't you shooting?" he yelled. "What's the
matter with you?" I'd warned him that if he did that three
times I'd leave, and this was the third time. We were out
on location with the cavalry, the railroad, thousands of
people. I told him to quit blowing off till he found out the
real cause of the trouble, but he persisted; so I said,
"Apparently you want to direct the picture", gave him the
micropone and left. He implored me to come back but I'd
had enough. It was two days before the end and I was
pretty tired.

Josef von Sternberg's contribution to *Duel in the Sun*
was as a sort of general assistant. He suggested lighting,
interviewed and tested actors, looked for locations—
anything that Selznick and I wanted him to do. He helped
in any way he could. He's a terribly nice, terribly likable
fellow, and Selznick and I both wanted to do something
for him.

He might, for example, have made suggestions concerning Jennifer Jones's clothes or her hair-style: things like
that. One night I had to leave and let him shoot a scene
I'd rehearsed of a sheriff (Charles Dingle) going through
a patio and opening doors in search of Lewt McCanles
(played by Gregory Peck).

But then he reverted to his old form of shooting many
takes so that was that. It's been claimed he had a lot to do
with the picture's colour design. Perhaps he did preliminary tests before I came on to it, but afterwards he
certainly had little to do with that aspect of it.

The reason for the three accredited cameramen—
Harold Rosson, Lee Garmes, and Ray Rennahan—was
because we had a strike in the middle of the film and had
to stop work for something like three to six weeks. Rosson
was our original cameraman, but when we resumed it was
with Garmes because Rosson was probably on another
film. All those flamboyant sunset effects were done by
Rennahan, who was Technicolor's man.

Jennifer Jones's climactic ride into the desert involved
shooting directly into the sun, an idea inspired by Orson
Welles's *Citizen Kane,* which had spotlights shining right
into the camera. The aim of that was to accentuate the
heat: the heat on the rocks, the heat on the desert, and
the heat of the atmosphere.

It *was* hot, too. We were on some jagged rocks about

twelve miles out of Tucson: I think Jennifer still has scars on her legs from crawling over those rocks. We did a few of her closeups in the studio but shot most of that sequence over a period of several days on a hilltop, about an hour's ride away from Tucson.

The ranch-house, "Spanish Bit", was built out in Arizona, but the narrow-gauge railroad scenes were done at Lasky Mesa on Camillo Ranch, about one hour from here: all this despite the fact that *Duel in the Sun* was set in Texas! But why go all the way to Texas when you can do it even better nearer home?

Next came *On Our Merry Way*, a synthetic hotchpotch of which I directed two episodes and George Stevens one, and then I went on to do a film I liked very much, *The Fountainhead*, based on Ayn Rand's novel.

Miss Rand wrote the screenplay herself, but not before other writers had made several previous attempts, spoiling the book in the process. I wanted her to adhere closely to the book, and she did. She's a very determined person. She knows exactly what she wants and is not easily persuaded. She agreed to work on the script only if they promised not to change it without her consent. Whenever actors wanted to change lines, we had to telephone her to come over. That helped stop a lot of actors changing lines, which was a benefit, I think, to the director.

The philosophy advanced by Ayn Rand in *The Fountainhead* was compatible with what I personally believe, inasmuch as I strongly hold that all inspiration and all life come to us directly from God without the intervention of orthodox institutions or intermediate channels of any kind. To that extent I think we're in direct communication with God.

Of course, that's an idealistic view that can be taken to the point of arrogance, but it's not essentially incompatible with Ayn Rand's philosophy.

I did greatly dislike *The Fountainhead*'s ending, however. It was silly to have an architect blow up a building just because they changed some of the facade.

"If you make a cut in this picture and I burn it," I asked Jack Warner, "will you forgive me?"

"Well, we won't," he replied, "but the judge might."

Originally I thought Gary Cooper, who was assigned to the picture before I came on to it, was miscast as the architect Howard Roark. I felt it should have been someone more arrogant, like Humphrey Bogart. But when I saw his performance again several years later, I came to accept his interpretation and thought he made a very good job of it. Patricia Neal I thought marvellous, splendid. I liked her tremendously.

Edward Carère designed those wonderful "modern" buildings used in *The Fountainhead*. Like Ayn Rand's book, they were heavily influenced by the work of Frank Lloyd Wright. In fact, Carère and I studied all that had been published about Wright and inspected all his buildings around here.

I planned to go out and see Wright himself and discuss the whole project, but Jack Warner heard about it at the last minute and stopped us, afraid that if I discussed the thing with Wright and didn't make a deal he might sue us later, claiming we'd stolen some of his ideas.

The set of the newspaper-office was actually an insurance office containing two hundred desks, while for the final scene atop the Roark Building in New York we used a process background shot from a helicopter and projected at an angle, while the cage with the people in it went by on a cable, and our camera shot it all from a great height on the sound-stage: quite a difficult technical thing.

My producer on *The Fountainhead* was Henry Blanke, with whom I made two other pictures, *Beyond the Forest* and *Lightning Strikes Twice*. I found him a charming fellow to work with and to get along with, except for his belief that women writers were infallible; for him they could do no wrong. On *The Fountainhead* it was Ayn Rand, on the other two it was Lenore Coffee.

I don't much care for *Beyond the Forest* for some reason or other, although it's become famous through being referred to in the opening scene of *Who's Afraid of Virginia Woolf?* It has a certain atmosphere—particularly in the exterior hunting sequence shot up at Lake Tahoe and in the ending when Rosa Moline lurches towards the train—but it's not among my favourite pictures. Still, I liked it a little better than *Lightning Strikes Twice*, which turned out terribly.

I had one or two run-ins with Bette Davis, who played Rosa Moline, and was told later that she'd tried—unsuccessfully—to have me taken off the picture.

"If he's still directing tomorrow," she said at one point, "either I won't be here or cancel my contract."

Well, I think at that time they were very anxious to

cancel her contract, so they jumped at it. They had an agreement there in about ten minutes.

My points of difference with Miss Davis were over terribly minor things. She's a pro, and she usually came and gave a good performance. But she's also terribly touchy and quick to take offence where none is intended.

I thought Jennifer Jones was very good in my next film, *Ruby Gentry*. That was rather like a Tennessee Williams story, with the characteristic mental heat and overcharged atmosphere of the Deep South. At first, Jennifer was very awkward handling guns for the final sequence in the swamp, but as it was shot in a studio and using blank cartridges, she soon became accustomed to them.

The scene in which the lovers drive their car into the moonlit sea was autobiographical and added to the script by me. That used to happen all the time in my part of Texas. Lovers would drive out to the shore, gaze at the moon and have a necking session, and by the time they wanted to move the tide had come up and they were stuck. We had to go all the way up to Pismo Beach near San Francisco to find a beach that you could drive along similar to the Texan one where I lived.

I was only mildly interested in *Man without a Star*, a potboiler done in four weeks, but I loved *War and Peace*, which came next. I thought we captured the book's atmosphere very well. I was really inspired, but then it's easy to be inspired by a great book. The recent Russian eight-hour version had an almost unlimited budget, but my *War and Peace* ran six months in Moscow, so they obviously liked it.

I wish I'd had Peter Ustinov as Pierre instead of Henry Fonda, but that was out of my hands. I also considered Paul Scofield for the part. Fonda was better than Scofield would have been, but I think Ustinov would have been great. It was of course inconceivable to have anyone other than Audrey Hepburn as Natasha, and among the supporting players I thought Oscar Homolka and Herbert Lom particularly outstanding.

The English cameraman Jack Cardiff—now a director—was brilliant. The Italian art director was probably the best I've ever worked with, and his compatriots[1]—the assistant director (who has since died), the costume design-

[1] King Vidor's *War and Peace* was shot in Italy. (Author's Note).

er, and all the rest—were collectively better than I've ever experienced here.

It's strange that of all my pictures *Solomon and Sheba* is spoken of least. I did half of it—two months—with Tyrone Power. More than once he told me: "This is the best part I've ever had, the best picture I've ever been in," and when we ran the rushes we had to agree: he was able to convey the character's vacillation between sex and religion, between sex and state obligation, so well that we thought we were going to have a simply marvellous movie.

Then Power died and was replaced by Yul Brynner, who was so cautious and inhibited at stepping into the part in those circumstances that *Solomon and Sheba* somehow turned into an unimportant, indifferent sort of picture. Its inherent unreality and phoniness were accentuated without Power's sincerity in the leading role. He was terribly interested in the part and was doing such a good job that it would have made all the difference to the finished film. It would be extremely interesting to compare *Solomon and Sheba* in its present form with the two months' footage we shot with Power: I'm sure it must be preserved somewhere.

We also had weather problems. I'd started shooting in September, but it was December by the time we came to re-shoot it and we could no longer go to the places I'd originally used, so we constantly had to cheat in matters of climate and landscape.

Since then I've done an experimental 25-minute 16 mm. film called *Truth and Illusion: An Introduction to Metaphysics*. It started when I simply wrote a narration that interested me and challenged myself to fit it to a film, using existing objects in nature, without animation techniques of any kind. I did the photography myself for very little money, and have only shown it to interested groups on request. Every time I see it I notice about half a dozen to a dozen things I'd like to change.

It represents an almost abstract attempt to illustrate philosophical thoughts and ideas with strictly photographed—not manufactured—images. What, it asks, is truth, and what is illusion? It draws its examples from obvious things like the movies' illusory "motion", and the way railroad tracks seem to converge to a point on the horizon.

I've also written two scripts. The first, on which I

worked a year, is on the life of Cervantes. It has since been filmed by Vincent Sherman in a greatly changed form, so different from my original conception that, on friends' advice, I withdrew from the project.

The other script is about Mary Baker Eddy. I haven't tried to push it too hard because it needs rewriting and because I prefer to wait until I can have Audrey Hepburn for the lead. I think she'd be perfect, although there are others who could possibly do it, too.

In addition, I've been preparing a film with Samuel Goldwyn Jr, based on a recently published novel called *Mr and Mrs Bojo Jones*. This is a contemporary story rather reminiscent of *The Crowd*, about a young small-town couple who marry because the girl gets pregnant. Some people might consider it just another *Peyton Place*, but I think the problem it treats is no less valid today than it was forty years ago when I made *The Crowd*, and I visualize it as almost a modern remake of that film.

Billy Wilder

*Almost alone among Hollywood directors, Billy Wilder
has succeeded in hanging on, through Hollywood's long
years of compromise, its increasingly desperate wooing of
the audience, to a corrosive misanthropy, a disenchanted
view of the public. If his most recent comedies have
sugared the pill, they have still come out with a philosophy
not calculated to please the nursing mothers of Podunk.
And his best films,* The Lost Weekend, *with its unsparing
portrait of drunkenness,* Double Indemnity, *a heartlessly
brilliant exploration of the criminal mind, and* Sunset
Boulevard, *cynical and cruel in its exposure of the vanity
of a faded film star, remain as tough and unsettling as
when they were made more than eighteen years ago.*

*One approaches Wilder with a slight sense of unease
then, and he isn't easily reached: his publicity man says he
is far too restless to sit down to a tape for more than five
minutes. His office, in the rather austere but friendly
atmosphere of the spartan Mirisch/UA outfit, is not at all
opulent, beige-and-brown as usual; and Wilder himself is
equally spartan: athletic and brisk in T-shirt and casual
California slacks. He looks at the tape-recorder uneasily,
but seems gradually to get used to its silent movement,
and, after the interview, examines it approvingly, even
announcing a decision to buy one like it himself. Genial
and relaxed while speaking, his only moves away are to
the telephone, and then only at the summoning of the
independent production chief, Walter Mirisch, boss of the
outfit for which he now works.*

I started as a newspaperman in Vienna, having quit
school and begun to work in my teens; then I went to

Berlin, which was at that time the dream of every middle-European journalist. In 1927 I ran into a group of young guys who were interested in making movies, I wrote a script, and—my God!—somehow we turned it into a film, *People on Sunday*. We borrowed money from the uncle of Robert Siodmak, the director. And Robert was the director for a very simple reason: when kids play football on a meadow the one who owns the football is the captain, and he owned the camera. The film cost five thousand marks to make. It was more *nouvelle vague* than a hippy picture! We were all dilettantes then. Eugen Shuftan was the cameraman and the only pro—he works in New York because he never could get a union ticket. He won the Oscar for *The Hustler*. Edgar G. Ulmer worked as Siodmak's assistant director, and Fred Zinnemann was Shuftan's assistant.

The film opened in a small cinema on the Kurfursten-damm. It was about young people having a good time in Berlin and it was talked about a lot. It represented a good way to make pictures: no unions, no bureaucracy, no studio, shot silent on cheap stock: we just "did it"! As a result of its success, we all got jobs at UFA, the huge German studios. I was considered an "up and coming young writer of twenty" in the commercial picture swim, and I'd write two, three, four pictures a month. I accumulated about a hundred silent picture assignments, and then, in 1929, when sound came in, I did scores more. I did vehicles for Kitty von Nagy, Ho Haberfeld, Lilian Harvey, and Willi Fritsch, a whole slew of stars, a version of *Emil and the Detectives*, and many, many more. I had my eye on Hollywood, as that was the proper progression for a writer; my mother had lived in America, and I had quite a few relatives here. I would have come here, Hitler or no Hitler, but I decided to come a little bit faster when he got into power!

I stopped over in France in 1933. Hitler had come into power on 30th January, and I left in March, just after the Reichstag fire. In Paris I made a film called *Mauvaise Graine* (no connection with the later *Bad Seed*), a story of kids, young automobile thieves, and Danielle Darrieux played the sister of one of the boys. We shot the picture in Paris and Marseilles, on a shoestring, with money put up by eight people.

We didn't use a single sound-stage: most of the interiors were shot in a converted garage, even the living-room set, and we did the automobile chase sequences without transparencies, live, on the streets, at speed, and it was very exhausting.

I sold a story to Columbia shortly afterwards, and got a contract with a one-way ticket and not much money. The story was *Pam-Pam,* about a gang of counterfeiters who live in an abandoned theatre. It's boarded up, its gone broke, and they make their phony money there, and sleep in the boxes and use the rain machine for a shower. An innocent, naïve girl from Scarsdale, New York, comes to the theatre wanting a job and the gang, pretending they are theatricals, give her some phony hundred dollar bills and ask her if she would go to the bank, bring eighty dollars back for each bill, and keep twenty dollars for herself. Finally, the gang steal a play and sets and try to make the idea of her being in a play come true. Ultimately I think the story was sold to Paramount and something similar was done.

I went to Mexico and waited until I got my immigration visa to the United States. Then I started writing original stories at Paramount; and I kind of starved for a little bit. I shared a room with Peter Lorre; we lived on a can of soup a day. And then I got a job at Paramount; they teamed me with Charles Brackett, and I stayed there for eighteen years.

We wrote several films for the director Mitchell Leisen, including *Midnight* and *Hold Back the Dawn,* and one for Sam Goldwyn, made into *Ball of Fire.* Paramount wouldn't buy several of my ideas, including *Sunset Boulevard* and *The Apartment*; they just didn't understand these themes; they weren't ready for them at the time.

The creative atmosphere at Paramount was absolutely marvellous: you just walked across the lot and there they were: von Sternberg and Gary Cooper and Dietrich and Leo McCarey and Lubitsch. It was an atmosphere of creativity: we made pictures then, we didn't just make deals. Today we spend eighty per cent of our time making deals and the other twenty per cent making pictures.

My first American directorial assignment was *The Major and the Minor,* about a girl, played by Ginger Rogers, who disguises herself as a twelve-year-old because she doesn't have the adult train fare home; she meets and falls in love with an army major, played by Ray Milland, who of course treats her as a child. I got the job after making myself rather unpopular as a writer: I would come on the set and they would chase me off it. I always tried to put them right on misinterpretations. I was known as "The Terror": they would say, "Keep Wilder off the stage; he's always raising hell; he wants everything done his way." The fact is that very few directors know how to read, how to interpret dialogue correctly, and they are too proud to ask if they don't understand a particular line. So lines tend to get thrown away. Arthur Hornblow, for whom Brackett and I had written a few pictures, saw my point and thought I had better direct my own scripts.

I was very careful; I did not set out to make a so-called "artistic" success straight away, I set out to make a commercial picture I wouldn't be ashamed of. My agent, Leland Hayward, brazenly approached Ginger Rogers, who was then something—she had just won the Academy Award for *Kitty Foyle*—and sold her on me as director.

It wasn't too difficult for her to imitate a girl of twelve then; after all this was 1941. Playing it, for her, was like Lemmon and Curtis playing girls in *Some Like it Hot*; it was on the verge of the impossible, but there was that willing suspension of shocked disbelief! Mrs Rogers played Ginger's mother for real, and Ginger played her own grandmother! My God, those were the great naïve days; now you couldn't do it any more! We're all too worried now about competing with that entertainment you get for free from a box to be spontaneous, to have fun any more. After all, if you can get a free throwaway newspaper under the door, you don't want to pay for one; do you? And on TV it's as though they are getting a piece by Walter Lippmann written ten years ago. They're not that interested now but they get it for free today, so they re-read it.

Next I made *Five Graves to Cairo*, set in North Africa during World War II, with Erich von Stroheim as Rommel. He was fascinating: *le grand seigneur* at all times. There was something very odd and yet noble and dignified about him. He wasn't a Von or anything like that, he had a very heavy accent from the rougher suburbs of Vienna, but it didn't matter; he had style.

He didn't resemble Rommel at all, but that didn't matter either: he gave the audience the proper sense of illusion, a correct impression of the character. Of course, he influenced me greatly as a director: I always think of my style as a curious cross between Lubitsch and Stroheim. I remember when he came over to make the picture, we had been shooting the tank stuff on location in Indio, in the desert. When I got back to Hollywood, the studio told me he was in town, in a place called Western Costumes, and they were fitting him into the uniform of the Desert Fox. I introduced myself politely and clicked my heels, and said, "Isn't it ridiculous, little me directing big Mr Stroheim?" And just to make him feel better, I added, "You know, the reason you aren't directing any more is you were always ten years ahead of your time." And he said, "Twenty." He was full of marvellous ideas. His makeup, for instance: it was black on the face and white on his head above the line of the cap—you see, he pointed out that Rommel was always in the sun, and when he took his cap off there would be no colour in the skin underneath.

He insisted on having two cameras slung around his neck. They had to be German; he even insisted on having film inside, saying: "The audience will sense if the films aren't inside; they'll feel they are merely props." Of course, he later contributed ideas to *Sunset Boulevard* as well: the idea that the butler he plays writes all the fan mail for the lost star Norma Desmond, for instance.

But then he could go too far. "Let me do a scene," he said, "where I'm washing and pressing my former wife Norma Desmond's panties. Please, I know I can do it." And I said, "Yes, I know you can, but I don't want to shoot it."

On *Double Indemnity*, adapted from the novel by James M. Cain, I worked with Raymond Chandler. I sat in a room with him and sorted it out; we did the whole thing in ten or twelve weeks.

Raymond was a kook, a crazy man, but he had a wonderful flair. I wanted to do the script with Cain himself, actually, but Cain was doing a Western for Twentieth Century-Fox, so Chandler seemed the best choice. It was, incidentally, the first time he had worked on a script, or been inside a studio.

We used as many locations for the film as possible: Los Feliz Boulevard—an old-fashioned area going towards Glendale—for the Barbara Stanwyck house, the railroad station, parts of downtown. The insurance office was a copy of the old Paramount offices in New York. I'd go in and kind of dirty up the sets a little bit and make them look worn. I'd take the white out of everything. I had John F. Seitz, the cameraman who had worked with Rex

Ingram and Rudolph Valentino, with me on the picture
and he helped me a great deal. I wanted that look that
Californian houses get, with the sun streaming through the
shutters and showing the dust. You couldn't photograph
that, so Seitz made some shreddings for me and they
photographed like motes in sunbeams. I like that kind of
realism . . . everything in Hollywood always looks like the
late Jayne Mansfield's bedroom, and it's ridiculous.

The whole film was deliberately underplayed, done very
quietly; if you have something that's full of violence and
drama you can afford to take it easy; it's only if you have
nothing that you have to "blow it up", to make the sparks
fly. I hate arty tricks; suddenly you're shooting a man
crossing a street and you take him from the ninth story of
a building, and you begin to think in the stalls, "It must be
an FBI man looking down from up there", and instead it's
just an arty cameraman. Why? Why shoot a scene from a
bird's eye view, or a bug's? I guess they call that kind of
thing "stylish" or "beautifully conceived". "What an eye!"
they say, "Shooting stuff through parking meters!" It's all
done to astonish the bourgeois, to amaze the middle-class
critic. It's the work of the kind of people who are impressed by the fancy setups you get in TV commercials;
you know, a man with his feet on a desk and you can see
the soles of his feet covering nine-tenths of the screen and
in between the two shoes you see a little bit of his face.
Why?

In *The Lost Weekend* I again went for a realistic
approach. Originally, I wanted Jose Ferrer to play the
part of the drunk: I had seen him as Iago to Paul
Robeson's Othello, and he was superb. But Paramount
told me to forget it. Buddy de Sylva, the studio boss, said
that if the drunk wasn't an extremely attractive man, who
apart from being a drunk could have been a hell of a nice
guy and wanted to be saved, then audiences wouldn't go
for it.

I wanted to make things like the nightmare of the bat
and the mouse and the scene when the drunk gets the d.t.'s
as realistic as the main action. We used the exterior of
Bellevue Hospital in New York and copied the alcoholic
ward down to the last detail. Harry and Joe's bar, where
the central figure Don Birnam gets drunk, was a pastiche
of 52nd Street dives, and Sam's bar, where Howard de
Silva was the barman, was based on P. J. Clark's bar on
55th Street where Charles Jackson, the novel's author,

drank, and we showed the apartment building where he lived with his brother.

I bought the book at a stall while changing trains with Leland Hayward on our way to New York, and I read it overnight and immediately called Charles Brackett from Grand Central. "Go in and see Buddy de Sylva," I said; "this is our next picture." He read it, talked to de Sylva, and called me a couple of days later saying, "They're not convinced." I came back, eager to make the very first picture where a drunk was not something funny. In those days an alcoholic was something you roared with laughter about.

Finally, we talked the studio into doing it and got Milland. He did well; a great part helps an actor. At first Paramount didn't want to do the film, but eventually they came round.

The bat and mouse sequence was wonderfully put together by the backroom boys at the studio. We may have old-fashioned directors, money-mad financiers, and stupid front offices, but we have a tremendous "backlot". All those guys, the technicians, the prop men, the special effects men, these are the strength of Hollywood. I assure you that if our outer space agencies had the brains to get six prop men and tell them, "Look, by a week from Tuesday we've got to be on the moon!", we'd *be* on the moon!

The part of the writer, gigolo to the old star in *Sunset Boulevard*, was originally written for Montgomery Clift (it was played by Bill Holden), and just before we were to start shooting he said he didn't want to play it, because he didn't want to be seen making love to an elderly woman. Very strange for a New York actor, whose audience consisted of elderly women!

Long before that, I had planned to do the picture with Mae West, on the burlesque side, but later it evolved into a tragic story. We considered Swanson, Mary Pickford, who needed the part like a hole in the head, and Pola Negri, who was trying for it; but Swanson was a lucky choice, I think.

The film caused a great stir: I've never seen so many prominent people at once in the projection-room at Paramount as I saw the first day they showed it. Word was out that this was a stunner, you see. After the picture ended there were violent reactions—from excitement to pure horror. I remember Barbara Stanwyck kneeling down in front of Miss Swanson and kissing the hem of her garment in one of those ridiculous adulation things, and I still remember Mr Louis B. Mayer shaking his fist and saying, "We should horsewhip this Wilder! We should throw him out of this town! He has dirtied the nest! He has brought disgrace on the town that is feeding him!" He was furious! I don't know what the hell was so anti-Hollywood in that picture. Louis B. Mayer lived in a kind of dream world, unfortunately.

We originally had a weird kind of framing sequence containing some of the best material I've ever shot, but when we previewed the picture in Chicago and in the suburbs of New York, people just screamed with laughter, so we cut it.

I still have the footage. We showed the corpse of a man being brought to the morgue downtown. In this particular section of the morgue are about eight people, including an elderly man, a young boy, and Bill Holden. And the corpses are telling each other the details of events leading to their deaths. The boy drowned, the elderly man retired from a little avocado grove in Tarzana and had a heart attack, and the Holden character tells the story. By the time Holden had arrived and they'd put the name tag on his big toe, people were helpless with mirth. So we chopped it off and the narrator's voice begins by saying, "This is Sunset Boulevard, and this is me; I'm quite dead." It was announced coldly, like the opening of a supermarket ... the star shot him dead in her swimming pool, the star who loved him. Of course it's illogical, but that doesn't matter; it's not boring. And as long as it's riveting, they will swallow it.

We had a shot of the corpse floating in the water of the pool, and the shot seemed to come from inside the pool itself. You can't, of course, really shoot through water at all, because if you do it acts as a mirror and shows you and the camera crew. After many experiments, we put a mirror at the bottom of the pool and poured in a lot of light. Then we shot down, and hiding the cameras was hard.

The Norma Desmond house was on the corner of Wilshire and Cranshaw, and it's now been torn down and replaced by Tidewater Oil. It was the house of the richest man in the world, Mr Paul Getty. We had to put the rats in the pool ... ugh! And for a card game, we had the old stars: Swanson, Anna Q. Nilsson, Buster Keaton (he really did play bridge) and "Jesus Christ", H. B. Warner.[1]

Ace in the Hole was an original idea; it was done with Lesser Samuels and Walter Newman; it was a takeoff on the Floyd Collins case of the twenties, about the man trapped in a cave, and the enormous sensation-hungry crowds that came to the spot. The picture was better than the fate it had; it was a big success in Europe but it was a bigger failure here. My mistake was in coaxing the American public into the theatre with the idea that they were going to get a cocktail, whereas instead they got a shot of vinegar. I remember the day after I read the reviews saying, "How could a newspaperman possibly behave like that? How could any director be as cynical as Wilder?" I was on Wilshire Boulevard, and I was very downhearted, and right in front of me I saw someone run over by a car. A cameraman came running up and I said, "Let's help him." And the cameraman said, "Not me, boy! I've got to get that picture in!" And off he went!

We showed the carnival that arrived and pitched tents and sold hot dogs and played tunes, all to exploit the man's incarceration. People criticized me for bad taste, but it all really happened. The audience unfortunately doesn't want to see reality. Maybe I was wrong; maybe I should have tried to get them out of the rut instead of showing it to them on the screen.

After *Ace in the Hole*, I began to make pictures based on plays. I actually don't much like doing that, because the challenge isn't there, but I kind of hope that the three versions I did were improvements on the originals: *Sabrina Fair*, *Stalag 17*, *Witness for the Prosecution*. In *Stalag 17* I directed another director, Otto Preminger, who played the commandant in a POW camp. He was fun, but he could never remember his lines, and every time he fluffed lines he said he would send me a jar of caviar. Soon I had shelves of them.

Friends of mine, Nichols and Zinnemann and Cukor, have been among those to get praise for adapting stage plays, but to give an Academy Award to a man who directs a play is like giving the removalists who took Michelangelo's *Pieta* from the Vatican to the New York

[1] Warner played Christ in Cecil B. De Mille's *King of Kings*, 1927. (Authors' Note.)

World's Fair a first award in sculpture. I did like *Witness for the Prosecution*, though; I directed the film because Marlene Dietrich asked me to. It made it easier for her, if I directed it, to get the part of the murderess in it. It was a tremendous experience, working with Laughton. And I was tremendously flattered to read the other day an interview with Agatha Christie in which she said it had been the only adaptation of her work she really liked.

The Spirit of St Louis, based on the Charles Lindbergh story, was tricky to make, especially because he's a very standoffish man; I know him quite well, and I'm very fond of him, but he's not easy to get through to. It was hard to explore things in his life which were not in the book, because he's rather a mysterious figure. The technical problems were enormous: we had to cover such a vast area, the flight from Long Island to Paris, which took in Newfoundland and Ireland, and we had to keep trying to keep in touch with Paul Mantz, who flew the plane, and you'd have to ground it to discuss the technical facts, and the weather didn't match. I've never done an outdoor picture before or since; I'm not an outdoor man; I've never done a Western.

I think I should confine myself to bedrooms, maybe. I was saying to Willy Wyler the other day: "I'm doing a picture where the boss is chasing a secretary round a desk. But I'm no fool, I'm going to have Andrew Marton shoot the chase sequence."

Some Like it Hot, the story of two boys who dress up as members of a girls' band in the twenties, was a very daring picture for its day. I only wish we had saved it until the sixties; it would have been a much bigger hit. Tony Curtis was shyer about getting into women's clothes than Jack Lemmon, who is an all-out clown and an extrovert ... Marilyn Monroe was very sensitive, difficult, and disorganized. She tried hard, but she couldn't help herself. In some cases you had to match shots from different takes to make it seem as though she were giving a performance; but there were stretches when she was absolutely phenomenal: one of the great comediennes. Once she started rolling, and that tiny kind of an inhibition disappeared, she was wonderful, as good as anyone. The metabolism had to be right with her; and if it was right, she was a marvellous thing to direct; but I was utterly dependent on her moods.

A lot of people wondered why we used the St Valentine's Day Massacre to start the picture. But we had to have something really powerful to force the boys to pretend to be girls, and to make it rational that, even if they were in love with Marilyn, they wouldn't take off their clothes and say, "Look, I'm a man!" So the fact that they're threatened with machine-guns supplied the reason. We needed the whole thing done in period to make it easy to swallow.

The Apartment and *Meet Whiplash Willie*[1], my last pictures, weren't really comedies. We sugar-coated them a little with a laugh here and there, but what I wanted to say was, human beings are human beings. Once again, I wanted the starkest realism and, unlike so many people, I like the larger canvas of the wide screens. In *The Apartment*, the apartment was small. I took the white out, and the office was built in exact perspective; we had tiny desks at the back with dwarfs and then tinier ones still—toys— with cut-out figures. Alexandre Trauner, the art director, is the best in the business, and he worked it all out brilliantly. In this picture, and in *One, Two, Three*, set in Germany, I wanted to say: "How corrupt we are, how money-mad we are! How shaky all our convictions are!" As someone says in *Meet Whiplash Willie*, "People will do anything for money. Except some people. They will do *almost* anything for money." I guess that's the theme of all my pictures, and it isn't just meant to refer to the American public, but to everybody. There's that terrifying fact that people are people, you know. I don't distinguish them by races or nationalities. I have a kind of philosophy; maybe it's cynical, but I have to be true to what I feel. There's nothing so brand new or so horrifyingly psychoanalytical in all this. If you can say something with a little verve, and rub them a little bit the wrong way, you're all right. Of course, my next picture is sure to be in bad taste, and I'm hoping the people financing it don't blow all the money. Try to entertain an audience and upset them a bit, and you haven't lost them. Have you?

---

[1] Called *The Fortune Cookie* in the U.S.A. and Australia.

Filmographies

ROBERT ALDRICH (Born 1918)
The Big Leaguer, 1953; World for Ransom, Apache, Vera Cruz, 1954; Kiss Me Deadly, The Big Knife, 1955; Autumn Leaves, Attack!, The Garment Jungle (co-director, uncredited), 1956; Ten Seconds to Hell, 1958; The Angry Hills, 1959; The Last Sunset, 1961; Sodom and Gomorrah, Whatever Happened to Baby Jane?, 1962; 4 for Texas, Hush, Hush, Sweet Charlotte, 1963; Flight of the Phoenix, 1965; The Dirty Dozen, 1966; The Legend of Lylah Clare; The Killing of Sister George, 1968; Too Late the Hero, 1969; The Grissom Gang, 1970.

CURTIS BERNHARDT (Born 1899)
Die Waise von Lowood, 1926; Das Letzte Fort, 1927-28; Schinderhannes, 1928; Die Frau nach der man sich sehnt, Die Letzte Kompagnie, Der Mann, der den Mord beging, 1931; Der Rebell, 1932; Der Tunnel, 1933; L'Or dans la Rue, 1934; The Dictator (producer), 1935; The Beloved Vagabond, 1936; Carrefour, The Girl in the Taxi, 1938; My Love Came Back, The Lady with Red Hair, 1940; Million Dollar Baby, 1941; Juke Girl, 1942; Happy Go Lucky, 1943; Devotion, 1943-6; Conflict, 1945; My Reputation, A Stolen Life, 1946; High Wall, Possessed, 1947; The Doctor and the Girl, 1949; Payment on Demand, Sirocco, The Blue Veil, 1951; The Merry Widow, 1952; Miss Sadie Thompson, 1953; Beau Brummel, 1954; Interrupted Melody, 1955; Gaby 1956; Stephanie in Rio, 1960; Damon and Pythias, 1961; Kisses for my President, 1964.

GEORGE CUKOR (Born 1899)
Grumpy, The Virtuous Sin, The Royal Family of Broad-

way (co-director), 1930; Tarnished Lady, Girls about Town, 1931; A Bill of Divorcement, What Price Hollywood, One Hour with You (co-director Lubitsch), Rockabye, 1932; Little Women, Dinner at Eight, Our Betters, 1933; David Copperfield, Sylvia Scarlett, 1935; Romeo and Juliet, 1936; Camille, 1937; Holiday, 1938; The Women, Zaza, 1939; Susan and God, The Philadelphia Story, 1940; Two-Faced Woman, A Woman's Face, 1941; Keeper of the Flame, Her Cardboard Lover, 1942; Gaslight, Winged Victory, 1944; Desire Me (co-director, uncredited), 1947; A Double Life, 1948; Edward My Son, Adam's Rib, 1949; Born Yesterday, A Life of Her Own, 1950; The Model and the Marriage Broker, 1951; The Marrying Kind, Pat and Mike, 1952; The Actress, 1952; It Should Happen to You, 1954; A Star is Born, 1955; Bhowani Junction, 1956; Les Girls, 1957; Wild is the Wind, 1958; Heller in Pink Tights, Song without End (co-director), 1959; Let's Make Love, 1960; The Chapman Report, Something's Got to Give (unfinished) 1962; My Fair Lady, 1963-4; Justine, 1969.

JOHN FRANKENHEIMER (Born 1930)
The Young Stranger, 1957; The Young Savages, 1960; The Manchurian Candidate, Birdman of Alcatraz, All Fall Down, 1962; Seven Days in May, 1963; The Train, 1964; Seconds, 1965; Grand Prix, The Extraordinary Seaman, 1967; The Fixer, 1968; The Gypsy Moths, 1969; The Horsemen, 1970.

ALFRED HITCHCOCK (Born 1899)
Number Thirteen, 1921; The Pleasure Garden, 1925; The Mountain Eagle, The Lodger, 1926; Downhill, Easy Virtue, The Ring, 1927; The Farmer's Wife, Champagne, 1928; The Manxman, Blackmail, 1929; Elstree Calling, Juno and the Paycock, Murder, 1930; The Skin Game, 1931; Rich and Strange, Number Seventeen, Lord Camber's Ladies, 1932; Waltzes from Vienna, 1933; The Man who Knew Too Much, 1934; The Thirty-Nine Steps, 1935; The Secret Agent, Sabotage, 1936; Young and Innocent, 1937; The Lady Vanishes, 1938; Jamaica Inn, 1939; Rebecca, Foreign Correspondent, 1940; Mr and Mrs Smith, Suspicion, 1941; Saboteur, 1942; Shadow of a Doubt, 1943; Lifeboat, 1944; Spellbound, 1945; Notorious, 1946; The Paradine Case, 1947; Rope, 1948; Under Capricorn, 1949; Stage Fright, 1950; Strangers on a

Train, 1951; I Confess, 1953; Dial M for Murder, Rear Window, 1954; To Catch a Thief, 1955; The Trouble with Harry, The Man who Knew Too Much, 1956; The Wrong Man, 1957; Vertigo, 1958; North by Northwest, 1959; Psycho, 1960; The Birds, 1963; Marnie, 1964; Torn Curtain, 1966; Topaz, 1968.

FRITZ LANG (Born 1890)
Halb-Blut, Der Herr der Liebe, Die Spinnen (Der Goldene See, Das Brillanten Schiff), Wandernde Bild, 1919; Vier um die Frau, 1920; Der Muede Tod, 1921; Doktor Mabuse, Der Spieler, 1922; Die Nibelugen, 1923-24; Metropolis, 1926; Spione, 1927; Frau im Mond, 1928; "M", 1931; Das Testament von Doktor Mabuse, 1932; Liliom, 1933; Fury, 1936; You Only Live Once, 1937; You and Me, 1938; The Return of Frank James, Western Union, 1940; Man Hunt, Confirm or Deny (co-director, uncredited), 1941; Moontide (co-director, uncredited), Hagmen Also Die, 1942; The Ministry of Fear, 1943; The Woman in the Window, 1944; Scarlet Street, 1945; Cloak and Dagger, 1946; Secret Beyond the Door, 1948; The House by the River, 1949; American Guerrilla in the Philippines (I Shall Return), 1950; Rancho Notorious, Clash by Night, 1951; The Blue Gardenia, 1952; The Big Heat, 1953; Human Desire, Moonfleet, 1954; While the City Sleeps, 1955; Beyond a Reasonable Doubt, 1956; Der Tiger von Eschnapur, Das Indische Grabmal, 1958; Die 1000 Augen des Doktor Mabuse, 1960.

ROUBEN MAMOULIAN (Born 1898)
The Beating on the Door, 1922; Applause, 1929; City Streets, 1931; Dr Jekyll and Mr Hyde, Love Me Tonight, 1932; The Song of Songs, Queen Christina, 1933; We Live Again, 1934; Becky Sharp, 1935; The Gay Desperado, 1936; High, Wide and Handsome, 1938; Golden Boy, 1939; The Mark of Zorro, 1940; Blood and Sand, 1941; Rings on Her Fingers, 1942; Summer Holiday, 1947; Silk Stockings, 1958.

LEWIS MILESTONE (Born 1895)
Seven Sinners, The Cave Man, 1925; The New Klondike, 1926; Two Arabian Knights, 1927; The Garden of Eden, The Racket, 1928; The Betrayal, New York Nights, 1929; All Quiet on the Western Front, Hell's Angels (co-director, uncredited), 1930; The Front Page, 1931; Rain,

1932; Hallelujah, I'm a Bum!, 1933; The Captain Hates the Sea, 1934; Paris in Spring, 1935; Anything Goes, The General Died at Dawn, 1936; Night of Nights, Of Mice and Men, Lucky Partners, 1940; My Life with Caroline, 1941; Edge of Darkness, The North Star, 1943; The Purple Heart, 1944; A Walk in the Sun, 1945; The Strange Love of Martha Ivers, Guest in the House (co-director, uncredited), 1946; Arch of Triumph, 1947; No Minor Vices, 1948; The Red Pony, 1949; Halls of Montezuma, 1950; Kangaroo, Les Misérables, 1952; Melba, 1953; They Who Dare, 1955; Pork Chop Hill, 1959; Ocean's Eleven, 1960; Mutiny on the Bounty, 1962.

VINCENTE MINNELLI (Born 1908)
Cabin in the Sky, 1943; Meet Me in St Louis, 1944; The Clock, Yolanda and the Thief, 1945; Ziegfeld Follies, Undercurrent, 1946; The Pirate, 1948; Madame Bovary, 1949; Father of the Bride, 1950; Father's Little Dividend, An American in Paris, 1951; The Bad and the Beautiful, The Story of Three Loves (one episode), 1952; The Band Wagon, 1953; The Long, Long Trailer, Brigadoon, 1954; The Cobweb, Kismet, 1955; Lust for Life, Tea and Sympathy, 1956; Designing Woman, 1957; Gigi, The Reluctant Debutante, 1958; Home from the Hill, Some Came Running, 1959; The Bells are Ringing, Four Horsemen of the Apocalypse, 1960; Two Weeks in Another Town, 1961; The Courtship of Eddie's Father, 1963; Goodbye Charlie, 1964; The Sandpiper, 1965; On a Clear Day You Can See Forever, 1969.

JEAN NEGULESCO (Born 1900)
Singapore Woman, 1941; The Mask of Dimitrios, The Conspirators, 1944; Three Strangers, Nobody Lives Forever, 1946; Deep Valley, 1947; Johnny Belinda, Road House, 1948; Britannia Mews, Three Came Home, 1949; Under My Skin, The Mudlark, 1950; Take Care of My Little Girl, Phone Call from a Stranger, 1951; Lydia Bailey, Lure of the Wilderness, The Last Leaf *from* O. Henry's Full House, 1952; Titanic, Scandal at Scourie, How to Marry a Millionaire, 1953; Three Coins in the Fountain, A Woman's World, 1954; Daddy Long Legs, The Rains of Ranchipur, 1955; Boy on a Dolphin, 1957; The Gift of Love, A Certain Smile, 1958; Count Your Blessings, 1959; Jessica, 1961; The Pleasure Seekers, 1962; The Invincible Six, 1969; Hello—Goodbye, 1970.

IRVING RAPPER (Born 1898)
Shining Victory, One Foot in Heaven, 1941; The Gay Sisters, Now Voyager, 1942; The Adventures of Mark Twain, 1944; The Corn is Green, Rhapsody in Blue, 1945; Deception, 1946; The Voice of the Turtle, 1947; Anna Lucasta, 1949; The Glass Menagerie, 1950; Another Man's Poison, 1951; Forever Female, Bad for Each Other, 1953; Strange Intruder, The Brave One, 1956; Marjorie Morningstar, 1958; The Miracle, 1959; Pontius Pilate, 1961; The Christine Jorgensen Story, 1970.

MARK ROBSON (Born 1913)
The Seventh Victim, 1943; The Ghost Ship, 1944; Isle of the Dead, Youth Runs Wild, 1945; Roughshod, Bedlam, 1946; Champion, Home of the Brave, 1949; Edge of Doom, My Foolish Heart, 1950; Bright Victory, 1951; I Want You, 1952; Return to Paradise, 1953; Hell Below Zero, Phffft!, The Bridges at Toko-Ri, 1954; Prize of Gold, Trial, 1955; The Harder They Fall, 1956; The Little Hut, Peyton Place, 1957; The Inn of the Sixth Happiness, 1958; From the Terrace, 1960; Nine Hours to Rama, The Prize, 1963; The Lost Command, 1965; Valley of the Dolls, 1967; Daddy's Gone A-Hunting.

JACQUES TOURNER (Born 1904)
Tout ça ne Vaut pas L'Amour, Toto, Vieux Garçon, Pour Etre Aimé, Les Filles de la Conceirge, 1931-34; They All Came Out, Nick Carter, Master Detective, 1939; Phantom Raiders, 1940; Doctors Don't Tell, 1941; Cat People, 1942; I Walked with a Zombie, Leopard Man, 1943; Days of Glory, Experiment Perilous, 1944; Canyon Passage, 1946; Out of the Past, 1947; Berlin Express, 1948; Easy Living, 1949; Stars in My Crown, The Flame and the Arrow, 1950; Circle of Danger, Anne of the Indies, 1951; Way of a Gaucho, 1952; Appointment in Honduras, 1953; Stranger on Horseback, Wichita, 1955; Great Day in the Morning, Nightfall, 1956; Night of the Demon, 1957; The Fearmakers, 1958; Timbuktu, Frontier Rangers, Mission of Danger (co-director, uncredited), Fury River (co-director, uncredited), 1959; The Giant of Marathon, 1960; The Comedy of Terrors, 1963; The City Beneath the Sea, 1965.

KING VIDOR (Born 1894)
The Turn in the Road, 1918; Better Times, The Other
Half, Poor Relations, The Jack-Knife Man, 1919; The
Family Hour, 1920; The Sky Pilot, Love Never Dies,
Conquering the Woman, Woman Wake Up, 1921; The
Adventure, Dusk to Dawn, Alice Adams, Peg O' My
Heart, 1922; The Woman of Bronze, Three Wise Fools,
Wild Oranges, Happiness, 1923; Wine of Youth, His Hour,
Wife of the Centaur, 1924; Proud Flesh, The Big Parade,
La Bohème, 1925; Bardelys the Magnificent, 1926; The
Crowd, The Patsy, Show People, 1928; Hallelujah!, 1929;
Not So Dumb, Billy the Kid, 1930; Street Scene, The
Champ, 1931; Bird of Paradise, Cynara, 1932; The Stran-
ger's Return, 1933; Our Daily Bread, The Wedding Night,
1934; So Red the Rose, 1935; The Texas Rangers, 1936;
Stella Dallas, 1937; The Citadel, 1938; Northwest Passage,
1939-40; Comrade X, 1940; H. M. Pulham, Esq, 1941; An
American Romance, 1944; Duel in the Sun, 1946; On Our
Merry Way (co-director), 1947; The Fountainhead, 1948;
Beyond the Forest, 1949; Lightning Strikes Twice, 1950;
Japanese War Bride, 1951; Ruby Gentry, 1952; Man
Without a Star, 1954; War and Peace, 1955; Solomon and
Sheba, 1959.

BILLY WILDER (Born 1906)
Mauvaise Graine (co-director, Alexandre Esway), 1933;
The Major and the Minor, 1942; Five Graves to Cairo,
1943; Double Indemnity, 1944; The Lost Weekend, 1945;
The Emperor Waltz, A Foreign Affair, 1948; Sunset Boulevard, 1950; The Big Carnival, 1951; Stalag 17, 1952; Sabrina Fair, 1954; The Seven-Year Itch, 1955; The Spirit
of St Louis, 1956; Love in the Afternoon, 1957; Witness
for the Prosecution, 1958; Some Like it Hot, 1959; The
Apartment, 1960; One, Two Three, 1961; Irma La Douce,
1963; Kiss Me, Stupid, 1964; Meet Whiplash Willie, 1967;
The Private Life of Sherlock Holmes, 1969.

INDEX

From the SIGNET Film Library

☐ **FOOL'S PARADE by Davis Grubb.** From the hapless adventures of three ex-convicts and the nefarious schemes of some marvelously colorful characters, Davis Grubb has created a warm and humorous tale in which good and evil meet head on in a rousing climax. "Consistently engaging and entertaining . . ."—**New York Times Book Review.** A Columbia Picture, starring Jimmy Stewart and George Kennedy. (#Q4642—95¢)

☐ **ON MAKING A MOVIE: BREWSTER McCLOUD by C. Kirk McClelland.** The day-by-day record of the time McClelland spent closely examining the entire complex technical process and complicated human drama of the creation of **Brewster McCloud.** It is a non-starry-eyed, irreverent and beautifully incisive revelation of moviemakers at work. (#Y4591—$1.25)

☐ **MOVIE COMEDY TEAMS by Leonard Maltin.** Author of **TV Movies,** Leonard Maltin has put together a thorough and scholarly study of movie comedy teams such as the Marx Bros., Ritz Bros., etc. Illustrated. (#W4453—$1.50)

☐ **TAKING OFF by Milos Forman, John Guare, Jean Carriere and John Klein.** The complete screenplay of one of 1971's best and most popular films, TAKING OFF centers around two concerned parents' search for their runaway sixteen-year-old daughter. Many photographs and an interview with Milos Forman are included. (#Q4706—95¢)

SIGNET Movie Tie-In Titles

☐ **2001: A SPACE ODYSSEY, a novel by Arthur C. Clarke** based on the screenplay by **Stanley Kubrick** and **Arthur C. Clarke.** A brilliant projection into the future, tracing man's lonely search among the stars for his intelligent equal, or master. Based on the MGM motion picture starring Keir Dullea and Gary Lockwood.

(#Q3580—95¢)

☐ **THE BROTHERHOOD by Lewis John Carlino.** The compelling drama of two brothers caught in the death-grip of the Mafia. A Paramount Picture starring Kirk Douglas.

(#T4990—75¢)

☐ **MAIDSTONE: A Mystery by Norman Mailer.** The complete screenplay, with stills, description of the filming and a major essay on filmmaking by the author-director-star of this revolutionary movie. (#W4782—$1.50)

☐ **THE PANIC IN NEEDLE PARK by James Mills.** The shocking inside story of life among New York City's dope addicts, recorded by a journalist who spent 60 days and nights in the desperate world of the junkie. A major motion picture starring Al Pacino and Kitty Winn.

(#Q4681—95¢)